THIRD EDITION

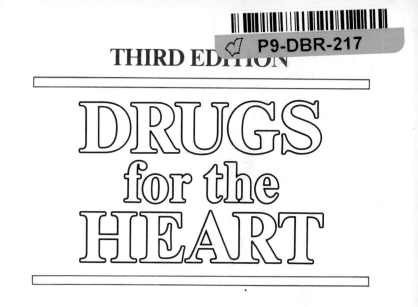

DRUGS
for the
HEART

Every effort has been made to check generic and trade names, and to verify drug doses. The ultimate responsibility for accuracy, however, lies with the prescribing physician. In no case can the institutions with which the authors are affiliated be held responsible for the views expressed in this book, which reflects the combined opinions of several authors. Please call any errors to the attention of the authors.

"When an approved treatment is considered for an unapproved indication, the physician must evaluate the safety of the medication, its value in related conditions, and the individual patient. What is asked is that he make a prudent decision based upon full knowledge of the available evidence."

Judge's instruction to jury

THIRD EDITION

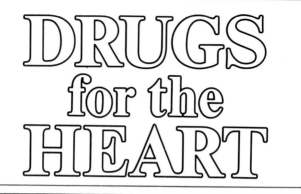

DRUGS for the HEART

Edited by

Lionel H. Opie, M.D., D.Phil., F.R.C.P.

Professor of Medicine
University of Cape Town
Cape Town, South Africa
Consultant Professor
Division of Cardiology
Stanford University Medical Center
Stanford, CA

With the collaboration of

Kanu Chatterjee, M.B., F.R.C.P.

Bernard J. Gersh, M.B.Ch.B., D.Phil., F.R.C.P.

Norman M. Kaplan, M.D.

Frank I. Marcus, M.D.

Philip A. Poole-Wilson, M.D., F.R.C.P.

Bramah N. Singh, M.D., D.Phil., F.R.C.P.

Edmund H. Sonnenblick, M.D.

Udho Thadani, M.B.B.S., M.R.C.P., F.R.C.P.(C.)

Foreword by

Eugene Braunwald, M.D.

1991
W.B. SAUNDERS COMPANY
Harcourt Brace Jovanovich, Inc.
Philadelphia   London   Toronto   Montreal   Sydney   Tokyo

W. B. Saunders Company
Harcourt Brace Jovanovich, Inc.

The Curtis Center
Independence Square West
Philadelphia, PA 19106

Library of Congress Cataloging-in-Publication Data

Drugs for the heart / edited by Lionel H. Opie, with the collaboration of
Kanu Chatterjee...[et al.]; foreword by Eugene Braunwald.—3rd ed.
p. cm.
Includes bibliographical references.
Includes index.
ISBN 0-7216-3278-5
1. Cardiovascular agents. I. Opie, Lionel H. II. Chatterjee, Kanu.
[DLNM: 1. Cardiovascular agents—adverse effects. 2. Cardiovascular
Agents—therapeutic use. 3. Heart—drug effects. QV 150 D7938]
RM345.D784   1991
615'.71—dc20
DNLM/DLC   90-9023

Editor: Richard Zorab
Designer: Paul Fry
Production Manager: Peter Faber
Manuscript Editor: Carol Florence
Illustration Coordinator: Brett MacNaughton
Indexer: Diana Witt
Cover Designer: Brett MacNaughton

Drugs for the Heart, third edition   ISBN 0-7216-3278-5

Printed in the United States of America.

Last digit is the print number: 9   8   7   6   5   4   3   2   1

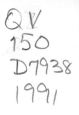
QV
150
D7938
1991

Contents

OTHER CARDIAC DRUGS

CHOICE OF DRUGS

Foreword

During the past decade, an extraordinary array of new cardiovascular drugs has become available, and both students and practitioners of medicine have difficulty deciding how to choose the proper drugs for their patients. Professor Opie's book provides a rational approach to this most important medical decision. This marvelous book is a concise yet complete presentation of cardiac pharmacology. It presents, in a very readable and eminently understandable fashion, an extraordinary amount of important information on the effects of drugs on the heart and circulation. Professor Opie and his colleagues have the unique ability to explain in a straightforward manner the mechanism of action of drugs without oversimplifying these complex matters. Simultaneously, his book provides important practical information to the clinician. This concise volume should be of value and interest to anyone who wishes to gain a clear understanding of cardiovascular therapeutics.

Eugene Braunwald, M.D.
Hersey Professor of Medicine
Harvard Medical School
Chairman, Department of Medicine
Brigham and Women's Hospital
Boston, Massachusetts

Preface

"Encouraged by the public reception of the former editions, the author has spared neither labour nor expense, to render this as perfect as his opportunities and abilities would permit. The progress of knowledge is so rapid, and the discoveries so numerous, both at home and abroad, that this may rather be regarded as a new work than as a re-publication of an old one. On this account, a short enumeration of the more important changes may possibly be expected by the reader."

William Withering, from Botany, *3rd Edition, 1801*

The last few years have seen a new and critical tendency in the evaluation of cardiac drug therapy. No longer is it sufficient to know that a drug has certain pharmacological qualities that can benefit individual patients. The new imperative is that any given mode of treatment should be able to decrease mortality, to lessen morbidity, and to enhance the quality of life. Treatment trials should ideally be placebo controlled. We have now entered the era of large-scale drug trials, especially those trials carried out in the acute phase of myocardial infarction (ISIS studies, GISSI study, TIMI and TAMI studies, as well as others). "Hard end-points" are also increasingly demanded in the evaluation of the therapy of hypertension and congestive heart failure. These major outcome trials are all evaluated in this new edition.

The overall form of this book remains a pocket-sized compendium based on the format of the ever-popular Michelin travel guides to Europe and North America. An important stylistic change is the introduction of two colors, designed to help the hard-pressed resident or equally busy practicing cardiologist who has to identify the best drug, its dose, and its side-effects at a moment's notice. While special care has been given to selection of new material, to keep the book pocket-sized, older material has had to be omitted. References have been completely updated to early 1990, including the most recent trial data given at the March meeting of the American College of Cardiology.

The next major change lies in the new arrangement of chapters, dividing cardiac drugs into three major categories: antianginal agents, antifailure agents, and other cardiac drugs, the latter including antihypertensives, antiarrhythmics, antithrombotics, and lipid-lowering agents. The new chapter devoted to antihypertensive drugs covers those agents established as being able to reduce both blood pressure and stroke. The more complex purposes of antihypertensives, including reduction of coronary disease, maintenance of quality of life, and avoidance of drug side-effects such as somnolence and impotence are also evaluated here. To compensate for the space required for the extra chapter, two previous chapters, namely those on angiotensin converting enzyme inhibitors and conventional vasodilators, have been amalgamated. As before, the end of the book answers the question "Which drug for which disease?". We have heard complaints that more detail is needed; however, our aim is not to provide a manual of cardiology. Rather, we wish to continue to provide a pocket-sized guide to cardiovascular drugs, designed to complement major textbooks such as those of Braunwald and Hurst.

A word about my co-authors. Though all but one are American, five of the eight have received British training, providing for the reader a point of view sensitive to the practical demands of the American resident or fellow, yet including the European viewpoint. The European practice of today becomes the American practice of tomorrow and vice versa. In the future, we propose obtaining a Japanese perspective as well. As before, meticulous attention has been paid to the recommendations of the Food and Drug Administration (FDA) of the USA, whose decisions usually reflect excellent judgment.

A final comment comes from the previous edition: "The best way to use this book is obvious—carry it with you, always! Don't hesitate to consult it in front of your patients, they appreciate your desire to be exact and to use the best possible drug in the optimal dose for their complaint."

The Lancet Editorial, 1980

(An Editorial from *The Lancet*, March 29, 1980, to introduce a series of articles on Drugs and the Heart)

Cardiovascular times are achanging. After a mere ten years' repose the medical Rip van Winkle would be thoroughly bewildered. For instance, there has been a big switch in attitudes to the failing heart. What would he make of those soft voices which now preach unloading or "afterload reduction"? Experience with beta-blockers has shown the fundamental importance of sympathetic activity in regulating cardiac contraction, and this activity can now be adjusted readily in either direction. Likewise, from calcium antagonists much has been discovered about the function of this ion at cellular level and its importance in the generation of necrosis and cardiac arrhythmia. New radionuclide and angiographic techniques have redirected attention to spasm in coronary arteries and fresh means to forestall it. Continuous ambulatory electrocardiography and special electrophysiological techniques have eased the assessment of arrhythmias, and, again, of drugs to stop or prevent them. Many new drugs have come on the scene, and increasingly they have been devised to act at specific points on pathways to cellular metabolism.

Dr. van Winkle apart, there may be one or two other physicians who regard with alarm the new flood of cardioactive drugs. For such as these, Professor Lionel Opie has written the series of articles which begin on the next page. As Professor Opie remarks, drugs should be given not because they *ought* to work but because they *do* work. We hope that this series will help stimulate the critical approach to cardiovascular pharmacology that will be much needed in the coming decade.

Acknowledgments

The rapid appearance of this revised edition has been made possible by the willing and unstinting co-operation of many people. I would like to thank my co-authors for generously sharing the expertise and clinical skills on which this book is based and for undertaking their meticulous updating of the earlier text. I extend a special welcome to Philip A. Poole-Wilson, Professor of Cardiology, National Heart and Lung Institute, London, joining us for the first time. Sadly, I say goodbye to two old friends—Tom Mackey, who for years guided this book through its birth and growth as an American offshoot of the original Lancet edition, and Don Harrison, previously Chief of Cardiology at Stanford and currently Senior Vice-President and Provost for Health Affairs at the University of Cincinnati. I thank Richard Zorab and the staff of W. B. Saunders for so efficiently dealing with the deadline and preparing such a well-produced book. The figures (my copyright unless otherwise stated) are based chiefly on the artistic skills of Jeanne Walker, an illustrator without peer. Professor Henry Wallman, previously of the Karolinska Institute, Stockholm, and now of Jerusalem, is thanked for interest, criticism, and careful proofreading. And, last but not least, my secretary June Chambers is thanked for prodigious patience and unfailing skills.

L. H. Opie
Cape Town, South Africa

Contributors

EUGENE BRAUNWALD, M.D. (FOREWORD)
> Hersey Professor of Medicine
> Harvard Medical School
> Chairman, Department of Medicine
> Brigham and Women's Hospital
> 75 Francis Street
> Boston, MA 02115

KANU CHATTERJEE, M.B., F.R.C.P.
> Professor of Medicine
> Lucie Stern Professor of Cardiology
> University of California, San Francisco
> Associate Chief, Cardiovascular Division
> Moffitt Hospital—Room 1186
> 505 Parnassus Avenue
> San Francisco, CA 94143-0124

BERNARD J. GERSH, M.B., Ch.B., D.Phil., F.R.C.P.
> Professor of Medicine
> Mayo Medical School
> Consultant in Cardiovascular Diseases and Internal Medicine
> Division of Medicine
> Mayo Clinic
> 500 First Street S.W.
> Rochester, MN 55905

NORMAN M. KAPLAN, M.D.
> Professor of Internal Medicine
> The University of Texas Health Sciences Center
> Southwestern Medical Center
> 5323 Harry Hines Boulevard
> Dallas, TX 75235-8852

FRANK I. MARCUS, M.D.
> Distinguished Professor of Medicine
> Cardiology Section
> Health Sciences Center
> University of Arizona
> Tucson, AZ 85724

LIONEL H. OPIE, M.D., D.Phil., F.R.C.P.
> Professor of Medicine
> University of Cape Town
> Cape Town, South Africa
> Consultant Professor
> Division of Cardiology
> Stanford University Medical Center
> Stanford, CA 94305

PHILIP A. POOLE-WILSON, M.D., F.R.C.P.
Professor of Cardiology
National Heart and Lung Institute
Dovehouse Street
London SW3 6LY
United Kingdom

BRAMAH N. SINGH, M.D., D.Phil., F.R.C.P.
Professor of Medicine
University of California, Los Angeles
Chief of Cardiology
Wadsworth Veterans Administration Hospital
Wilshire and Sautelle Boulevards
Los Angeles, CA 90073

EDMUND H. SONNENBLICK, M.D.
Chief, Division of Cardiology
Olson Professor of Medicine
Albert Einstein College of Medicine
1300 Morris Park Avenue
Bronx, NY 10461

UDHO THADANI, M.B.B.S., M.R.C.P., F.R.C.P.(C.)
Professor of Medicine
University of Oklahoma Health Sciences Center
Director of Clinical Research
Vice Chief, Cardiology Section
Oklahoma Memorial Hospital and Veterans Administration
    Center
P.O. Box 26901
Oklahoma City, OK 73190

Commonly Used Abbreviations

ACE inhibitor = angiotensin converting enzyme inhibitor
AMI = acute myocardial infarction
BP = blood pressure
CHF = congestive heart failure
LVF = left ventricular failure
LVH = left ventricular hypertrophy

L.H. Opie
E.H. Sonnenblick
N.M. Kaplan
U. Thadani

1

β-Blocking Agents

β-Adrenergic receptor antagonist agents remain a cornerstone in the therapy of all stages of ischemic heart disease, with the possible exception of Prinzmetal's variant angina, caused by coronary spasm. β-blockers are established agents for post-infarction management. β-blockers retain their position among basic therapies for numerous other conditions, including arrhythmias and hypertrophic cardiomyopathy (Table 1–1). For hypertension, however, β-blockers are now increasingly challenged by the calcium antagonists and angiotensin converting enzyme (ACE) inhibitors, although the new vasodilatory β-blockers may in due course regain lost ground in the therapy of hypertension.

The β-Adrenoceptor and Signal Transduction

The β-receptors classically are divided into the β_1-receptors found in heart muscle and the β_2-receptors of bronchial and vascular smooth muscle. There also are sizeable populations of β_2-receptors in the myocardium. Some metabolic β-receptors cannot easily be classified. Situated on the cell membrane, the β-receptor is part of the adenylate cyclase (AC) system (Fig. 1–1). The G-protein system links the receptor to AC, when the G-protein is in the stimulatory configuration (Gs). The link is interrupted by the inhibitory form (Gi), the formation of which results from muscarinic stimulation following vagal activation. When activated, AC produces cyclic adenosine (AMP) from monophosphate adenosine triphosphate (ATP). Cyclic AMP is the intracellular messenger of β-stimulation; among its actions is the opening of calcium channels to promote a positive inotropic effect and increased re-uptake of cytosolic calcium into the sarcoplasmic reticulum (relaxing, or lusitropic, effect). In the sinus node the pacemaker current is increased (positive chronotropic effect), while the rate of conduction is accelerated (positive dromotropic effect). The effect of a given β-blocking agent depends not only on the way it is absorbed, bound to plasma proteins, and on its metabolites, but also on the extent to which it inhibits the β-receptor (lock and key fit). To the extent that any given β-blocker also has some capacity to activate its receptor, the agent is also an agonist; hence, the term partial agonist activity (PAA), also called intrinsic sympathomimetic activity (ISA), as epitomized in pindolol.

PHARMACOLOGIC PROPERTIES

β-Blocker Generations

First generation agents, such as propranolol, nonselectively block all the β-receptors (both β_1 and β_2). Second generation agents such as

TABLE 1–1 SUMMARY OF CARDIAC INDICATIONS FOR SELECTED β-BLOCKERS

Indications (Alphabetical Order)	Acebutolol	Atenolol	Celiprolol	Labetalol	Metoprolol	Nadolol	Propranolol	Xamoterol
Angina pectoris	+	++	+	+	++	++	++	0
Arrhythmias	++	+	0	0	++	+	++	0
CHF, mild to moderate	0	0	0	0	+	0	0	++
Dissecting aneurysm	0	+	0	+	+	0	++	0
Fallot's tetralogy	0	0	0	0	0	0	++	0
Hypertension	++	++	++	++	++	++	++	0
Hypertensive crisis (IV therapy)	0	+	0	++	+	0	+	0
Hypertrophic cardiomyopathy	0	+	0	0	+	0/+	++	0
Left ventricular hypertrophy	+	+	(+)	(+)	+	+	+	0
Mitral stenosis	0	+	0	0	+	+	++	0
Mitral valve prolapse	0	+	0	0	+	0	++	0
Myocardial infarction and follow-up	(+)	++	0	(+)	++	0	++	0
Pheochromocytoma	0	0	0	++	0	0	0	0
Prolonged QT, congenital	0	0	0	0	0	0	++	0
Silent myocardial ischemia	(+)	++	(+)	+	++	++	++	0

0 = no good evidence for use without excluding potential benefit; (+) = reasonable evidence for efficacy in limited studies; + = good evidence for efficacy; ++ = excellent evidence for efficacy or agent approved for indication in USA; CHF = congestive heart failure; IV = intravenous.

All agents licensed for use in USA and UK except celiprolol. Xamoterol is licensed in the UK but only for mild to moderate CHF; it is contraindicated in severe CHF (see ref. 82).

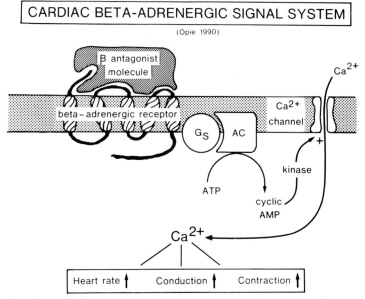

FIGURE 1–1. The cardiac β-adrenoceptor and signaling system. The β-antagonist molecule interacts with the β-receptor, whose molecular structure recently has been revealed and the amino acid sequence characterized. In the presence of the stimulatory form of the G-protein (Gs), adenylate cyclase (AC) converts ATP to cyclic AMP, which, acting via a protein kinase, enhances phosphorylation of the calcium channel and permits more calcium to enter through the calcium channel during voltage-induced depolarization. Such calcium releases much more from the sarcoplasmic reticulum (calcium-induced calcium release) to increase cytosolic calcium, heart rate, conduction, and contraction, as well as the rate of relaxation (the latter by phosphorylation of the protein phospholamban in the sarcoplasmic reticulum).

atenolol and metoprolol have relative selectivity when given in low doses for the β_1 (largely cardiac) receptors. Third generation agents have additional vasodilatory properties, acting through a variety of mechanisms, chiefly β_2 ISA, which stimulates the blood vessels to relax. Other marked differences between β-blockers lie in the pharmacokinetic properties, with half-lives varying from about 10 minutes to over 30 hours, and in the different degrees of lipid or water solubility. Hence the side-effect pattern may vary from agent to agent. Nonetheless, there is no evidence that any of these ancillary properties has any compelling therapeutic advantage, although for the individual patient the art of minimizing β-blocker side-effects may be of great importance. For example, a patient with chronic obstructive airway disease needs a cardioselective agent, whereas a patient with early morning angina needs a long-acting blocker. Likewise, a patient with cold extremities might benefit from a vasodilatory agent.

Nonselective Agents (β_1 plus β_2-Blockers)

The prototype β-blocker is propranolol, which still is used more than any other agent. By blocking β_1-receptors it achieves its effects on heart rate, conduction, and contractility, yet by blocking β_2-receptors it tends to cause smooth muscle contraction with risk of bronchospasm in predisposed individuals. This same quality might, however, explain the benefit in migraine when vasoconstriction could inhibit the attack. Among the nonselective blockers, nadolol and sotalol are much longer acting and lipid-insoluble.

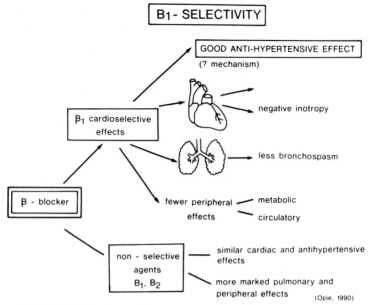

FIGURE 1–2. β-antagonist agents may be either cardioselective or noncardioselective. In general, note several advantages of cardioselective β-blockers. There may be occasional disadvantages, as in acute infarction-associated hypokalemia.

Cardioselective Agents (β_1-Selectivity)

Cardioselective agents (atenolol, metoprolol, acebutolol, and celiprolol) are preferable in patients with chronic lung disease, asthma or chronic smoking, peripheral vascular disease, and insulin-requiring diabetes mellitus (Fig. 1–2). Cardioselectivity varies among agents. As judged by bronchospasm in asthmatics (fall in forced expiratory volume), atenolol is somewhat more cardiospecific than metoprolol, and both are more so than acebutolol.[4] Cardioselectivity declines or is lost at high doses. No β-blocker is completely safe in the presence of asthma; low-dose cardioselective agents can be used with care in patients with bronchospasm, chronic lung disease, or chronic smoking. In angina and hypertension, cardioselective agents are just as effective as noncardioselective agents. In acute myocardial infarction (AMI) complicated by stress-induced hypokalemia, nonselective blockers theoretically should be better antiarrhythmics than β_1-selective blockers.[15]

Vasodilatory β–Blockers

INTRINSIC SYMPATHOMIMETIC ACTIVITY (PARTIAL AGONIST ACTIVITY)

β-Blockers with ISA lower resting heart rate and cardiac output to a lesser extent than those without ISA.[77] **Pindolol** is the β-blocker with the most ISA and nonselective β-blocking qualities. **Acebutolol** has less ISA, which in clinical practice is not enough to distinguish it from metoprolol.[39] The effect of a β-blocker with ISA on resting heart rate depends on the degree of sympathetic stimulation at rest and the relative ratios of β_1 or β_2 agonism. β_1-stimulation acts chiefly on the heart, β_2 on the peripheral arterioles and the bronchi. Pindolol has both β_1 and β_2 agonist activity with β_2 greater than β_1. **Celiprolol**, under evaluation, has chiefly β_2 agonism. If the resting sympathetic tone is high, a β-blocker with β_1 ISA reduces the resting heart rate. If the sympathetic activity is low, the heart rate either does not decrease or may increase. With a high degree of cardioselective ISA, such as with xamoterol (in Europe), the agent becomes more of an agonist than an antagonist with dominant inotropic qualities, and the antihypertensive effect is lost.[18] When there is bronchospasm, a β-blocker with high ISA, such as pindolol, may diminish β-blockade–induced spasm, although cardioselectivity is more desirable because ISA may lessen the bronchodilator effects of β_2-stimulants such as albuterol (Proventil) or salbutamol (Ventolin). As with β-blockade, ISA may be selective for β_1- or β_2-receptors or may be nonselective. ISA introduces a quality of potential β-receptor stimulation that is probably useful in patients with hypertension because of peripheral vasodilation; in elderly patients, in whom fatigue might be caused by limitation of cardiac output; or in black patients, in whom vasodilation appears to improve the antihypertensive effect. In patients with ischemic heart disease, however, a slower heart rate might be better, and ISA is a potential disadvantage.

Another potential disadvantage of ISA is the stimulation of the central nervous system at night, when sympathetic tone is low, causing sleep impairment.[57]

Added α-Blocking Activity

Labetalol is a combined α- and β-blocking agent that causes less bronchospasm and vasoconstriction than propranolol, lowers the blood pressure more rapidly, and works better than propranolol in black hypertensives.[6] These advantages are bought at the cost of two potential side-effects—postural hypotension with high doses and occasional retrograde ejaculation (α-blockade relaxes the bladder neck sphincter and is used in the therapy of prostatism). Besides α-blockade, labetalol may possess significant ISA.[29] Labetalol is a more powerful β-blocker than α-blocker (β:α ratio 3:1 after oral, and 7:1 after intravenous (IV) dosage), so that a high dose may be required for adequate α-blockade. A standard dose of labetalol (200 mg 2x daily) was as effective as atenolol (100 mg daily) in controlling angina in patients with coexisting hypertension.[14] For angina without hypertension, the efficacy of labetalol is not well documented. Intravenous labetalol is also effective for severe hypertension and is well-tested in pregnancy hypertension (IV or oral). Even oral labetalol leads to a rapid fall of blood pressure, in contrast to propranolol or other conventional β-blockers.

Combined Vasodilatory–β-Blocking Molecules

Bucindolol, a developmental drug, has a hydralazine-like moiety built into the molecule.

Celiprolol is a highly cardioselective agent with β_2 agonism and a non-specific vasodilatory quality (see page 21).

MEMBRANE STABILIZING ACTIVITY (MSA)

MSA, as in propranolol, is important experimentally because in high concentrations certain β-blockers have a quinidine-like, membrane-stabilizing effect on the action potential. Such activity is not relevant to clinical practice. In overdose, this property is potentially hazardous.

Pharmacokinetic Properties

The plasma half-life of **propranolol** (Table 1-2) is only 3 hours, but continued administration saturates the hepatic process that removes propranolol from the circulation; the active metabolite 4-hydroxy-propranolol is formed, and the effective half-life then becomes longer. The biologic half-life of propranolol and metoprolol (and all other

TABLE 1–2 PROPERTIES OF VARIOUS β-ADRENOCEPTOR ANTAGONIST AGENTS, NONSELECTIVE VERSUS CARDIOSELECTIVE AND VASODILATORY AGENTS

Generic Name (Trade Name)	ISA	Plasma Half-life (hr)	Lipid† Solubility	First-pass Effect	Loss by Liver or Kidney	Plasma Protein Binding (%)	Usual Dose for Angina	Usual Doses as Sole Therapy for Mild/Moderate Hypertension	IV Dose (Caution)
Noncardioselective									
Propranolol* (Inderal)	–	1–6	+++	++	Liver	90	120–140 mg/day, 3–4 divided doses; but 80 mg 2x daily usually adequate. Start as for hypertension.	Start with 10–40 mg 2x daily to lessen side-effects. Mean 160–320 mg/day, 1–2 doses; usually 120 mg 2x daily[1]	1–10 mg* (0.1 mg/kg)
(Inderal-LA)	–	8–11	+++	++	Liver	90	80–320 mg 1x daily	80–320 mg 1x daily	–
Oxprenolol* (Trasicor)	++	2	++	++	Liver	80	As propranolol; mean 160 mg/day	160–800 mg/day; mean 260 mg/day. 444 mg, 2–3 divided doses	1–12 mg
Timolol* (Blocadren)	–	4–5	+	+	L,K	60	15–45 mg (in 3–4 divided doses)	20–60 mg/day = 160–480 mg propranolol, 2–3 doses/day	0.4–1 mg
Nadolol* (Corgard)	–	16–24	0	0	Kidney	20	80–240 mg 1x daily; mean 100 mg	40–560 mg/day; mean 110 mg/day single dose	–
Sotalol (Sotacor)	–	15–17	0	0	Kidney	5	240–480 mg/day single dose	80–320 mg/day; mean 190 mg	10–20 mg
Penbutolol* (Levatol)	+	27	+++	++	Liver	98	Not studied	10–20 mg daily[1]	–
Cardioselective									
Acebutolol* (Sectral)	++	8–12 (diacetolol)	0 (diacetolol)	++	L,K	15	200–400 mg 3x daily; 900 mg optimal	400–1200 mg/day; can be given as a single dose	12.5–50 mg

(Trade name)									
Atenolol* (Tenormin)	–	6–9	0	0	Kidney	10	100 mg 1x daily; 25 mg 2x daily nearly as effective	50–200 mg/day as single dose; usual dose 100 mg. Flat dose-response curve	5–10 mg*
Betaxolol* (Kerlone)	–	15	++	++	L,K	50	10–20 mg 1x daily (use pending approval)	10–20 mg once daily	–
Metoprolol* (Lopressor) (Betaloc)	–	3	+	++	Liver	15	50–100 mg 2 or 3x daily; mean total 200 mg	50–400 mg/day; mean about 250 mg in 1 or 2 doses	5–15 mg*
Vasodilatory β-blockers, nonselective									
Carteolol* (Cartrol)	+	5–6	0/+	0	Kidney	20–30	Not evaluated	2.5–10 mg as single dose	–
Labetalol* (Trandate) (Normodyne)	–	3–4	+++	++	Liver	90	As for hypertension	300–600 mg/day in 3 doses; top dose 2400 mg/day	1–2 mg/kg* for severe HT
Pindolol* (Visken)	+++ $\beta_1\beta_2$	4	+	+	L,K	55	2.5–7.5 mg 3x daily	10–30 mg/day; mean 21 mg (some on diuretics); single dose	–
Vasodilatory β-blockers, selective									
Celiprolol** (Selecor)	+β_2	6–8	0/+	0	Chiefly kidneys; also L	? low	400 mg once daily	400 mg once daily	–

[†] Octanol-water distribution coefficient (pH 7.4, 37°C) where $0 = <0.5$; $+ = 0.5$–2.0; $++ = 2$–10; $+++ = >10$; L = liver; K = kidney; HT = hypertension; data sources, see previous editions and Frishman and Sonnenblick[82] and Physician's Desk Reference (1990).

* Approved by FDA.

** Pending approval for hypertension by FDA.

[1] Schoenberger.[71]

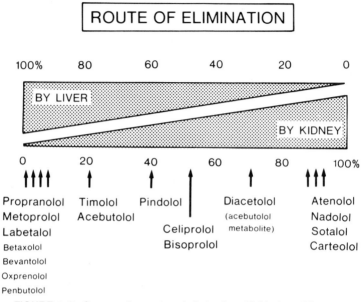

FIGURE 1–3. Comparative routes of elimination of β-blockers. Those most hydrophilic and least lipid-soluble are excreted unchanged by the kidneys. Those most lipophilic and least water-soluble are largely metabolized by the liver. Note that the metabolite of acebutolol, diacetolol, is largely excreted by the kidney, in contrast to the parent compound. (For derivation of figure, see previous edition. Estimated data points for acebutolol and newer agents added). (Figure copyright L.H. Opie.)

β-blockers) exceeds the plasma half-life considerably, so that **2× daily dosage is effective even in angina pectoris.** Clearly, the higher the dose of any β-blocker, the longer the biologic effects. Longer-acting compounds, such as nadolol, sotalol, atenolol, and slow-release propranolol (Inderal-LA) should be better for hypertension and ordinary angina, whereas shorter-acting drugs, such as metoprolol or ultrashort-acting IV esmolol, are preferable in unstable angina and threatened infarction, when hemodynamic changes may call for withdrawal of β-blockade.

PROTEIN BINDING

Propranolol is highly bound, as are pindolol and labetalol. Hypoproteinemia calls for lower doses of such compounds.

First-pass liver metabolism is found especially with the highly lipid-soluble compounds, such as propranolol, labetalol, and oxprenolol; acebutolol, metoprolol, and timolol have only modest lipid-solubility, yet with hepatic clearance; first-pass metabolism varies greatly among patients and alters the dose required. In liver disease or low-output states the dose should be decreased. First-pass metabolism produces active metabolites with, in the case of propranolol, properties different from those of the parent compound. Acebutolol produces large amounts of diacetolol, also cardioselective with ISA, but with a longer half-life and chiefly excreted by the kidneys (Fig. 1-3).[1]

IDEAL KINETICS

Lipid-insoluble hydrophilic compounds (**atenolol, sotalol, nadolol**) are excreted only by the kidneys (Fig. 1–3) and have low brain pene-

TABLE 1–3 CENTRAL EFFECTS OF β-BLOCKERS

Drug	Ref	Subjects	Daily dose (mg)	Duration	Effects
Propranolol	1	Healthy	160	1 wk	Insomnia
	2	Hypertensives	80–160	2–4 wk	Increased depression, anger, confusion, fatigue
Pindolol	1	Healthy	20	1 wk	Insomnia
Dilevalol	3	Hypertensives	600	8 wk	Less fatigue, less depression
Atenolol	2	Hypertensives	50–100	2–4 wk	*Vs placebo:* less anxiety, hostility, inertia, depression; however, more fatigue *vs propranolol:* less of all of above except fatigue
	1	Healthy	100	1 wk	No insomnia
	5	Hypertensives	100	2 wk	Modest sedation
	6	Hypertensives	100	2 wk	Decreased performance of complex tasks
	7	Hypertensives	50–100	12 wk	Improved memory and performance of complex tasks, though not as good as enalapril
Metoprolol	1	Healthy	200	1 wk	Insomnia
	5	Hypertensives	150	2 wk	Modest sedation, but less than with atenolol
	6	Hypertensives	150	2 wk	Improved capacity for complex tasks; better than atenolol

1 Kostis and Rosen.[57]
2 Conant, et al.[41]
3 Schoenberger, et al.[72]
4 Gengo, et al.[48]
5 Streufert, et al.[75]
6 Herrick, et al.[53]
7 Drew, et al.[44]

tration. In patients with renal or liver disease, the simpler pharmaco-kinetic patterns of lipid-insoluble agents make dosage easier. As a group, these agents have low protein binding (Table 1-2).

Renal Effects

β-Blockers that reduce the cardiac output (nonvasodilatory agents) will tend to lessen renal blood flow. However, the glomerular filtration rate (GFR) is unchanged because of renal autocompensation. Only with propranolol is there firm evidence that the GFR can fall. Ultimately β-blockers are usually excreted by the kidneys, so that in renal failure the dose may have to be altered, especially in the case of water-soluble agents excreted by the kidneys. In general, agents highly metabolized by the liver can be given in an unchanged dose. There continues to be no firm evidence (contrary to claims) that some β-blockers such as nadolol are better at maintaining glomerular filtration rates in patients with renal impairment. All β-blockers reduce circulating **renin** levels,[77] an effect that may contribute to but does not fully explain the antihypertensive action. High ISA (as in pindolol) reduces this effect. Thus, in general, the more the heart rate falls with a β-blocker, the more the renin falls. The antihypertensive action of β-blockers is not directly related to the antirenin effect.

TABLE 1–4 β-BLOCKADE: CONTRAINDICATIONS AND CAUTIONS

Cardiac

Absolute: Severe bradycardia, high-degree heart block, overt left ventricular failure (exception: some cardiomyopathies).

Relative: Treated heart failure, cardiomegaly without clinical failure (not a contraindication in hypertensive heart disease), Prinzmetal's angina (unopposed alpha-spasm), high doses of other agents depressing SA or AV nodes (verapamil, diltiazem, digitalis, antiarrhythmic agents); in angina, avoid sudden withdrawal (dangerous in unreliable patient).

Pulmonary

Absolute: Severe asthma or bronchospasm. No patient may be given a β-blocker without questioning for past or present asthma. Fatalities have resulted when this rule is ignored.

Relative: Mild asthma or bronchospasm or chronic airway disease. Use agents with cardioselectivity plus $β_2$-stimulants (by inhalation). High ISA also protects, but results in loss of sensitivity to $β_2$-stimulation.

Central Nervous

Absolute: Severe depression (avoid propranolol).

Relative: Vivid dreams: avoid highly lipid-soluble agents (propranolol) and pindolol; avoid evening dose. Visual hallucinations: change from propranolol. Fatigue (all agents; try change of agent). If low cardiac output is cause of fatigue, try vasodilatory β-blockers. Impotence: rare (try change of agent). Psychotropic drugs (with adrenergic augmentation) may adversely interact with β-blockers.

Peripheral Vascular, Raynaud's Phenomenon

Absolute: Active disease: gangrene, skin necrosis, severe or worsening claudication.

Relative: Cold extremities, absent pulses, Raynaud's phenomenon. Avoid nonselective agents (propranolol, sotalol, nadolol); prefer vasodilatory agents.

Diabetes Mellitus

Relative: Insulin-requiring diabetes: nonselective agents decrease reaction to hypoglycemia; use selective agents — atenolol, metoprolol (acebutolol more doubtful). β-blockers may increase blood sugar by 1.0–1.5 mmol/L and impair insulin sensitivity; hence caution in family history of diabetes. Adjust control accordingly.

Renal Failure

Relative: In general, renal blood flow falls. Reduce doses of all except pindolol.

Liver Disease

Relative: Avoid agents with high hepatic clearance (propranolol, oxprenolol, timolol, acebutolol, metoprolol). Use agents with low clearance (atenolol, nadolol, sotalol, or pindolol). If plasma proteins low, reduce dose of highly bound agents (propranolol, pindolol).

Pregnancy Hypertension

β-blockade increasingly used, but may depress vital signs in neonate and cause uterine vasoconstriction. Labetalol and atenolol best tested. Avoid diuretics — low blood volume.

Surgical Operations

β-blockade may be maintained throughout, provided indication is not trivial; otherwise stop 24–48 hours beforehand. May protect against anesthetic arrhythmias. Use atropine for bradycardia, β-agonist for severe hypotension.

Age

β-blockade, found by some to be less effective in hypertension in the elderly, is increasingly used especially in combination with diuretics. Watch pharmacokinetics and side-effects.

Smoking

In hypertension, nonselective β-blockade is not effective in reducing coronary events in smoking men. Selective agents may be better. In general, smoking interferes with efficacy of propranolol.[60]

Hyperlipidemia

β-blockers may have unfavorable effects on the blood lipid profile, especially nonselective agents. It is thought that there are less unfavorable effects with selective agents. Vasodilatory agents, especially those with ISA, may have mildly favorable effects.

*ISA = intrinsic sympathomimetic activity.

Central Effects

An attractive hypothesis is that the lipid-soluble β-blockers (epitomized by propranolol) with their high brain penetration are more likely to cause central side-effects. This hypothesis can explain why propranolol, pindolol, and metoprolol cause insomnia, whereas atenolol does not (Table 1-3). Furthermore, an extremely detailed comparison of propranolol and atenolol showed that atenolol, which is not lipid-soluble, causes far fewer central side-effects than does propranolol.[41] On the other hand, the lipid-solubility hypothesis does not explain why metoprolol, moderately lipid-soluble, appears to interfere less with some complex psychologic functions than does atenolol and may even enhance some aspects of psychologic performance.[75] The hypothesis has to be modified to take account of the fact that eventually even lipid-insoluble β-blockers penetrate the cerebrospinal fluid, and, once there, the longer-acting atenolol may stay longer than the shorter-acting metoprolol. It should be noted that overall the cardioselective β-blockers atenolol and metoprolol appear to be remarkably, but not totally, free of central side-effects. The intriguing possibility remains that these agents can actually improve certain aspects of central function.

Side-effects of β-Blockers (Table 1-4)

The three major mechanisms are (1) smooth muscle spasm (bronchospasm and cold extremities), (2) exaggeration of the cardiac therapeutic actions (bradycardia, heart block, excess negative inotropic effect), and (3) central nervous penetration (insomnia, depression). The **mechanism of fatigue** is not clear. When compared with propranolol, however, it is reduced by use of either a cardioselective β-blocker or a vasodilatory agent, so that both central and peripheral hemodynamic effects may be involved. When patients are appropriately selected, double-blind studies show no differences between a cardioselective agent such as **atenolol** and placebo.[28] This may be because atenolol does not penetrate the brain and should have lesser effects on bronchial and vascular smooth muscle than propranolol. When **propranolol** is given for hypertension, the rate of serious side-effects (bronchospasm, cold extremities, worsening of claudication) leading to withdrawal of therapy is about 10%.[28] The rate of withdrawal with atenolol is considerably lower (about 2%) but when it comes to dose-limiting side-effects, both agents can cause cold extremities, fatigue, dreams, worsening claudication, and bronchospasm. Heart failure, although a theoretical hazard with β-blockade therapy, is in fact rare when the correct contraindications are observed. Clearly if β-blockade is given to patients who are already severely ill, the risk of side-effects is increased.[5]

QUALITY OF LIFE

In the famous "quality of life" study,[42] propranolol induced considerably more central effects than did the ACE inhibitor captopril, which is not surprising in view of the major central side-effects of propranolol (Table 1-3). However, atenolol with its far fewer central side-effects compares favorably with the ACE inhibitor enalapril.[53] Whether atenolol or metoprolol would give a better quality of life with a formal evaluation needs to be tested, and the results might depend on the test used. For example, the patient given atenolol sleeps better, performs less well on complex cognitive tasks, but may have improved memory when compared with placebo.[41,53]

During **exercise**, β-blockade reduces the total work possible by about 15% and increases the sense of fatigue. Vasodilatory β-blockers

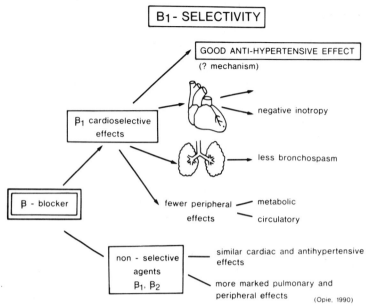

FIGURE 1–4. Effects of β-blockade on ischemic heart. β-blockade has a beneficial effect on the ischemic myocardium, unless (1) the preload rises substantially as in left heart failure or (2) there is vasospastic angina, in which spasm may be promoted in some patients. Note the recent proposal that β-blockade diminishes exercise-induced vasoconstriction.

may be an exception. Sometimes side-effects found with one β-blocker may be avoided by switching to another. Impotence is a side-effect quite frequently complained of in middle-aged men, who in any case are prone to this problem once hypertensive labeling has occurred, as their self-esteem is diminished. Most package inserts give a rate of impotence of about 1% for any given agent. Speculatively, a change to a β-blocker with ISA and reassurance might do the trick.

DRUG INTERACTIONS

Cimetidine reduces hepatic blood flow and therefore increases blood levels of propranolol (but not of agents such as atenolol, sotalol, and nadolol, which are not metabolized in the liver). Verapamil may raise blood levels of metoprolol.[21] Nonsteroidal anti-inflammatory drugs (NSAIDs) such as indomethacin attenuate the antihypertensive effects of β-blockers and of thiazide diuretics.[32]

ANGINA PECTORIS

β-blockade reduces the oxygen demand of the heart (Fig. 1–4) by reducing the double product (heart rate x blood pressure) and depressing contractility. Of these, the most important and easiest to measure is the reduction in heart rate. In addition, an aspect frequently neglected is the increased oxygen demand resulting from left ventricular dilation, so that any accompanying failure needs active therapy. Besides decreasing the oxygen demand, it is now becoming apparent that β-blockade improves the supply side of the equation by lessening exercise-induced vasoconstriction and improving myocardial perfusion as a result of the increased diastolic time (reviewed by Opie[63]) (Fig. 1-4).

The list of **contraindications** and side-effects of β-blockers is formidable (Table 1-4). **The most important contraindication is asthma or a past history of asthma;** several fatalities or near fatalities have been reported with the first dose of noncardioselective agents, and even selective agents can be given only under supervision.

All β-blockers are potentially equally effective in angina pectoris (Table 1-1), and the choice of drug matters little in those who do not have concomitant diseases. In the case of early morning angina, the ultralong-acting compound nadolol is better than atenolol.[17] But about 20% of patients do not respond to any β-blocker,[30] because of (1) underlying severe obstructive coronary artery disease, responsible for angina at a low level of exertion and at heart rates of 100 beats/min or lower; or (2) an abnormal increase in left ventricular (LV) end-diastolic pressure resulting from an excess negative inotropic effect and a resultant decrease in subendocardial blood flow. Although it is conventional to adjust the dose of a β-blocker to secure a resting heart rate of 55-60 beats/min, rates below 50 beats/min may be acceptable provided that heart block is avoided and there are no symptoms. In the case of the vasodilatory β-blockers, it may not be possible or desirable to achieve low resting heart rates, because reduction of the afterload plays an increasingly larger role in reducing the myocardial oxygen demand. Nonetheless, in general, vasodilatory β-blockers have not been well tested against angina. Reduction in exercise-induced tachycardia during β-blockade therapy is an important determinant of the response to therapy of effort angina with all β-blockers, and the aim should be an exercise heart rate of less than 100 to 110 beats/min.

Combination Therapy of Angina Pectoris

β-Blockers are often combined with nitrate vasodilators and calcium antagonists in the therapy of angina. Such triple therapy is not necessarily the best and has been decried by Packer.[65] Of the possible β-blocker–calcium antagonist combinations, that with nifedipine is hemodynamically the soundest, as the tendency to tachycardia with nifedipine and related compounds is antagonized by the β-blocker, whereas the nifedipine-like compounds contribute vasodilation to the mechanism of antianginal effect. β-blockers should only be combined with verapamil and diltiazem with caution, as extreme bradycardia or atrioventricular (AV) block may occasionally occur and, in the case of verapamil, a marked negative inotropic effect is possible.[74] In any case, the benefits of adding β-blockade to high doses of diltiazem are questionable and fatigue often results.[45] Therefore the decision to add a calcium antagonist to β-blocker–nitrate therapy requires, first of all, a knowledge of the hemodynamics of the combination β-blocker–calcium antagonist (see Fig. 3–6), a careful examination of the cardiovascular system, and a certain amount of judicious guesswork. Of the combinations, β-blocker–nifedipine is likely to be simplest, β-blocker–diltiazem is almost as simple but without much increased benefit, and that with verapamil is most likely to cause problems.[74]

IMPAIRED LV FUNCTION

In angina pectoris with abnormal LV function, β-blockade may decrease angina at the cost of lessening exercise tolerance because of increased LV size and wall tension; digitalis and diuretics can prevent the clinical deterioration and reverse the cardiac enlargement.[3] However, as the positive inotropic effect of digitalis should theoretically increase the myocardial oxygen demand, the current trend is to treat such patients by diuretics combined with ACE inhibitors. Theoretically, vasodilatory β-blockers should depress myocardial function less. An alternative is the combination of nifedipine with a β-blocker when the LV impairment results from hypertension.

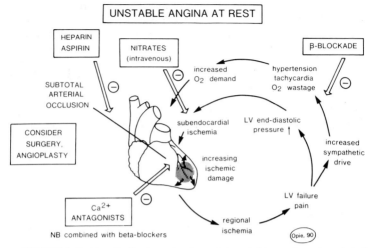

FIGURE 1–5. Hypothetical mechanisms for unstable angina at rest and proposed therapy. Increasing emphasis is being placed on the role of anti-thrombotics and antiplatelet agents. β-Blockade may be particularly effective in the presence of sympathetic activation with increased heart rate and blood pressure. Calcium antagonists, especially nifedipine, should be used with care, and nifedipine should be used only in combination with β-blockade.

β-Blockade Withdrawal

When β-blockers are suddenly withdrawn, angina may be exacerbated, sometimes resulting in myocardial infarction. All patients with ischemic heart disease must be severely warned not to stop β-blocker therapy abruptly, unless resting in bed, when a sudden stop seems to be safe. In the case of poorly compliant patients, the use of a β-blocker with added ISA such as pindolol appears to lessen withdrawal effects. Treatment of the withdrawal syndrome is by reintroduction of β-blockade.

Unstable Angina with Threat of Myocardial Infarction

Unstable angina is an all-purpose term, including a large number of clinical entities. In view of the complex etiology, different therapies may be appropriate (Fig. 1–5). Short-lived attacks of chest pain at rest, although falling into the overall syndrome, may have a very different connotation from increasingly severe and prolonged pain with threat of myocardial infarction, the sense in which the term unstable angina is now increasingly used. At present, partial coronary thrombosis or platelet aggregation is seen as the basic pathology in threatened infarction, so that antithrombotic therapy by heparin or aspirin is basic. β-blockade therapy is standard, especially in patients with elevated blood pressure and heart rate. Logically, the lower the heart rate, the less the risk of recurrent ischemia. Hence, standard blockers are preferred to the vasodilatory agents. The actual objective evidence favoring the use of β-blockers in unstable angina is limited to one placebo-controlled trial.[55] Patients who were not on prior β-blockade were randomized either to metoprolol or nifedipine, or to the combination. Patients on prior β-blockade were randomized to placebo or nifedipine. "Of all the treatments studied, only the addition of nifedipine to previous maintenance with a β-blocker was clearly beneficial," as judged by recurrent ischemia or myocardial infarction · at 48 hours. In the case of β-blockade alone, statistical proof of a reduction in recurrent ischemia was not achieved. An important conclusion of this study was a trend to increased complications with nifedipine alone, which is therefore relatively contraindicated in unstable angina in the absence of β-blockade.[50,55]

In patients with crescendo angina or prolonged ischemic chest pain poorly relieved by nitroglycerin and without evidence of Prinzmetal's angina, propranolol (initial dose 40 mg, increased to 80 mg 3x daily) is as effective as the calcium antagonist diltiazem (initial dose 60 mg, followed by 120 mg also 3x daily).[31]

In patients with unstable angina, once the acute phase is over, coronary angiography is likely to lead to coronary artery bypass grafting or to angioplasty in selected patients. Occasionally acute intervention is attempted when pain does not respond to standard therapy.

Prinzmetal's Variant Angina

β-Blockade is commonly held to be ineffective and even harmful, supposedly because of enhanced coronary spasm from unopposed α-receptor activity. On the other hand, there is good evidence for the benefit of calcium antagonist therapy. Nonetheless, it must be pointed out that Robertson and colleagues[70] studied only six patients and in only half of the observations was there clearcut exaggeration by propranolol. Furthermore, Guazzi and co-workers[52] have reported relief of variant angina with propranolol (mean dose 391 mg daily). However, in the case of exercise-induced attacks in patients with variant angina, there is good evidence, obtained from a prospective randomized study in 20 patients, that nifedipine is considerably more effective than propranolol.[59] Some evidence favoring the possibility that propranolol could act as a coronary vasodilator is given by Gaglione and colleagues.[47]

Cold Intolerance and Angina

During exposure to severe cold, effort angina may occur more easily.[66] Conventional β-blockade by propranolol is not as good as vasodilatory therapy by nifedipine. Speculatively, vasodilatory β-blockers may also be better than propranolol.

Mixed or Double-Component Angina

Much has been made of the possibility that coronary spasm contributes to the symptomatology of mixed or double-component angina where, in addition to ordinary effort angina, there is angina at rest. However, in a double-blind comparison of atenolol 100 mg daily, nifedipine 60 mg daily, and isosorbide mononitrate 80 mg daily, atenolol was the best overall agent and was as effective as nifedipine in abolishing nocturnal ST-segment changes.[69] Likewise, propranolol (80 mg 4x daily) was more effective than nifedipine (20 mg 4x daily) in double-component angina as assessed by the incidence of silent and symptomatic ischemic episodes.[43]

Silent Myocardial Ischemia

Increasing emphasis is now placed on the importance of silent myocardial ischemia in patients with angina. Nonetheless, large-scale studies regarding the prognostic significance of silent ischemia are still missing. β-blockers are very effective in reducing the frequency and number of episodes of silent ischemic attacks and are probably superior to nitrates and calcium antagonists.[40,56,62] In a very recent study comparing propranolol with diltiazem and nifedipine in silent ischemia, only propranolol was better than placebo[73] (see p 263).

ACUTE MYOCARDIAL INFARCTION

In AMI without obvious clinical contraindications, very early IV β-blockade in patients is now increasingly used despite occasional unpredictable hemodynamic effects. The risk of ventricular fibrillation (VF) may be lessened;[24,27] infarct size may be variably reduced by up to 30%.[11,22] Theoretically, IV β-blockade is of most use in about the first 4 hours of the onset, when VF might be most prevalent. For this use against VF, a nonselective agent like propranolol is probably best (Inderal, 0.5-mg increments IV up to a total of 0.1 mg/kg[24]), although no formal comparisons exist between selective and nonselective agents. Early IV metoprolol (Lopressor, 5 mg every 5 min to a total of 15 mg) followed by 100 mg 2x daily for 3 months lessens VF[27] and decreases mortality.[54] The massive ISIS (the name of the river in Oxford, England) trial shows that about 150 patients need to be treated by early IV β-blockade (atenolol 5–10 mg) followed by oral therapy for 1 week to save one life;[12] the mechanism was probably by prevention of cardiac rupture. Most of the benefit is achieved on the first day, at least in the case of atenolol. In the USA, metoprolol and atenolol are the only β-blockers licensed for IV use in AMI.

Recently the widespread use of thrombolytic agents within the first 6 hours of AMI has overshadowed the possible benefits of early IV β-blockade. In the TIMI-2 study, the addition of IV metoprolol to thrombolytic therapy improved the outcome.[76] Although further control studies are required, the combination might be attractive in decreasing reperfusion injury.[64]

Postinfarct Follow-up

In the postinfarct phase, β-blockade reduces the risk of sudden death and reinfarction. Timolol, propranolol, metoprolol, and atenolol[25] are all effective, while β-blockers such as oxprenolol with ISA are ineffective.[33] Nonetheless, in higher risk postinfarct patients, acebutolol reduced total and vascular mortality.[35a]

The only outstanding questions are (1) whether low risk patients should be given β-blockade, which seems pointless because of their already excellent prognosis; (2) which β-blocker should be used—here it is safest to stick to those with documented efficacy and follow-up; (3) when to start—taking together the data on metoprolol and timolol, it seems reasonable to start either by early IV β-blockade or as soon as the patient's condition allows, but optimally once the patient has stabilized at about 1 to 2 weeks; and (4) for how long should β-blockade be continued? In the absence of data to prove this point, and bearing in mind the risk of β-blockade withdrawal in patients with angina, many clinicians continue β-blockade administration forever once a seemingly successful result has been obtained. Yet unless adequate stratification of risk is undertaken post-infarct, many patients have to be treated for a long time before there is any benefit (an estimated 30 patient-years of treatment for 1 extra year of life).[23] The high risk patients who should benefit most also have the most contraindications to β-blockade.[10] Because β-blockers are effective post infarct and calcium antagonists (exception, verapamil) are not, β-blockers are preferred therapy in post-infarct patients with angina or hypertension, although these categories of patients have not been studied in detail, nor are there any good comparisons between β-blockers and calcium antagonists.

β-BLOCKERS FOR HYPERTENSION

Despite their widespread use, the exact mechanism whereby β-blockers lower blood pressure remains an open question. An early

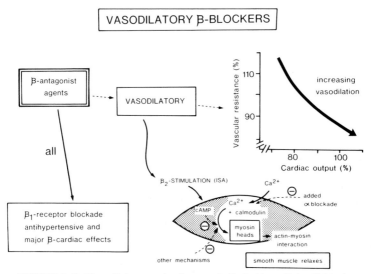

FIGURE 1–6. Vasodilatory mechanisms and effects. Vasodilatory β-blockers decrease the cardiac output less as the systemic vascular resistance falls. Vasodilatory mechanisms include α-blockade, nonspecific mechanisms, and intrinsic sympathomimetic activity (ISA). ISA increases sympathetic tone when it is low, as at night, and increases nocturnal heart rate, which might be disadvantageous in nocturnal angina or unstable angina. (Figure copyright L.H. Opie.)

fall of cardiac output is clearly one factor. The peripheral vascular resistance initially increases, later to fall to normal or somewhat below, while agents with added vasodilatory qualities, such as high degrees of ISA, specifically decrease the systemic vascular resistance (Fig. 1–6).[77] The presumed site of action causing the later fall in the vascular resistance with the conventional nonvasodilatory blockers is inhibition of the presynaptic β-receptor (see Fig. 5–2).

Of the large number of β-blockers now available, all have been shown to be antihypertensive. Of those available, atenolol, acebutolol, and nadolol come closest to the ideal pharmacologic profile. Vasodilatory blockers may be better for those susceptible to symptomatic bradycardia or cold extremities, or in the elderly or in black patients. On the other hand, in hypertension with angina, a slower heart rate would seem preferable.

Can β-blockade reduce coronary mortality in hypertensives, as in the case of post-infarct management? In the recently published MAPHY trial,[81] it was claimed that prolonged treatment with a cardioselective β-blocker metoprolol reduced mortality when compared with a diuretic. However, the β-blocker–treated patients did not have a lower coronary death rate than seen in other trials; rather, the diuretic-treated group had a higher rate (see also Chap. 7).

ARRHYTHMIAS

Both supraventricular and ventricular arrhythmias may respond to β-blocker therapy (Fig. 1–7). The possible cardiodepressant effects of β-blockers argue against their use for arrhythmias when there are numerous alternative agents. In AMI, however, the desirable combination of a proven effect against VF and the possibility of reduction of infarct size has led to the increasing use of IV β-blockade, although such use is still very far from general. Post infarction, one of the beneficial mechanisms of action of β-blockade is by prevention of sudden death, which may reflect an antifibrillatory mechanism. In the therapy of supraventricular tachycardias, verapamil and adenosine

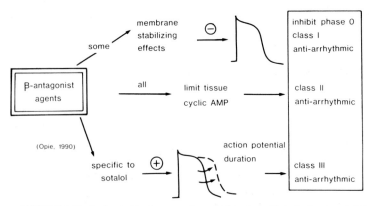

FIGURE 1–7. Antiarrhythmic properties of β-blockers. Note that only sotalol has a Class-III antiarrhythmic effect. It is questionable whether the membrane stabilizing effects of propranolol and related agents confer additional antiarrhythmic properties.

are now standard, although IV esmolol is better than verapamil in achieving sinus rhythm in acute onset atrial fibrillation or in atrial flutter.[67] β-blockers are particularly effective in arrhythmias caused by increased circulating catecholamines (early phase AMI, pheochromocytoma, anxiety, anesthesia, postoperative states, and some exercise-related arrhythmias) or by increased cardiac sensitivity to catecholamines (thyrotoxicosis) and in the arrhythmias of mitral valve prolapse. In severe ventricular tachycardia or fibrillation, long-term β-blockade therapy was successful in most patients, especially those with an LV ejection fraction exceeding 45% and, surprisingly, in the absence of coronary disease.[37] Among β-blockers used for ventricular arrhythmias, sotalol with added Class III activity may be best at the risk of occasional torsades de pointes.

In **chronic atrial fibrillation** without LV failure, β-blockade can be used to reduce ventricular response rate. In **digitalis-induced tachyarrhythmias**, propranolol is licensed for its effect.

IV DOSAGE

With the ECG and blood pressure monitored and with atropine at hand, some β-blockers may be given slowly IV over 5 to 20 minutes (see Table 1-2). The ultrashort-acting agent **esmolol,** with a half-life of only 9 minutes, is increasingly used for this purpose, especially when the LV status is not clear or when there is some other question about the possible tolerance to β-blockade.

OTHER CARDIAC INDICATIONS

In **hypertrophic obstructive cardiomyopathy**, propranolol is standard therapy, although it is increasingly challenged by verapamil and disopyramide. High-dose propranolol (average 462 mg/day)[7] is thought to reduce ventricular arrhythmias. Lower dose β-blockade (mean, 280 mg propranolol or equivalent per day)[19] has been ineffective against the arrhythmias; amiodarone therapy may be required in patients at risk of sudden death.[20]

In **congestive cardiomyopathy**, low-dose β-blockade may also be added very cautiously to conventional therapy, especially when there is resting tachycardia. This indication remains highly controversial, although increasingly supported. In a recent sophisticated study, there was deterioration in two-thirds of the patients with dilated cardiomyopathy on long-term treatment with metoprolol when the drug was withdrawn, and an improvement on drug readministration. Furthermore, long-term metoprolol caused a moderate up-regulation of ventricular β-receptors.[79]

In **congestive heart failure**, in the large trial comparing digoxin with **xamoterol** in patients with mild to moderate heart failure, mostly of a nonspecified etiology, xamoterol increased work performance, decreased symptoms, and appeared to be better than digoxin.[49] The reason for the difference between the benefit in mild-to-moderate heart failure and the harm in severe heart failure is not understood and makes it difficult to use this drug.[82]

In **mitral stenosis** with sinus rhythm, β-blockade benefits by decreasing resting and exercise heart rates, thereby allowing longer diastolic filling and improved exercise tolerance.[16] In mitral stenosis with chronic atrial fibrillation, β-blockade may have to be added to digoxin to obtain sufficient ventricular slowing during exercise (see p 269). Occasionally β-blockers, verapamil, and digoxin are all combined.

In **mitral valve prolapse**, β-blockade is the standard procedure for control of associated arrhythmias.

In **dissecting aneurysms**, in the hyperacute phase, IV propranolol has been standard, although it could be replaced by esmolol. Thereafter, oral β-blockade is continued.

In **Fallot's tetralogy**, propranolol 2 mg/kg 2x daily is usually effective against the cyanotic spells, probably acting by inhibition of right ventricular contractility.

In **congenital QT-prolongation**, propranolol is standard therapy. It is thought that an imbalance between the left and right stellate ganglion may play a role in the QT-prolongation.

In general, β-blockade is seen as an effective means of reducing **left ventricular hypertrophy** in hypertension. An example is the decreased total wall thickness and increased radius to thickness ratio, found echocardiographically after 50 weeks of treatment by atenolol.[35]

Cardioprotection

The only proven case for cardioprotection by β-blockade is in postinfarct patients. No such studies exist in angina. In hypertension (p 170), the MAPHY study[81] suggests better cardioprotection by a cardioselective blocker than by diuretic therapy in smokers. Further evidence supporting the protective role of β-blockade is given by a retrospective case analysis study.[68]

NONCARDIAC INDICATIONS FOR β-BLOCKADE

Thyrotoxicosis

Together with antithyroid drugs or radioiodine, or as the sole agent before surgery,[34] β-blockade is now commonly used in thyrotoxicosis, although the hypermetabolic state is not decreased. β-blockade controls tachycardia, palpitations, tremor, and nervousness and reduces the vascularity of the thyroid gland, thereby facilitating operation.[34] In **thyroid storm**, IV propranolol can be useful at a rate of 1 mg/min (to a total of 5 mg at a time); circulatory collapse is a risk, so that β-blockade should be used in thyroid storm only if LV function is normal, as shown by conventional noninvasive tests. Because control of tachycardia is important, the choice of agent usually falls on those without ISA (see ISA, p 4). A cardioselective agent is advisable when there is bronchospasm.

Anxiety States

Although propranolol is most widely used in anxiety (and is licensed for this purpose in several countries, including the USA), probably all β-blockers are effective, acting not centrally but by a reduction of peripheral manifestations of anxiety such as tremor and tachycardia.[13] In a recent double-blind study of anxiety in hypertensive patients (not the same as nonhypertensive patients presenting with anxiety), atenolol was considerably better than propranolol.[41]

Other Central Nervous System Indications

Atenolol and propranolol are very effective in **postalcoholic withdrawal syndrome**.[58]

In **subarachnoid hemorrhage**, early treatment by propranolol with long-term follow-up appeared to be beneficial,[80] although the study design was imperfect.

In acute stroke, on the contrary, atenolol or propranolol not only failed to benefit the patient but increased mortality. In contrast, patients taking β-blockers at the start of the stroke appeared to have some protection.[36]

Glaucoma

The use of local timolol eye solution (Timoptic in USA, Timoptol in UK) is established for open-angle glaucoma; care needs to be exerted with occasional systemic side-effects such as sexual dysfunction,[8] bronchospasm, and cardiac depression. **Betaxolol** is a new, cardioselective long-acting β-blocker that has been introduced recently in the USA for glaucoma and, in its oral form, as an antihypertensive.

Migraine

Propranolol (80–240 mg daily) reduces the incidence of migraine attacks in 60% of patients, as do some other β-blockers without ISA,[26] a quality that presumably inhibits the beneficial vasoconstriction. The antimigraine effect is prophylactic, not for attacks once they have occurred. If there is no benefit within 4 to 6 weeks of top doses, propranolol should be discontinued.

OVERDOSE OF β-BLOCKERS

Bradycardia may be countered by IV atropine 1 to 2 mg; if serious, temporary transvenous pacing may be required. When an infusion is required, glucagon (2.5–7.5 mg/hr) is the drug of choice, because it stimulates formation of cyclic AMP by bypassing the occupied β-receptor. Logically an infusion of amrinone should help cyclic AMP to accumulate. Alternatively, dobutamine is given in doses high enough to overcome the competitive β-blockade (15 μg/kg/min). In patients without ischemic heart disease, an infusion (up to 0.10 μg/kg/min) of isoproterenol may be used.

NEW β-BLOCKERS

Of the large number of β-blockers in development, the ideal agent for hypertension or angina might have (1) advantageous pharmacokinetics (lipid-insolubility); (2) cardioselectivity; and (3) long duration of action. Vasodilatory properties should be of benefit in the treatment of hypertension, but might be a disadvantage in the treatment of certain types of angina such as unstable angina at rest.

Betaxolol (Kerlone) is a new, long-acting, lipid-soluble cardio-selective β-blocker (oral dose 10–40 mg once daily) now available in the USA for hypertension.

Bevantolol, a cardioselective agent, is moderately lipid-soluble, undergoes hepatic metabolism without the formation of active meta-bolites, and does not accumulate in renal disease. The usual dose is 150 to 300 mg daily given as one or two doses for hypertension or angina.[46]

Bisoprolol (Emcor, Monocor) is a highly selective agent, thought to be more selective than atenolol, licensed for hypertension and angina in the United Kingdom. The dose is 5 to 10 mg once daily with an average of 10 mg. In a double-blind comparison of bisoprolol 10 to 20 mg daily with atenolol 50 to 100 mg daily, there was a slightly higher response rate with bisoprolol, especially in regular smokers.[38]

Carteolol (Cartrol) is a nonselective β-blocker with moderate ISA, low lipid-solubility, and a half-life similar to that of atenolol. In hypertension (for which it is licensed in the USA), the initial dose is 2.5 mg as a single daily dose, which may be increased to 10 mg daily. Because of predominant renal excretion, the dose is decreased in renal impairment.

Celiprolol (pending approval in USA as Selecor) is a highly cardioselective β-blocker with low lipid-solubility and a half-life similar to that of atenolol. The ancillary properties include partial β_2-agonist activity (β_2 ISA) and direct vasodilation. In hypertension, it is significantly better than enalapril in reducing exercise-induced blood pressure increases, and is as good with resting blood pressure.[51] In effort angina, it is as good as atenolol (400 mg celiprolol vs 100 mg atenolol) when given once daily, but acts with less suppression of heart rate at rest and during exercise.[61] Its cardioselectivity is at least as good as that of atenolol, and probably better.[78] It is claimed to be lipid neutral or possibly even able to induce favorable changes in blood lipids.

Dilevalol is an isomer of labetalol without α-blocking activity but with marked vasodilatory β_2 ISA. Although promising in the treatment of hypertension,[72] it has been withdrawn because of potential hepatotoxicity.

Esmolol (Brevibloc) is an ultrashort-acting cardioselective β-blocker with a half-life of 9 minutes, rapidly converted to inactive metabolites by blood esterases. The dose range is 50 to 400 mg/kg/min intravenously,[9] and full recovery from β-blockade occurs within 30 minutes in patients with a normal cardiovascular system. The indications of esmolol are situations in which on-off control of β-blockade is desired, as in supraventricular tachycardia[2] or perioperative tachy-cardia, or perioperative or emergency hypertension. In recent-onset atrial fibrillation or flutter, esmolol is better than verapamil in conversion to sinus rhythm.[67] Exploratory uses are in unstable angina and AMI, when the hemodynamic effects of β-blockade may be uncertain.

Penbutolol (Levatol). There are two optical isomers of propranolol—only the *l*-form is β-blocking whereas both possess membrane-stabilizing activity (MSA). Thus the ratio of β-blockade to MSA is increased by penbutolol, which has only the *l*-isomer and also has modest ISA, similar to acebutolol. It is highly lipid-soluble and liver metabolized. In the treatment of mild-to-moderate hypertension, the usual initial dose is 20 mg once daily with a flat dose-response curve. In the UK, it is marketed in a combination tablet (penbutolol 40 mg, furosemide 20 mg, as Lasipressin).

CONCLUSIONS

β-blockade is very effective treatment, alone or combined with other drugs, in 70 to 80% of patients with classic angina, or 50 to 70%

of those with mild to moderate hypertension; black hypertensives respond less well, unless vasodilatory blockers are used. Propranolol (Inderal) is likely to remain the gold standard because it is still so widely used and licensed for so many different indications, including angina, hypertension, arrhythmia, migraine, anxiety states, and postinfarct follow-up. However, propranolol is not β_1-selective. Being lipid-soluble, propranolol has a high brain penetration and undergoes extensive hepatic first-pass metabolism. Propranolol also has a short half-life, so that it must be given 2x daily (4x daily, still sometimes used, is bad practice because it leads to poor patient compliance).

Although propranolol is still the most widely used β-blocker, we see no particular advantages for this drug with its high lipid-solubility and high first-pass metabolism, unless there is the coexistence of hypertension with some other condition in which experience with propranolol is greater than with other β-blockers (e.g., cardiomyopathy, migraine, or essential tremor).

Other compounds are increasingly used because of specific attractive properties: cardioselectivity (atenolol, metoprolol, acebutolol, celiprolol, and betoxol); lipid-insolubility and no hepatic metabolism (atenolol, nadolol, sotalol); long action (nadolol greater than sotalol greater than atenolol); ISA to help avoid myocardial depression (pindolol, acebutolol, celiprolol); added α-blockade to achieve more arterial dilation (labetalol); and superior antiarrhythmic properties (sotalol, not in the USA). New β-blockers under evaluation include the highly cardioselective agents celiprolol and bisoprolol, and the newly released β-blockers include the nonselective agents penbutolol and carteolol. It is clear that not all of these agents will have a wide market. Every clinician should become thoroughly familiar with only a limited number of β-blocking agents, one of which must be cardioselective. Where side-effects are encountered, they can sometimes be avoided by a switch to another β-blocker. Generally, if one agent in adequate dose will not work, neither will another; nor should one β-blocker be added to another in the hope of improved therapeutic response, with the exception sometimes of a better response to vasodilatory β-blockers, especially in black hypertensives. Probably smokers also respond better to the vasodilatory agents. As concluded in previous editions of this book, in clinical practice the differences between existing β-blockers are often relatively slight and hardly justify the vast commercial pressures applied in competitive promotion. In specific patients, ancillary properties such as cardioselectivity, long half-life, and vasodilation may be required.

REFERENCES

References from Previous Editions

1. Abernethy DR, Arendt RM, Greenblatt DJ: Am Heart J 109:1120–1125, 1985
2. Byrd RC, Sung RJ, Marks J, et al: J Am Coll Cardiol 3:394–399, 1984
3. Crawford MH, LeWinter MM, O'Rourke RA, et al: Ann Intern Med 83:449–455, 1975
4. Decalmer PBS, Chatterjee SS, Cruickshank JM, et al: Br Heart J 40:184–189, 1978
5. Douglas-Jones AP, Baber NS, Lee A: Eur J Clin Pharmacol 14:163–166, 1978
6. Flamenbaum W, Weber MA, McMahon FG, et al: J Clin Hypertens 1:56–69, 1985
7. Frank MJ, Abdulla AM, Canedo MI, et al: Am J Cardiol 42:993–1001, 1978
8. Fraunfelder FT, Meyer SM: JAMA 253:3092–3093, 1985
9. Gorczynski RJ, Quon CY, Krasula RW, et al: In Scriabine A (ed): New Drugs Annual: Cardiovascular Drugs, Vol 3. New York, Raven Press, 1985, pp 99–119

10. Hansteen V, Moinichen E, Lorentsen E, et al: Br Med J 284:155–160, 1982
11. International Collaborative Study Group. N Engl J Med 310:9–15, 1984
12. ISIS-1 Group. Lancet II:57–65, 1986
13. James I, Savage I: Am Heart J 108:1150–1155, 1984
14. Jee LD, Opie LH: Am J Cardiol 56:551–554, 1985
15. Johansson BW, Dziamski R: Drugs 28 (suppl 1):77–85, 1984
16. Klein HO, Sareli P, Schamroth C, et al: Am J Cardiol 56:598–601, 1985
17. Kostis JB, Lacy CR, Krieger SD, et al: Am Heart J 108:1131–1136, 1984
18. Leonetti G, Sampieri L, Cuspidi C, et al: J Hypertens 3 (suppl 3):S243–S245, 1985
19. McKenna WJ, Chetty S, Oakley CM, et al: Am J Cardiol 45:1–5, 1980
20. McKenna WJ, Harris L, Rowland E, et al: Am J Cardiol 54:802–810, 1984
21. McLean AJ, Knight R, Harrison PM, et al: Am J Cardiol 55:1628–1629, 1985
22. MIAMI Trial Research Group. Eur Heart J 6:199–226, 1985
23. Mitchell JRA: Br Med J 285:1140–1148, 1982
24. Norris RM, Barnaby PF, Brown MA, et al: Lancet 2:883–886, 1984
25. Olsson G, Rehnqvist N, Sjogren A, et al: J Am Coll Cardiol 5:1428–1437, 1985
26. Ryan RE: Am Heart J 108:1156–1159, 1984
27. Ryden L, Ariniego R, Arnman K, et al: N Engl J Med 308:614–618, 1983
28. Simpson WT: Postgrad Med J 53 (suppl 3):162–167, 1977
29. Tadepalli AS, Novak AS: J Cardiovasc Pharmacol 8:44–50, 1986
30. Thadani U, Davidson C, Singleton W, et al: Am J Med 68:243–250, 1980
31. Theroux P, Taeymans Y, Morissette D, et al: J Am Coll Cardiol 5:717–722, 1985
32. Webster J: Drugs 30:32–41, 1985
33. Yusuf S, Peto R, Lewis JA, et al: Prog Cardiovasc Dis 27:335–371, 1985
34. Zonszein J, Santangelo RP, Mackin JF, et al: Am J Med 66:411–416, 1979

New References

35. Allen JW, Kaiser PJ, Montenegro A: Effects of atenolol on left ventricular hypertrophy and early left ventricular function in essential hypertension. Am J Cardiol 64:1157–1161, 1989
35a. APSI Investigators: Acebutolol and the secondary prevention in high risk post-MI patients (APSI). J Am Coll Cardiol 15:214A, 1990
36. Barer DH, Cruickshank JM, Ebrahim SB, Mitchell JRA: Low dose beta-blockade in acute stroke (BEST trial): an evaluation. Br Med J 296:737–741, 1988
37. Brodsky MA, Allen BJ, Luckett CR, et al: Antiarrhythmic efficacy of solitary beta-adrenergic blockade for patients with sustained ventricular tachyarrhythmias. Am Heart J 118:272–280, 1989
38. Bühler FR, Berglund G, Anderson OK, et al: Double-blind comparison of the cardioselective beta-blockers bisoprolol and atenolol in hypertension: The Bisoprolol International Multicenter Study (BIMS). J Cardiovasc Pharmacol 8 (suppl 11):S122–S127, 1986
39. Carlsen JE, Kober L, Heeboll-Nielsen NC: A randomised comparison of acebutolol and metoprolol in 215 patients with hypertension. Lack of importance of intrinsic sympathomimetic activity and solubility for adverse effects. Drug Investigation 1:29–33, 1989
40. Cohn PF, Lawson WE: Effects of long-acting propranolol on A.M. and P.M. peaks in silent myocardial ischemia. Am J Cardiol 63:872–873, 1989
41. Conant J, Engler R, Janowsky D, et al: Central nervous system side effects of beta-adrenergic blocking agents with high and low lipid solubility. J Cardiovasc Pharmacol 13:656–661, 1989
42. Croog SH, Levine S, Testa MA, et al: The effect of antihypertensive therapy on the quality of life. N Engl J Med 314:1657–1664, 1986
43. DeCesare N, Bartorelli A, Fabbiocchi F, Folli A, Loaldi A, et al: Superior efficacy of propranolol versus nifedipine in double-component angina, as related to different influences on coronary vasomotility. Am J Med 87:15–21, 1989
44. Drew PJT, Barnes JN, Evans SJW: The effect of acute beta-adrenoceptor blockade on examination performance. Br J Clin Pharmacol 19:783–786, 1985
45. El-Tamimi H, Davies GJ, Kaski J-C, et al: Effects of diltiazem alone or with isosorbide dinitrate or with atenolol both acutely and chronically for stable angina pectoris. Am J Cardiol 64:717–724, 1989

46. Frishman WH, Goldberg RJ, Benfield P: Bevantolol. A preliminary review of its pharmacodynamic and pharmacokinetic properties, and therapeutic efficacy in hypertension and angina pectoris. Drugs 35:1–21, 1988

47. Gaglione A, Hess OM, Corin WJ, et al: Is there coronary vasoconstriction after intracoronary beta-adrenergic blockade in patients with coronary artery disease? J Am Coll Cardiol 10:299–310, 1987

48. Gengo FM, Huntoon L, McHugh WB: Lipid-soluble and water-soluble beta-blockers. Comparison of the central nervous system depressant effect. Arch Intern Med 147:39–43, 1987

49. German and Austrian Xamoterol Study Group: Double-blind placebo-controlled comparison of digoxin and xamoterol in chronic heart failure. Lancet 1:489–493, 1988

50. Gerstenblith G, Ouyang P, Achuff SC, et al: Nifedipine in unstable angina: a double-blind randomized trial. N Engl J Med 306:885–889, 1982

51. Ghiringhelli S, Cozzi E, Tsialtas D: Hemodynamic effects of celiprolol at rest and during exercise: a comparison with enalapril. Cardiovasc Drugs Ther 2:211–218, 1988

52. Guazzi M, Fiorentini C, Polese A, et al: Treatment of spontaneous angina pectoris with beta-blocking agents. A clinical, electrocardiographic, and haemodynamic appraisal. Br Heart J 37:1235–1245, 1975

53. Herrick A, Waller P, Berkin K, et al: Comparison of enalapril and atenolol in mild to moderate hypertension. Am J Med 86:421–426, 1989

54. Hjalmarson A, Elmfeldt D, Herlitz J, et al: Effect on mortality of metoprolol in acute myocardial infarction. Lancet 2:823–827, 1981

55. Holland Interuniversity Nifedipine/Metoprolol Trial (HINT) Research Group: Early treatment of unstable angina in the coronary care unit: a randomised, double-blind, placebo-controlled comparison of recurrent ischaemia in patients treated with nifedipine or metoprolol or both. Br Heart J 56:400–413, 1986

56. Imperi GA, Lambert CR, Coy K, et al: Effects of titrated beta-blockade (metoprolol) on silent myocardial ischemia in ambulatory patients with coronary artery disease. Am J Cardiol 60:519–524, 1987

57. Kostis JB, Rosen RC: Central nervous system effects of beta-adrenergic blocking drugs: the role of ancillary properties. Circulation 75:204–212, 1987

58. Kraus ML, Gottlieb LD, Horwitz RI, Anscher M: Randomized clinical trial of atenolol in patients with alcohol withdrawal. N Engl J Med 313:905–909, 1985

59. Kugiyama K, Yasue H, Horio Y, et al: Effects of propranolol and nifedipine on exercise-induced attack in patients with variant angina: Assessment by exercise thallium-201 myocardial scintigraphy and quantitative rotational tomography. Circulation 74:374–380, 1986

60. Materson BJ, Reda D, Freis ED, Henderson WG: Cigarette smoking interferes with treatment of hypertension. Arch Intern Med 148:2116–2119, 1988

61. McLenachan JM, Wilson JT, Dargie HJ: Importance of ancillary properties of beta-blockers in angina: A study of celiprolol and atenolol. Br Heart J 59:685–689, 1988

62. Mulcahy D, Keegan J, Cunningham D, et al: Circadian variation of total ischaemic burden and its alteration with anti-anginal agents. Lancet 2:755–759, 1988

63. Opie LH. Pharmacology of acute effort angina: Cardiovasc Drugs Ther 3 (suppl 1):257–270, 1989

64. Opie LH: Reperfusion injury and its pharmacologic modification. Circulation 80:1049–1062, 1989

65. Packer M: Combined β-adrenergic and calcium entry blockade in angina pectoris. N Engl J Med 320:709–718, 1989

66. Peart I, Bullock RE, Albers C, Hall RJC: Cold intolerance in patients with angina pectoris: effect of nifedipine and propranolol. Br Heart J 61:521–528, 1989

67. Platia EV, Michelson EL, Porterfield JK, Das G: Esmolol versus verapamil in the acute treatment of atrial fibrillation or atrial flutter. Am J Cardiol 63:925–929, 1989

68. Psaty BM, Koepsell TD, LoGergo JP, et al: β-blockers and primary prevention of coronary heart disease in patients with high blood pressure. JAMA 261:2087–2094, 1989

69. Quyyumi AA, Crake T, Wright CM, et al: Medical treatment of patients with severe exertional and rest angina: Double-blind comparison of β-blocker, calcium antagonist, and nitrate. Br Heart J 57:505–511, 1987

70. Robertson RM, Wood AJJ, Vaughn WK, Robertson D: Exacerbation of vasotonic angina by propranolol. Circulation 65:281–285, 1982
71. Schoenberger JA: Usefulness of penbutolol for systemic hypertension. Am J Cardiol 63:1339–1342, 1989
72. Schoenberger JA, Wallin JD, Gorwit JI, et al: A multicenter double-blind study of the efficacy and safety of once and twice daily dilevalol compared to propranolol. Am J Hypertens 2:840–846, 1989
73. Stone PH, Gibson RS, Glasser SP, et al: Comparison of diltiazem, nifedipine, and propranolol in the therapy of silent ischemia (abstract). Circulation 80 (suppl II):II-267, 1989
74. Strauss WE, Parisi AF: Combined use of calcium channel and β-adrenergic blockers for the treatment of chronic stable angina. Ann Intern Med 109:570–581, 1988
75. Streufert S, DePadova A, McGlynn T, et al: Impact of β-blockade on complex cognitive functioning. Am Heart J 116 311–315, 1988
76. TIMI Study Group: Comparison of invasive and conservative strategies after treatment with intravenous tissue plasminogen activator in acute myocardial infarction: Results of the thrombolysis in myocardial infarction (TIMI) Phase II Trial. N Engl J Med 320:618–627, 1989
77. Van den Meiracker AH, Man in 't Veld AJ, Ritsema van Eck HJ, et al: Hemodynamic and hormonal adaptations to β-adrenoceptor blockade: A 24-hour study of acebutolol, atenolol, pindolol, and propranolol in hypertensive patients. Circulation 78:957–968, 1988
78. Van Zyl AI, Jennings AA, Bateman ED, Opie LH: Comparison of respiratory effects of two cardioselective β-blockers, celiprolol and atenolol, in asthmatics with mild to moderate hypertension. Chest 95:209–213, 1989
79. Waagstein F, Caidahl K, Wallentin I, et al: Long-term beta-blockade in dilated cardiomyopathy. Effects of short- and long-term metoprolol treatment followed by withdrawal and readministration of metoprolol. Circulation 80:551–563, 1989
80. Walter P, Neil-Dwyer G, Cruickshank JM: Beneficial effects of adrenergic blockade in patients with subarachnoid hemorrhage. Br Med J 284:1661–1664, 1982
81. Wikstrand J, Warnold I, Olsson G, et al: Primary prevention with metoprolol in patients with hypertension: Mortality results from the MAPHY study. JAMA 259:1976–1982, 1988
82. Xamoterol Study Group: Xamoterol in severe heart failure. Lancet 336:1–6, 1990

Review

83. Frishman WH, Sonnenblick EH: β-adrenergic blocking drugs. In Hurst JW, Schlant RC, Rackley CE, et al (eds): The Heart, 7th ed. New York, McGraw-Hill Information Services, 1990, pp 1712–1731

Book

84. Cruickshank JM, Prichard BNC: Beta-blockers in clinical practice. Edinburgh, Churchill-Livingstone, 1987

U. Thadani
L. H. Opie

2

Nitrates

"As often true in matters of the heart, absence (nitrate-free intervals) makes the heart grow fonder (more nitrate responsiveness)."[56]

MECHANISM OF ACTION

In 1933 Sir Thomas Lewis held that the effect of amyl nitrite was probably due mainly to its powerful dilatation of the coronary vessels, rather than to its effect in lowering the blood pressure, as originally suggested by Lauder Brunton in Scotland in 1867. As time went on, the important role of nitrate-induced venodilation came to be recognized. Currently, emphasis is on the endothelial-derived relaxation factor (EDRF), now known to be nitric oxide (NO). Nitrates provide an exogenous source of NO in the vascular cells, thereby inducing coronary vasodilation even when production of NO is impaired by coronary artery disease. Chronic use of nitrates produces tolerance, which is a significant clinical problem, probably resulting from impaired production of NO in the vessel wall. The main focus of current clinical work is on strategies to minimize or prevent the development of tolerance. The major proposal is that a nitrate-free interval allows blood levels to fall and thereby to restore nitrate responsiveness.

Vasodilatory Effects, Coronary and Peripheral

A distinction must be made between antianginal and vasodilator properties. Nitrates (1) redistribute blood flow along collateral channels and from epicardial to endocardial regions and (2) relieve coronary spasm and dynamic stenosis, especially at epicardial sites,[2] acting in part on the coronary arterial constriction induced by exercise.[38] Thus, nitrates are "effective" vasodilators for angina; dipyridamole and many other vasodilators are not and may increase angina by diverting blood from the ischemic area—a "coronary steal" effect.

The peripheral hemodynamic effects of nitrates cannot, however, be ignored, because nitrates reduce the afterload, and especially the preload, of the heart (Fig. 2–1). Hence, nitrates are now being used not only to treat angina pectoris but also to unload the heart in left ventricular (LV) failure and in selected cases of myocardial infarction.

Vascular Receptors

The cellular mechanism of these vascular effects may be as follows. An intact vascular endothelium is required for the vasodilatory effects of some other agents (thus serotonin physiologically vasodilates but constricts when the endothelium is damaged). Nitrates vasodilate whether or not the endothelium is intact. The postulated "nitrate

ACTION OF NITRATES ON CIRCULATION

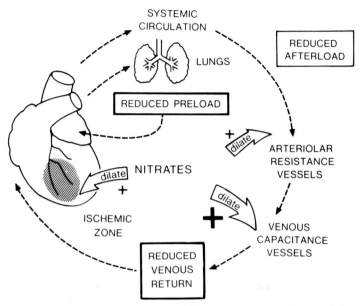

FIGURE 2–1. Schematic diagram of effects of nitrates on the circulation. The major effect is on the venous capacitance vessels, with additional coronary and peripheral arteriolar vasodilatory benefits. (Figure copyright L.H. Opie.)

receptor" is therefore likely to be situated on the myocyte rather than on the endothelium. Nitrates, after entering the vessel wall, are eventually converted to the NO group, which is thought to stimulate guanylate cyclase to produce cyclic GMP (Fig. 2–2). The cyclic nucleotide thus formed causes vasodilation as cell calcium falls either by inhibition of calcium ion entry or by promotion of calcium exit. Sulfhydryl (SH) groups are required for the formation of NO and the stimulation of guanylate cyclase. Vascular tolerance occurs when the SH groups are oxidized by excess exposure to nitrates. Nitroglycerin powerfully dilates when injected into an artery, an effect that is probably limited in humans by reflex vasoconstriction in response to preload reduction.[14] Hence, nitrates are better venous dilators than arteriolar dilators.

Oxygen Demand

Nitrates increase the venous capacitance, causing pooling of blood in the peripheral veins and thereby a reduction in venous return and in ventricular volume, to lessen the stress on the myocardial wall and to reduce the oxygen demand. Furthermore, a modest fall in arterial pressure also reduces the oxygen demand, although this is offset by a reflex increase in heart rate. The latter can be attenuated by concurrent β-blockade. The beneficial effect of nitrates in congestive heart failure (CHF) depends on venodilation.

PHARMACOKINETICS

Nitroglycerin (glyceryl trinitrate) is absorbed from the skin and oral mucosa and, less readily, from the gut.

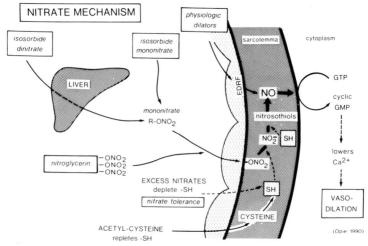

FIGURE 2–2. Effects of nitrates in generating NO and stimulating guanylate cyclase to cause vasodilation. Note role of cysteine cascade in stimulating guanylate cyclase, and role of SH depletion in nitrate tolerance. Note that mononitrates bypass hepatic metabolism. EDRF=endothelial-derived relaxation factor; SH=sulfhydryl; GTP=guanosine triphosphate; GMP=guanosine monophosphate. (For further details, see Fung[36] and Ignarro.[39])

Sublingual nitroglycerin has incomplete bioavailability, but clinical effects start within a minute or two and last up to an hour (Table 2-1); peak blood levels occur at 2 minutes, and the half-life is 7 minutes.

Nitroglycerin ointment is slow in its onset of action. The effects persist for 4 to 6 hours, the amount of nitroglycerin absorbed depending on the surface area covered by the ointment.

Nitroglycerin patches containing nitroglycerin in a reservoir or matrix form give plasma levels that are fairly constant from 2 to 24 hours or longer. Although the nitroglycerin content of the patches is variable (see Table 2-1), the amount of nitroglycerin delivered over 24 hours is dependent upon the surface area covered by the patch rather than the content of nitroglycerin.[15] The total nitroglycerin delivered over a 24-hour period is 0.5 mg/cm^2 from Transderm Nitro and Nitro-Dur patches and 0.625 mg/cm^2 from Nitrodisc patches. Recent studies emphasize the inevitability of tolerance development if constant, and especially high, nitrate blood levels are maintained, so that intermittent therapy is now advocated.

Nitroglycerin spray releases 0.4 mg per dose, and the vial contains 200 doses.

Isosorbide dinitrate is absorbed from the oral mucosa and gut, with slower onset and longer action; after liver metabolism, active mononitrate metabolites are ultimately excreted by the kidney, with a half-life of about 10 hours. Significant accumulation of intact isosorbide dinitrate occurs in plasma after 4x daily dosing at 30 mg, 60 mg, and 120 mg for 1 week.[13] The elimination half-life is about 30 minutes after a sublingual dose, and 1.5 to 4 hours after oral dosing.[13] Metabolites of isosorbide dinitrate (i.e., 2- and 5-mononitrates) also contribute to its action. The effect of the first dose persists for 6 to 8 hours, but the duration of effects and peak effects are attenuated during 4x a day therapy.[28]

Mononitrates (not yet available in the USA) are logical successors to isosorbide dinitrate, because the latter's activity depends on hepatic conversion to mononitrates (see Fig. 2–2). Thus with mononitrates the potentially variable effect of liver metabolism can be avoided; mononitrates have a high bioavailability with less variation in their effect when there is a fixed dose. Plasma levels of isosorbide-5–

mononitrate reach their peak between $\frac{1}{2}$ and 2 hours before being excreted by the kidney, partially unchanged and partially as an inactive glucuronide metabolite, with an elimination half-life of 4 to 6 hours. After the first dose its clinical efficacy is about 6 to 8 hours after a 20-mg dose and correlates with its plasma concentration.[21] In contrast, during chronic twice daily therapy there is a poor correlation between plasma concentrations and antianginal effects.[58]

SHORT-ACTING NITRATES FOR ACUTE EFFORT ANGINA

Sublingual nitroglycerin is very well established in the therapy of angina of effort (Table 2-2), yet may be ineffective, frequently because the patient has not received proper instruction. When angina starts, the patient should rest in the sitting position (standing promotes syncope, lying down enhances venous return and heart work) and take sublingual nitroglycerin (0.3–0.5 mg) every 3 minutes until the pain goes or a maximum of 4 to 5 tablets have been taken. **Nitroglycerin spray** or **buccal nitroglycerin** are alternative means of oral administration.

Isosorbide dinitrate may be given **sublingually** (5 mg) to abort an anginal attack and then exerts antianginal effects for about 1 hour. Because the dinitrate requires hepatic conversion to the mononitrate, the onset of antianginal action must be slower than with nitroglycerin. After **oral** ingestion, hemodynamic and antianginal effects persist for several hours.[27] Single doses of isosorbide dinitrate confer longer protection against angina than can single doses of sublingual nitroglycerin (see Table 2-1).

(Isosorbide mononitrate is not available as a sublingual preparation for acute relief of angina).

Side-effects and Failure of Nitrate Therapy (Table 2-3)

Causes of failure are increasing severity of angina or development of nitrate-resistant myocardial ischemia; loss of potency of tablets; incorrect route of administration (some sublingual preparations should not be taken orally, and vice versa); arterial hypoxemia, especially in chronic lung disease (caused by increased venous admixture); and non-compliance, usually because of headaches. Dry mucous membranes impair oral absorption. Nitrates are more effective if taken before the expected onset of anginal pain. When nitrates are less effective than expected owing to tachycardia, combination with β-blockade gives better results. A wrong diagnosis may be made, because nitrates sometimes relieve the pain of esophageal spasm and renal or biliary colic. During prophylactic therapy with long-acting nitrates, tolerance is a frequent cause of apparent failure.

LONG-ACTING NITRATES FOR ANGINA PROPHYLAXIS

Long-acting nitrates are not continuously effective if regularly taken over a prolonged period.

Isosorbide dinitrate (oral preparation) is frequently given in the prophylaxis of angina. An important question is whether regular therapy with isosorbide dinitrate gives long-lasting protection against angina. Improvement in exercise tolerance for up to 3 hours during acute therapy and for up to 5 hours during sustained therapy with isosorbide dinitrate has been reported.[8] In a critical placebo-controlled study, exercise duration improved significantly for 6 to 8 hours after single oral doses of 15 to 120 mg isosorbide dinitrate, but for only

TABLE 2–1 NITRATE PREPARATIONS: DOSES, PREPARATIONS, AND DURATION OF EFFECTS

Compound	Route	Preparation and Dose	Duration of Effects and Comments
Amyl nitrite	Inhalation for diagnosis	2–5 mg	10 sec–10 min
Nitroglycerin (trinitrin, TNT, glyceryl trinitrate)	(a) Sublingual	0.3–1.5 mg, as needed Tablets—usually 0.3, 0.5, or 0.6 mg	1 1/2 min–1 hr; peak blood levels at 2 min (1/2-time of 7 1/2 min)
	(b) Spray	0.4 mg/metered dose, as needed	Effects apparent within 5 min, duration of effects not known
	(c) Percutaneous	2% ointment 15x15 cm or 12.5–40 mg	3–4 hr
	(d) Transdermal patches: Nitrodur, Transderm-Nitro, Nitrodisc, Minitran	7.5–10 mg/12hr or 16 mg/14hr	Effects start within 1–2 hr, last 8–12 hr during intermittent therapy. Not effective during continuous therapy
	(e) Oral; sustained-release	2.6 mg, 1–2 tablets 3x daily	4–8 hr
	(f) Intravenous	0.3–12.0 mg/hr when urgent 0.1 mg bolus (care; lower dose for new sets). Tridil 0.5 mg/ml Nitrostat, or Nitrol IV 0.8 mg/ml	In unstable angina, increasing doses often are needed During intracoronary infusion and 30 min post infusion high K^+ in some preparations may cause VF

Drug	Route	Dose	Notes
Isosorbide dinitrate (=sorbide nitrate) Isordil *Isordil Tembids	(a) Sublingual	5–15 mg	Onset 5–10 min, effect up to 60 min
	(b) Oral	5–80 mg 2–3x daily (top dose 480 mg daily)	Exercise time raised for 2–8 hr (see text for tolerance)
	(c) Spray	1.25 mg on tongue	Rapid action 2–3 min
	(d) Chewable	5 mg as single dose	Exercise time raised for 2 min–2½hr
	(e) Oral; sustained-release*	40 mg once or 2x daily	2–6 hr free from angina
	(f) Intravenous	1.25–5.0 mg/hr (care; absorbed into tubing)	May need increasing doses for unstable angina at rest
	(g) Ointment	100 mg/24 hr	Not effective during continuous therapy
Isosorbide-5-mononitrate (not in USA)	Oral	10–40 mg 2x daily eccentric dosage	6–10 hr
	Sustained-release	40–100 mg 1x daily	Claimed efficacy up to 9 hr during chronic use, depending on preparation
Pentaerythritol tetranitrate	(a) Sublingual	10 mg as needed	45 min; classified as "possibly effective" in USA
Erythrityl tetranitrate	(a) Sublingual	5–10 mg as needed	10–45 min
	(b) Oral	10–30 mg 3x daily; chew before swallowing	Effects begin after 20–30 min. Not intended for acute attacks

For references, see previous editions. For tolerance with isosorbide mononitrate, see Wisenberg et al[165] and Thadani et al.[60-62]
*Duration of hemodynamic effects has been most closely studied, but there is good correlation between such effects and antianginal action.

TABLE 2–2 PROPOSED STEP-CARE FOR ANGINA OF EFFORT

1. General therapy: History and physical examination to exclude valvular disease, anemia, hypertension, thromboembolic disease, and heart failure. Check risk factors for coronary artery disease (smoking, hypertension, blood lipids, diabetes). Must stop smoking.

2. Nitrates, short/long-acting, given **intermittently** as needed to control pain.

3. **Intermittent** short/long-acting nitrates plus beta-adrenergic blocker
   or
   Intermittent short/long-acting nitrates plus calcium antagonist, preferably verapamil or diltiazem.
   (For prophylactic long-acting nitrates, see below.)

4. **Intermittent** short/long-acting nitrates plus calcium antagonists plus beta-blocker (triple therapy).

5. Consider bypass surgery after failure to respond to medical therapy or for left main stem lesion or for triple vessel disease. Even response to medical therapy does not eliminate need for investigation.

6. In selected patients, PTCA may be attempted at any stage, especially for highly symptomatic single-vessel disease.

As an alternative to steps 3 and 4, replace intermittent long-acting nitrates with **prophylactic long-acting nitrates** taken regularly, while trying to avoid nitrate tolerance (low eccentric dose), in which case intermittent short-acting nitrates are still used as needed.

PTCA = Percutaneous transluminal angioplasty.

2 hours when the same doses were given repetitively 4x daily.[28] Marked tolerance to the antianginal effects of 30 mg 4x daily can develop during sustained therapy,[50] despite much higher plasma isosorbide dinitrate concentrations during sustained than during acute therapy.[28] Currently, eccentric dosage schedules are advised to avoid tolerance (see Table 2-4).

Transdermal nitroglycerin patches are designed to permit the timed release of nitroglycerin over a 24-hour period. Despite initial claims of 24-hour efficacy, almost all subsequent studies have failed to show prolonged improvement. The decisive study (which may never be published) was a multicenter FDA-monitored trial evaluating chronic patch therapy in 562 patients, using patches that delivered up to 105 mg of nitroglycerin over a 24-hour period. There was no improvement in treadmill exercise duration measured at 4 and 24 hours after patch application when compared with placebo.[63] Furthermore, in a British trial on 427 men, 5-mg nitroglycerin patches had no antianginal effect and actually decreased the quality of life as judged by the psychosocial score.[35] However, eccentric dosage schedules of patches do work (see Table 2-4).

Nitroglycerin paste may be used for nocturnal angina or angina at rest. Clearly, its nocturnal use should not be combined with eccentric therapeutic schedules, which work by providing a nocturnal nitrate-free interval (see Table 2-4). For convenience, nitroglycerin paste is applied to the skin of the chest. In AMI, it can be wiped off in the event of an adverse reaction.

Mononitrates have been compared with dinitrates in only a few clinical trials. The mean incidence of attacks of angina and use of nitroglycerin during the mononitrate therapy was lower than during medication with slow-release dinitrate or with placebo.[23] On the whole, the dosage and effects of mononitrates are similar to those of isosorbide dinitrate. Nitrate tolerance, likewise a potential problem,[25,61,62] can be prevented or minimized when the drug is given twice daily in an eccentric pattern (see Table 2-4).

TABLE 2–3 PRECAUTIONS AND SIDE-EFFECTS IN USE OF NITRATES

Precautions

Nitrate tablets should be kept in airtight containers and stored in cold. Some nitrates are inflammable (especially the spray).

Serious Side-effects

Syncope and hypotension from reduction of preload and afterload; alcohol or co-therapy with vasodilators may enhance. Treat by recumbency. **Tachycardia** frequent, but unexplained bradycardia occasionally arises in acute myocardial infarction. Hypotension may cause cerebral ischemia. Prolonged high dosage can cause **methemoglobinemia**; treat by intravenous methylene blue. High-dose IV nitrates can induce **heparin resistance**.

Other Side-effects

Headaches frequently limit dose. Facial flushing. Sublingual nitrates may cause halitosis.

Contraindications

In angina caused by **hypertrophic obstructive cardiomyopathy**, nitrates may exaggerate outflow obstruction and are contraindicated except for diagnosis. **Cardiac tamponade** or constrictive pericarditis; the already compromised diastolic filling may be aggravated by reduced venous return.

Relative Contraindications

Acute inferior myocardial infarction with right ventricular involvement; fall in filling pressure may lead to hemodynamic and clinical deterioration. In **cor pulmonale** and arterial hypoxemia, nitrates decrease arterial O_2 tension by venous admixture. Although **glaucoma** is usually held to be a contraindication, there is no objective evidence to show any increase in intraocular pressure (possible exception: amyl nitrite).[30] In **mitral stenosis**, nitrates may reduce the preload excessively.

Tolerance

Shown experimentally and clinically. Continuous therapy and high-dose frequent therapy leads to tolerance that low-dose interval therapy may avoid. Cross-tolerance established.

Withdrawal Symptoms

Established in munitions workers, in whom withdrawal may precipitate symptoms and sudden death. Some evidence for a similar clinical syndrome. Therefore, only gradually discontinue long-term nitrate therapy. With eccentric dose schedules (see Table 2–4) there is a low rate of recurrent pain in the nitrate-free interval.

CAUSES OF FAILURE OF LONG-ACTING PREPARATIONS

During therapy with long-acting preparations, two of the chief causes of failure are (1) the development of tolerance, treated by gradually decreasing the dose and the frequency of drug administration until there is a nitrate-free interval (see section on tolerance); and (2) worsening of the disease process, treated by combination therapy while excluding aggravating factors such as hypertension, atrial fibrillation or anemia, and considering surgical intervention.

NITRATES FOR MIXED ANGINA AND SILENT ISCHEMIA

"**Mixed**" **or double-component angina** means the combination of nocturnal and effort angina. In a double-blind comparison of a β-blocker (atenolol 100 mg daily), a calcium antagonist (nifedipine 20 mg 3x daily), and isosorbide mononitrate (40 mg twice daily), the β-blocker was best overall, although equal control of nocturnal ST-segment

TABLE 2–4 INTERVAL THERAPY FOR EFFORT ANGINA BY ECCENTRIC NITRATE DOSAGE SCHEDULES DESIGNED TO AVOID TOLERANCE

Preparation	Dose	Reference
Isosorbide dinitrate	30 mg at 7 am, 12 noon, 5 pm	50
Isosorbide dinitrate sustained-release (Tembids)	80 mg at 8 am, or 8 am and 12 noon	57
Isosorbide mononitrate	20 mg at 8 am and 3 pm	60
Isosorbide mononitrate, controlled-release (Astra preparation)	60 mg at 8 am	65
Isosorbide mononitrate slow-release (Knoll-Pharma Schwartz preparation)	50 and 100 mg once daily ineffective	61
Transdermal nitrate patches	1) 7.5–10 mg per 12 hr patches removed after 12 hr	33 63
	2) Maximum tolerated dose 16 mg mean, over 14 hr	56
	3) About 6 mg/14 hr ineffective	64
Phasic-release nitroglycerin patch	15 mg, most released in first 12 hr	51

changes was achieved by all three agents. Pain relief was similar with nifedipine and isosorbide.[52]

In **silent myocardial ischemia**, although nitrates are effective,[52] there is the same risk of development of tolerance as with overt angina, as judged by a study with transdermal nitroglycerin.[46]

NITRATES FOR UNSTABLE ANGINA AT REST

"The one setting in which intermittent nitrate therapy does not have a role is the treatment of the hospitalized patient with unstable ischemic symptoms with or without myocardial infarction."[53]

In the therapy of unstable angina, it is presumed that upward titration of the dose of IV nitrate can overcome tolerance, as in the case of AMI.[41]

IV nitroglycerin is very effective in the management of patients with unstable angina, although there is surprisingly little objective evidence of such efficacy in properly controlled trials. IV therapy allows more rapid titration to an effective dose and permits rapid reversal of hemodynamic effects if an adverse reaction occurs. The usual initial starting dose is 5 to 10 µg/min, which can be titrated up to 200 µg/min or occasionally higher up to 1000 µg/min, depending on the clinical course and aiming at the relief of anginal pain, or in patients who are already pain-free at a fall of mean blood pressure of 10%, the infusion being maintained for up to 36 hours.[18] IV nitroglycerin exceeding 350 µg/min may induce heparin resistance.[32]

IV isosorbide dinitrate, infused in patients with repetitive episodes of angina at rest at a rate of 1.25 to 5.0 mg/hr, relieves pain and reduces the incidence of ischemic episodes as judged by spontaneous ST-deviations[9] with few side-effects. Why the IV route is so much more effective than the oral route is not well understood. However, the blood levels are almost 10x higher for equivalent doses given IV than when given orally,[26] stressing the poor bioavailability of oral isosorbide dinitrate, due to extensive presystemic metabolism.

Nitrate patches and **nitroglycerin ointment** are still frequently used in unstable angina at rest despite any good evidence that the development of tolerance can be avoided. As there is no role for intermittent nitrate therapy in unstable angina, eccentric dosage schedules cannot be used. IV therapy, which can be titrated upwards as needed, is far better for control of pain.

ACUTE MYOCARDIAL INFARCTION

Here there is an obvious dilemma. Overall evidence suggests that IV nitrates reduce mortality,[66] acting by reduction of infarct size, infarct expansion, and infarct-related complications.[40] On the other hand, marked hypotensive episodes can occur, especially in patients with acute inferior myocardial infarction with right ventricular involvement who are highly dependent on the preload.[34] Logically, the combination of nitrates with other agents tending to produce hypotension, such as β-blockers or thrombolytic agents, requires caution. Whereas the beneficial effects of thrombolytic agents and β-blockers in AMI are now well established in large trials, nitrate trials have been conducted on relatively small numbers of patients. Hence IV nitrates in AMI should be reserved for patients with ongoing anginal pain, for those with LV failure or severe hypertension, or when the differential diagnosis between early transmural AMI and Prinzmetal's angina is not clear. **Low-dose therapy is preferred.** An initial dose of nitroglycerin of 5 µg/min is increased by 5 to 20 µg/min every 5 minutes in the first 30 minutes until the mean blood pressure is reduced by 10% in normotensive patients and by 30% in hypertensive patients.[41] Thereafter, buccal nitroglycerin (1 to 3 mg 3x daily at 5-hour intervals with prolonged washout) is titrated to reduce the blood pressure by 10% for 6 weeks, to give improved LV function at 6 months.[41a]

CONGESTIVE HEART FAILURE

Both short- and long-acting nitrates are used in the therapy of acute and chronic heart failure. Their dilating effects are more pronounced on veins than on arterioles, so they are best suited to patients with raised pulmonary wedge pressure and clinical features of pulmonary congestion.

In **acute pulmonary edema** from various causes, including AMI, nitroglycerin can be strikingly effective, with some risk of precipitous falls in blood pressure and of tachycardia or bradycardia. Sublingual nitroglycerin in repeated doses of 0.8 to 2.4 mg every 5 to 10 minutes can relieve coarse rales and dyspnea within 15 to 20 minutes, with a fall of LV filling pressure and a rise in cardiac output.[5] IV nitroglycerin, however, is usually a better method to administer nitroglycerin, as the dose can be rapidly adjusted upward or downward, depending on the clinical and hemodynamic response. Little has been reported on the combination of nitrates with conventional therapy in acute pulmonary edema.

In **severe CHF**, nitrates may be used as the sole vasodilator agent (as in mitral stenosis[4]) or added to converting enzyme inhibitors or hydralazine (for combination with hydralazine, see Chapter 5). Isosorbide dinitrate (orally 40 mg 4x daily), given to 16 patients with severe CHF, increased the maximal exercise duration when compared with placebo.[11]

The dinitrate was effective over a 2-month period in one study,[12] and a dose of 40 mg 4x daily was better than placebo during 3 months of treatment in another study.[17] Because of the lack of a deliberate nitrate-free interval, the potential effect of nitrate therapy was almost certainly blunted. Eccentric dosing, designed to counter periods of expected dyspnea (at night, anticipated exercise) seems a better policy. Oral isosorbide dinitrate, 20 to 80 mg 4x daily, can be added to digitalis and diuretics[6] and to hydralazine in chronic oral therapy of heart failure[7,20] with beneficial hemodynamic and symptomatic effects. **Tolerance** is a definite risk with sustained therapy and in one study was treated by discontinuation of therapy for 36 hours.[3]

Nitrate patches have given variable results. Tolerance is inevitable with sustained-release patches.[44] **IV nitroglycerin** (6.4 µg/kg/min) produces tolerance with continuous but not with interrupted infusions.[49]

NITRATE TOLERANCE

Now that there is overwhelming evidence for the existence of nitrate tolerance if blood nitrate levels are continuously maintained, **interval therapy** with eccentric dosage has become standard (see Table 2-4). Arguments against sustained-release preparations are so strong that such preparations should no longer be used unless, for example, patches are removed at night. Yet the use of interval therapy and the nitrate-free interval leads to the risk of rebound angina,[33] so that a more logical long-term approach is to examine the mechanism of tolerance with the ultimate aim of maintaining the efficacy of nitrate therapy over 24 hours.

Vascular sulfhydryl depletion is the currently favored theory. SH groups, derived from cysteine, are required for the intracellular formation of NO, the active moiety stimulating guanylate cyclase (see Fig. 2–2). The NO thus formed oxidizes intracellular SH groups and thiol depletion results. Acetylcysteine may counteract tolerance either by providing SH groups with formation of intracellular S-nitrothiols or by forming extracellular thiols, which could enter the vascular cells.[37] When N-acetylcysteine fails, the explanation may be an excess dosage of nitrates, especially in experimental studies, or else the existence of non-vascular mechanisms of tolerance.

Speculatively, **high- and low-affinity nitrate receptors** might exist. During the treatment of unstable angina, increasing doses of IV nitrates may be required to relieve pain and to achieve hemodynamic effects. If vascular levels of SH groups were really the crucial rate-limiting factor, it would seem unlikely that higher doses of nitrates could overcome tolerance.

Non-vascular mechanisms of tolerance also exist. In congestive heart failure, nitrate tolerance is accompanied by increased circulating levels of renin,[49] thereby suggesting neurohumoral activation with increased plasma norepinephrine levels.[48] N-acetylcysteine only partially reverses tolerance. The proposal is that such neurohumoral activation contributes to the development of nitrate tolerance.[42,49]

Prevention of Tolerance

Interval dosing with low eccentric doses is the most commonly used and simplest procedure.[54] In effort angina, many studies now show that tolerance can be avoided by interval dosing, which may explain why some nitrate efficacy seems to be kept during chronic sustained oral therapy (seesaw blood levels) in contrast to loss of efficacy with nitrate patches (sustained blood levels).

Upward adjustment of the dose appears to work in unstable angina and acute myocardial infarction, where nitrate-free intervals are contraindicated because of the risk of rebound. **Rapidly increasing blood nitrate levels** may overcome tolerance. For example, with established nitrate tolerance, sublingual nitrate can still have some therapeutic effect, albeit diminished.[54] Thadani and colleagues[59] measured blood levels during mononitrate therapy and found that, even when trough levels were high, a further rapid increase was associated with therapeutic benefit.

Phasic delivery systems are a logical development to achieve therapeutic benefit with nitrate patches even when they are left on for 24 hours.[51]

Sulfhydryl donors, such as N-acetylcysteine, are still investigational. In a particularly impressive study, Packer and coworkers[49] used a relatively high dose of N-acetylcysteine, 200 mg/kg, and achieved partial reversal of tolerance with oral dosage. In contrast, Parker and colleagues[50] failed to revert tolerance with a single IV administration of acetylcysteine.

Angiotensin-converting enzyme inhibitors are increasingly being tested, with captopril the favorite because it would not only antagonize neurohumoral activation but also provide SH groups.[43]

Nitrate Cross-Tolerance

Long- and short-acting nitrates frequently are combined. In patients already receiving isosorbide dinitrate, addition of sublingual nitroglycerin gives a further small (10%) therapeutic effect.[16] Hypotensive effects of sublingual nitroglycerin or sublingual isosorbide dinitrate are, however, rapidly attenuated during chronic therapy with oral isosorbide dinitrate.[3,27] Logically, tolerance to long-acting nitrates should cause cross-tolerance to short-acting nitrates, as shown for the capacitance vessels of the forearm,[19] coronary artery diameter,[47] and on exercise tolerance during IV nitroglycerin therapy.[67] Cross-tolerance to sublingual nitroglycerin (no change in BP, heart rate) is proposed as a simple clinical test for nitrate tolerance.[31]

Nitrate tolerance may attenuate the therapeutic effects, especially in the case of long-acting nitrates. A nitrate-free interval should be built into the dose regimen whenever possible. Yet because of the wide variations in the dose-response curves, each patient merits specific evaluation of the optimal dose.

COMBINATION THERAPY FOR ANGINA

β-**blockade and nitrates** are often combined in the therapy of angina (see Table 2-2). Both β-blockers and nitrates decrease the oxygen demand, and nitrates increase the oxygen supply; β-blockade cancels the tachycardiac effect of nitrates. β-blockade tends to increase heart size, and nitrates to decrease it. Anginal patients on β-blockers are better able to withstand pacing-stress when nitroglycerin is added,[24] and patients already receiving beta-blockade respond no less well than others to nitroglycerin.[10] The combination of isosorbide dinitrate (mean daily dose 90 mg) and β-blockade (propranolol mean dose 120 mg/day) is more effective than β-blockade by itself,[22] although less effective than the combination propranolol-nifedipine.

Calcium antagonists and nitrates are also often combined. For example, in a double-blind trial of 47 patients with effort angina, verapamil 80 mg 3x daily decreased the use of nitroglycerin tablets by 25% and prolonged the exercise time by 20%.[1] Nifedipine, when added to propranolol and titrated to the maximum tolerated dose (mean 77 mg/day) and then given for 3 weeks, was more effective in effort angina than isosorbide dinitrate likewise titrated and given.[22] Combination of verapamil or diltiazem with long-acting nitrates is usually preferable to nitrates with nifedipine, because of the powerful and sometimes excessive pre- and afterload reduction achieved by the latter combination. In contrast, nifedipine combines better with β-blockers.

Nitrates, β-blockers, and calcium antagonists may also be combined as triple therapy, frequently deemed to be maximal. Yet sometimes such therapy is less effective than only two of the components, possibly because of excess hypotension.[29] Because of individual variations among patients, some will tolerate one type of combination therapy better than another, so that triple therapy should not be automatic when dual therapy fails.

NEW ANTIANGINAL AGENTS

Molsidomine acts by release of vasodilatory metabolites such as SIN-1 formed during first-pass liver metabolism. These metabolites bypass the cysteine-dependent metabolic cascade and, therefore, should provide substantial protection from tolerance. However, strict comparisons with nitrates are not yet available. In a dose of 2 mg 3x daily, this agent is widely used in Germany.

Nicorandil is a nicotinamide nitrate, acting chiefly by dilation of the large coronary arteries, as well as by reduction of pre- and afterload. It has a double cellular mechanism of action, both acting as a potassium channel activator and having a nitrate-like effect,[55] which may explain why experimentally it causes less tolerance than nitrates. It is widely used as an antianginal agent in Japan in a dose of 10 to 20 mg 12-hourly.[45]

SUMMARY

Nitrates act by venodilation and relief of coronary vasoconstriction (including that induced by exercise) to treat anginal attacks. Their unloading effects also benefit patients with backward CHF and high LV filling pressures. Newer nitrate preparations are not a substantial advance over the old, especially not the nitrate patches, which clearly predispose to tolerance by sustained blood nitrate levels. Mononitrates, not yet available in the USA, are a modest advance over dinitrates because they eliminate variable hepatic metabolism, on which the action of the dinitrates depends. Yet with all nitrate preparations the fundamental problem of potential tolerance remains. During the treatment of effort angina by isosorbide dinitrate or mononitrate, substantial evidence suggests that eccentric doses with a nitrate-free interval go far to avoid tolerance. For unstable angina at rest, a nitrate-free interval is not possible, and short-term treatment for 24 to 48 hours with IV nitroglycerin is frequently effective with, however, higher and higher doses often required to overcome tolerance. In AMI, the use of IV nitrates is returning, bringing with it the risk of hypotension, especially in inferior infarctions or during co-therapy with β-blockers or thrombolytic agents. During the treatment of CHF, tolerance also develops, so that nitrates are best reserved for specific problems such as acute LV failure, nocturnal dyspnea, or anticipated exercise. Two new antianginal agents, molsidomine and nicorandil, may yet solve the problem of tolerance to the nitrate vasodilators.

REFERENCES

References from Previous Editions

1. Andreasen F, Boye E, Christoffersen P, et al: Eur J Cardiol 2:443–452, 1975
2. Badger RS, Brown BG, Gallery CA, et al: Am J Cardiol 56:390–395, 1985
3. Blasini R, Froer KL, Blumel G, et al: Herz 7:250–258, 1982

4. Bornheimer JF, Kim JS, Sambasivan V, et al: Am Heart J 104:1288–1293, 1982

5. Bussmann W-D, Schupp D: Am J Cardiol 41:931–936, 1978

6. Cohn JN: In Cohn JN, Rittinghausen R (eds): Mononitrates. Berlin, Springer-Verlag, 1985, pp 299–305

7. Cohn JN, Archibald DG, Phil M, et al: N Engl J Med 314:1547–1552, 1986

8. Dahany DT, Burwell DT, Aronow WS, et al: Circulation 55:381–387, 1977

9. Distante A, Maseri A, Severi S, et al: Am J Cardiol 44:533–539, 1979

10. Fox KM, Dyett JF, Portal RW, et al: Eur J Cardiol 5:507–515, 1977

11. Franciosa JA, Nordstrom LA, Cohn JN: JAMA 240:443–446, 1978

12. Franciosa JA, Cohn JN: Am J Cardiol 45:648–654, 1980

13. Fung HL, McNiff EF, Ruggirello D, et al: Br J Clin Pharmacol 11:579–590, 1981

14. Imaizumi T, Takeshita A, Ashihara T, et al: Circulation 72:747–752, 1985

15. Karim A: Angiology 34:11–22, 1983

16. Lee G, Mason DT, DeMaria AN: Am J Cardiol 41:82–87, 1978

17. Leier CV, Huss B, Margorien D, et al: Circulation 67:817–822, 1983

18. Lin S-G, Flaherty JT: Am J Cardiol 56:742–748, 1985

19. Manyari DE, Smith ER, Spragg J: Am J Cardiol 55:927–931, 1985

20. Massie B, Chatterjee K, Werner J, et al: Am J Cardiol 40:794–801, 1977

21. Maclean D, Feely J: Br Med J 286:1127–1130, 1983

22. Morse JR, Nesto RW: J Am Coll Cardiol 6:1395–1401, 1985

23. Muller G, Hacker W, Schneider B. Klin Wochenschr 61:409–416, 1983

24. Schang SJ Jr, Pepine CJ. Br Heart J 40:1221–1228, 1978

25. Tauchert M, Jansen W, Osterspey A, et al. Z Kardiol 72 (suppl 3):218–228, 1983

26. Taylor T, Chasseaud LF: In Lichtlen PR, Engel H-J, Schrey A, et al (eds): Nitrates. III: Cardiovascular effects. Berlin, Springer-Verlag, 1981, pp 40–46

27. Thadani U, Fung HL, Darke AC, et al: Circulation 62:491–502, 1980

28. Thadani U, Fung HL, Darke AC, et al: Am J Cardiol 49:411–419, 1982

29. Tolins M, Weir K, Chesler E, et al: J Am Coll Cardiol 3:1051–1057, 1984

30. Whitworth CG, Grant WM: Arch Ophthalmol 7:492–497, 1964

New References

31. Amidi M, Shaver JA: Sublingual NTG test for detection of nitrate tolerance in patients with coronary artery disease (abstract). Circulation 80 (suppl II):II–214, 1989

32. Becker RC, Corrao JM, Baker SP, et al: Nitroglycerin-induced heparin resistance: A qualitative defect in antithrombin III (abstract). Circulation 80 (suppl II):II–52, 1989

33. DeMots H, Glasser SP: Intermittent transdermal nitroglycerin therapy in the treatment of chronic stable angina. J Am Coll Cardiol 13:786–793, 1989

34. Ferguson JJ, Diver DJ, Boldt M, Pasternak RC: Significance of nitroglycerin-induced hypotension with inferior wall acute myocardial infarction. Am J Cardiol 64:311–314, 1989

35. Fletcher A, McLoone P, Bulpitt C: Quality of life on angina therapy: A randomized controlled trial of transdermal glyceryl trinitrate against placebo. Lancet 2:4–8, 1988

36. Fung H-L: Pharmacokinetics and pharmacodynamics of organic nitrates. Am J Cardiol 60:4H–9H, 1987

37. Fung H-L, Chong S, Kowaluk E, et al: Mechanisms for the pharmacologic interaction of organic nitrates with thiols: Existence of an extracellular pathway for the reversal of nitrate vascular tolerance by N-acetylcysteine. J Pharmacol Exp Ther 245:524–530, 1988

38. Gage JE, Jess DM, Murakami T, et al: Vasoconstriction of stenotic coronary arteries during dynamic exercise in patients with classic angina pectoris: Reversibility by nitroglycerin. Circulation 73:865–876, 1986

39. Ignarro LJ: Biological actions and properties of endothelium-derived nitric oxide formed and released from artery and vein. Circ Res 65: 1–21, 1989

40. Jugdutt BI, Warnica JW: Intravenous nitroglycerin therapy to limit myocardial infarct size, expansion, and complications: Effect of timing, dosage and infarct location. Circulation 78:906–919, 1988

41. Jugdutt BI, Warnica JW: Tolerance with low dose intravenous nitroglycerin therapy in acute myocardial infarction. Am J Cardiol 64:581–587, 1989

41a. Jugdutt BI, Neiman JC, Michorowski BL, et al. Persistent improvement in left ventricular geometry and function by prolonged nitroglycerin therapy after anterior transmural acute myocardial infarction. J Am Coll Cardiol 15:214A, 1990

42. Katz RJ: Mechanisms of nitrate tolerance. A Review. Cardiovasc Drugs Ther 4:247–252, 1989

43. Levy WS, Katz RJ, Buff L, Wasserman AG: Nitroglycerin tolerance is modified by angiotensin converting enzyme inhibitors (Abstract). Circulation 80 (suppl II):II–214, 1989

44. Lindvall K, Eriksson SV, Lagerstrand L, Sjogren A: Efficacy and tolerability of transdermal nitroglycerin in heart failure. Eur Heart J 9:373–379, 1988

45. Meany TB, Richardson P, Camm AJ: Exercise capacity after single and twice-daily doses of nicorandil in chronic stable angina pectoris. Am J Cardiol 63:66J–70J, 1989

46. Nabel EG, Barry J, Rocco MB, et al: Effects of dosing intervals on the development of tolerance to high dose transdermal nitroglycerin. Am J Cardiol 63:663–669, 1989

47. Naito H, Matsuda Y, Shiomi K, et al: Effects of sublingual nitrate in patients receiving sustained therapy of isosorbide dinitrate for coronary artery disease. Am J Cardiol 64:565–568, 1989

48. Olivari MT, Carlyle PF, Levine TB, et al: Hemodynamic and hormonal response to transdermal nitroglycerin in normal subjects and in patients with congestive heart failure. J Am Coll Cardiol 2:872-878, 1983

49. Packer M, Lee WH, Kessler PD, et al: Prevention and reversal of nitrate tolerance in patients with congestive heart failure. N Engl J Med 317:799–804, 1987

50. Parker JO, Farrell B, Lahey KA, et al: Effect of intervals between doses on the development of tolerance to isosorbide dinitrate. N Engl J Med 316:1440–1444, 1987

51. Parker JO: Antianginal efficacy of a new nitroglycerin patch. Eur Heart J 10 (suppl A):43–49, 1989

52. Quyyumi AA, Crake T, Wright CM, et al: Medical treatment of patients with severe exertional and rest angina:Double blind comparison of beta-blocker, calcium antagonist, and nitrate. Br Heart J 57:505–511, 1987

53. Reichek N: Intermittent nitrate therapy in angina pectoris. Eur Heart J 10 (suppl A):7–10, 1989

54. Rudolph W, Dirschinger J, Reiniger G, et al: When does nitrate tolerance develop? What dosages and which intervals are necessary to ensure maintained effectiveness? Eur Heart J 9 (suppl A):63–72, 1988

55. Sakai K: Nicorandil: Animal pharmacology. Am J Cardiol 63:2J–10J, 1989

56. Schaer DH, Buff LA, Katz RJ: Sustained antianginal efficacy of transdermal nitroglycerin patches using an overnight 10-hour nitrate-free interval. Am J Cardiol 61:46–50, 1988

57. Silber S, Vogler AC, Krause K-H, et al: Induction and circumvention of nitrate tolerance applying different dosage intervals. Am J Med 83:860–870, 1987

58. Thadani U, Hamilton SF, Olson E, et al: Duration of effects and tolerance of slow-release isosorbide-5-mononitrate for angina pectoris. Am J Cardiol 59:756–762, 1987

59. Thadani U, Prasad R, Hamilton SF, et al: Usefulness of twice-daily isosorbide-5-mononitrate in preventing development of tolerance in angina pectoris. Am J Cardiol 42:58–65, 1987

60. Thadani U, Whitsett TL: Pharmacokinetic-pharmacodynamic relationship of the organic nitrates. Clin Pharmacokinetics 15:32–43, 1988

61. Thadani U, Bittar N, Doyle R, et al: Nitrate tolerance: Do "critical" trough plasma levels exist to prevent tolerance (abstract)? Circulation 80 (suppl II):II–215, 1989

62. Thadani U, Friedman R, Jones JP, et al: Nitrate tolerance: Eccentric versus concentric twice daily therapy with isosorbide-5-mononitrate in angina pectoris. Circulation 80 (suppl II):II–216, 1989

63. Transdermal Nitroglycerin Cooperative Study. Presentation to Food and Drug Administration Cardiovascular and Renal Drugs Advisory Committee, Bethesda, Maryland, January 26, 1988

64. Waters DD, Juneau M, Gossard D, et al: Limited usefulness of intermittent nitroglycerin patches in stable angina. J Am Coll Cardiol 13:421–425, 1989

65. Wisenberg G, Roks C, Nichol P, Goddard MD: Sustained effect of and lack of development of tolerance to controlled-release isosorbide-5-mononitrate in chronic stable angina pectoris. Am J Cardiol 64:569–576, 1989

66. Yusuf S, Collins R, MacMahon S, Peto R: Effect of intravenous nitrates on mortality in acute myocardial infarction: An overview of the randomised trials. Lancet 1:1088–1092, 1988
67. Zimrin D, Reichek N, Bogin KT, et al: Antianginal effects of intravenous nitroglycerin over 24 hours. Circulation 77:1376–1384, 1988

Reviews

Abrams J: Interval therapy to avoid nitrate tolerance: Paradise regained? Am J Cardiol 64:931–934, 1989

Flaherty JT. Nitrate tolerance: A review of the evidence. Drugs 37:523–550, 1989

Parker JO: Intermittent transdermal nitroglycerin therapy in the treatment of chronic stable angina. J Am Coll Cardiol 13:794–795, 1989

Thadani U, Whitsett T, Hamilton SF: Nitrate therapy for myocardial ischemic syndrome: Current perspectives including tolerance. Curr Problems in Cardiol 13:725–784, 1988

L.H. Opie

3

Calcium Channel Antagonists (Calcium Entry Blockers)

The calcium antagonists (or calcium entry blockers) have now become one of the standard first-line treatments for essential hypertension and, together with β-blockers and nitrates, have become established therapy for angina pectoris. Their effectiveness and low side-effect profile has made these agents among the most widely used cardiovascular drugs. The three first-generation calcium antagonists—verapamil, nifedipine, and diltiazem—(in historical order of appearance) are the three patriarchs, according to Braunwald.[140] Their progeny, the second-generation calcium antagonists, of which more and more are currently becoming available in the USA and Europe, are chiefly nifedipine-like agents (dihydropyridines), with improved kinetic qualities, such as longer half-lives and, for some, greater vascular selectivity with less direct negative inotropic effects.

PHARMACOLOGIC PROPERTIES

Calcium Channels: L- and T-Types

The most important property of calcium antagonists (= calcium entry blockers = slow channel blockers) is selectively to inhibit the inward calcium current (Fig. 3–1) in those tissues where the action potential has a dominant calcium-dependent upstroke, not fired by a fast sodium signal, as in vascular smooth muscle and nodal tissue (sinus and AV nodes). Previously, the term "slow channel blocker" was used, but now it is realized that the calcium current develops much faster than previously believed and that there are at least two types of calcium channels, the L and the T. The conventional calcium channel, long known to exist, is now termed the **L-channel,** which is blocked by calcium antagonists and increased by catecholamines. The newly described **T-type channel** appears at more negative potentials than the L-type and probably plays a role in the initial depolarization of sinus and AV nodal tissue. The function of the L-type is to maintain the action potential plateau, thereby admitting the substantial amount of calcium ions required for initiation of contraction via calcium-induced calcium release from the sarcoplasmic reticulum. Specific blockers for T-type calcium channels are not yet available, but can be expected to inhibit the sinus and AV nodes profoundly.

Cellular Mechanism: β-Blockade Versus Calcium Antagonists. Both calcium antagonists and β-blockade have a negative inotropic effect, whereas only calcium antagonists relax vascular and other smooth muscle (Fig. 3–2). Calcium antagonists "block" the entry of calcium through the calcium channel in both smooth muscle and myocardium, so that less calcium is available to the contractile appa-

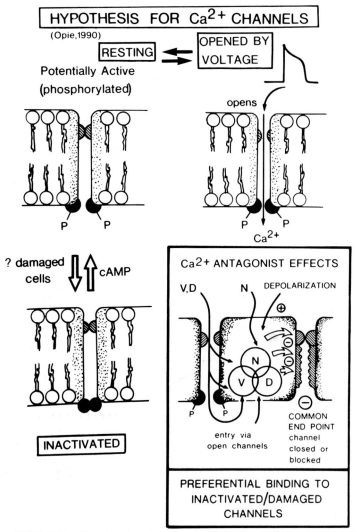

FIGURE 3–1. Drawing of calcium channel, based on multiple concepts.[140] N = nifedipine (i.e., dihydropyridine)-binding site; V = verapamil-binding site, and D = diltiazem-binding site. (This is a schematic visual aid that will need further modification.)

ratus in both tissues. The result is vasodilation and a negative ino- tropic effect; the latter is usually modest and is overridden, especially in the case of nifedipine, by peripheral vasodilation.

β-Blockade has contrasting effects on smooth muscle and on the myocardium. Whereas it tends to promote smooth muscle contrac- tion, β-blockade impairs myocardial contraction (negative inotropic effect). In explaining this difference, a fundamental difference lies in the regulation of the contractile mechanism by calcium ions in these two tissues. In the myocardium, calcium ions interact with troponin C to allow actin-myosin interaction; β-stimulation enhances the entry of calcium ions via the slow channel, as well as the rate of uptake in the sarcoplasmic reticulum, so that calcium ions rise and fall more rap- idly; hence both contraction and relaxation are speeded up as cyclic AMP forms under β-stimulation. Furthermore, the peak force of con- traction is enhanced. β-Blockade opposes all these effects.

In smooth muscle (see Fig. 3–2), calcium ions regulate the contrac- tile mechanism by interaction with calmodulin to form calcium- calmodulin, which then stimulates myosin light chain kinase (MLCK)

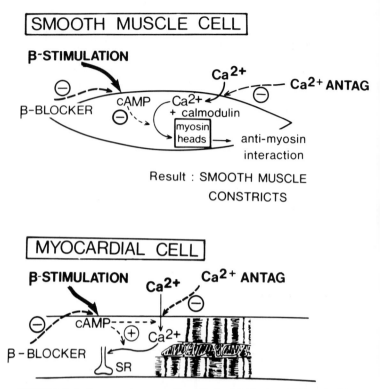

FIGURE 3–2. Proposed comparative effects of ß-blockers (BB) and calcium antagonists (Ca²⁺ antag) on smooth muscle and myocardium. The opposing effects on vascular smooth muscle are of critical therapeutic importance. MLCK = myosin light chain kinase. SR = sarcoplasmic reticulum.

to phosphorylate the myosin light chains to allow actin-myosin inter-action. Cyclic AMP inhibits the MLCK. β-Blockade, by inhibiting the effect of cyclic AMP, removes the inhibition on MLCK and, therefore, promotes contraction in smooth muscle. In addition, a further mechanism is that β-blockade may permit unopposed α-induced vasoconstriction.

Major Indications for Calcium Antagonists

Angina. Common to the effects of all types of calcium antagonists is the inhibition of the L-calcium current in arterial smooth muscle, occurring at relatively low concentrations of the agents (Table 3-1). Hence coronary vasodilation is a major common property. Although the antianginal mechanisms are many and varied, the shared effects are (1) coronary vasodilation, which is of importance not only in vasospastic angina, but also in classic effort angina in which exercise induces coronary vasoconstriction, as recently described; and (2) afterload reduction due to blood-pressure reduction. In addition, in the case of diltiazem, slowing of the sinus node is important, and in the case of verapamil the negative inotropic effect is important.

Hypertension. It is increasingly realized that the calcium antago-nists are excellent antihypertensive agents. Nifedipine and all the dihydropyridines (DHPs) decrease peripheral vascular resistance in low concentrations, and verapamil and diltiazem have similar effects.

Supraventricular Tachycardia. Verapamil (and diltiazem to a lesser extent) inhibits the AV node, which explains the effect in supraventricular tachycardias; nifedipine and other DHPs lack this effect at clinical doses.

Post-infarct Follow-up. As a group, the calcium antagonists are

TABLE 3–1   RELATIVE EFFECTS OF THE THREE PROTOTYPICAL CALCIUM ANTAGONISTS IN EXPERIMENTAL PREPARATIONS COMPARED WITH THERAPEUTIC LEVELS IN HUMANS

	Verapamil	Diltiazem	Nifedipine
Therapeutic level in humans			
ng/ml	80–400	50–300	15–100
molecular weight	455	415	346
molar value	$2–8 \times 10^{-7}$	$1–7 \times 10^{-7}$	$0.3–2 \times 10^{-7}$
protein binding	about 90%	about 85%	about 95%
molar value, corrected for protein binding	$2–8 \times 10^{-8}$	$1–5 \times 10^{-8}$	$0.3–1 \times 10^{-8}$
Isolated coronary artery contraction, molar 50% inhibition	10^{-7}	10^{-7}	10^{-8}
Negative inotropic effect, different isolated preparations, molar	$10^{-8}–10^{-6}$	$10^{-7}–10^{-4}$	10^{-7}
Slowing of sinus rate by 20% (isolated atria)	10^{-6}M	10^{-8}M	10^{-5}M
VSM contraction (portal vein), molar	4×10^{-7}	6×10^{-7}	4×10^{-8}
Ratio VSM vs negative inotropic effect	1.4	7	14
Inhibition of experimental ischemic-reperfusion injury, molar	$10^{-7}–10^{-6}$	10^{-7}	$10^{-8}–10^{-7}$
Relative effect on AV node versus contractile force	6.5:1	20:1	1:1

VSM = vascular smooth muscle. Molar=moles per liter.
For data sources, see Table 1–5 (Opie,[140] pp 50–51).

not protective in the post-infarct period and may even have harmful effects, especially in the presence of pre-existing left ventricular failure.[114] In a prospective unpublished trial in which patients with heart failure were excluded, verapamil decreased cardiac mortality and re-infarction.

Side-Effects

Class side-effects are those dependent on vasodilation (flushing, headaches, pedal edema). Peripheral vasodilation usually offsets the direct negative inotropic effect, especially in the case of nifedipine and the DHPs, yet CHF can be precipitated by all. An important finding with nifedipine is that beneficial vasodilatory effects dominate at low doses which give medium blood levels of the drug, whereas with high doses harmful negative inotropic effects come into play.[81]

Differences Between the Calcium Antagonists

Why different calcium antagonists have different effects on nodal and vascular tissues is still unknown; however, they are structurally different. Verapamil is a papaverine derivative, nifedipine a dihydropyridine, and diltiazem is a benzothiazine. Despite their clinical similarities, verapamil and diltiazem interact with different binding sites;[140] both depress nodal tissue as well as vascular tissue. Dihydropyridines such as nifedipine bind to a third site and have little clinical effect on nodal tissue. Clinically, each of the first-generation calcium antagonists—verapamil, nifedipine, and diltiazem—has a

TABLE 3–2 PROTOTYPICAL CALCIUM ANTAGONISTS: COMPARATIVE INDICATIONS

Condition	Verapamil	Diltiazem	Nifedipine
Chronic stable angina of effort	++	++	+/++[a]
Angina with hypertension	++	++	++
Angina with heart failure	+/-	+	++
Angina at rest, Prinzmetal's angina	++	++	++
Unstable angina (threatened infarction)	+	+	0
Unstable angina already treated by β-blockade	+	+	++
Infarction, non-Q-wave*	0/+	+	0
Postinfarct, no LVF*	++	+	0
Severe hypertension	+	+	++
Hypertension (2nd or 3rd line therapy)	+	+	++
Hypertension, first-line monotherapy	++	+	+
Combination with β-blockade (angina, hypertension)	+	+	++
Supraventricular tachycardia,** acute IV use	++	+	0
Supraventricular tachycardia,** oral prophylaxis	++	++	0
Chronic atrial fibrillation or flutter** (+ digitalis)	++	++	0
Raynaud's phenomenon*	0/+	++	+++
Hypertrophic cardiomyopathy*	++	+	0/+
Hypertrophic obstructive cardiomyopathy*	++	+	0

+++ = strongly indicated, in the author's opinion.
++ = indicated, in the author's opinion.
+   = marginal positive effect.
0   = no effect.
−   = negative effect.
[a]   = careful titration needed.
*   = not approved in USA.
** = only verapamil approved in USA.

slightly different spectrum of clinical activity (Table 3-2). Their common denominator is their ability to block the calcium channel, which results in their vasodilatory effect. They are virtually exchangeable when used for coronary artery spasm; all may be used for mild to moderate hypertension and for angina of effort, albeit acting through a mixture of mechanisms.

VERAPAMIL

Introduced in Europe in 1963 and more recently in the USA, verapamil (Isoptin; Calan) remains the prototype of calcium antagonists and the one that has been most extensively studied experimentally and clinically. Although it was originally used as an antianginal and antihypertensive agent, these properties were soon overshadowed by a dramatic effect in supraventricular arrhythmias[52] **so that only recently has the wide therapeutic potential of verapamil again come to be appreciated** (Fig. 3–3). The use of this agent in angina, and especially in hypertension, is increasing. Its role in obstructive cardiomyopathy is also reasonably well defined. Post-infarct protection has just been demonstrated.

Pharmacologic Properties

Electrophysiologically, verapamil inhibits the action potential of the upper and middle nodal regions, where depolarization is

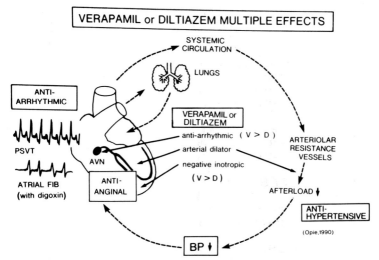

FIGURE 3–3. Verapamil and diltiazem have a broad spectrum of therapeutic effects. PSVT = paroxysmal supraventricular tachycardia.

Ca^{2+}-mediated. Verapamil thus inhibits one limb of the re-entry circuit, which is believed to underlie most paroxysmal supraventricular tachycardias. Increased AV block and the increase in effective refractory period of the AV node explain the reduction of the ventricular rate in atrial flutter and fibrillation. On electrophysiologic grounds, one might expect verapamil not to be very effective in ventricular arrhythmias except in certain uncommon forms.

Hemodynamically, verapamil combines arteriolar dilation with a direct negative inotropic effect. The cardiac output and left ventricular (LV) ejection fraction do not increase as expected following peripheral vasodilation,[7] which may be an expression of the negative inotropic effect. Peripheral vasodilation generally overcomes the direct depressant effect of verapamil on the sinus node so that the heart rate is unchanged or variably altered.

Pharmacokinetics. The hemodynamic effects (hypotension) of IV verapamil are short-lived, with a peak at 5 minutes and loss of activity by 10 to 12 minutes; but the peak effect on the AV node occurs at 10 to 15 minutes and lasts up to 6 hours, suggesting preferential binding by nodal tissues. When given IV for acute hypertension, 5 mg starts to reduce blood pressure within 1 minute.[80] Oral verapamil takes 2 hours to act and peaks at 3 hours. Therapeutic blood levels (80–400 ng/ml) are seldom measured.[15] The elimination half-life usually is 3 to 7 hours, but it increases significantly during chronic administration and in patients with liver or advanced renal insufficiency. Despite nearly complete absorption of oral doses, bioavailability is only 10 to 20% (high first-pass liver metabolism). Ultimate excretion of the parent compound, as well as the active hepatic metabolite norverapamil, is 75% by the kidneys and 25% by the gastrointestinal (GI) tract. Verapamil is 87 to 93% protein-bound, but no interaction with warfarin has been reported. When verapamil and digoxin are given together, their interaction causes digoxin levels to rise, probably due to a reduction in the renal clearance of digoxin.[33]

Norverapamil is a hepatic metabolite of verapamil, which appears rapidly in the plasma after oral administration of verapamil and in concentrations similar to those of the parent compound; like verapamil, norverapamil undergoes delayed clearance during chronic dosing.

Dose (Table 3-3). The usual **oral dose** of the standard preparation is 80 to 120 mg 3x daily; large differences of pharmacokinetics among individuals mean that dose titration is required. Lower or higher doses may therefore be needed; the highest reported daily dose is

TABLE 3–3 PROTOTYPICAL CALCIUM ANTAGONISTS: INDICATIONS AND DOSAGE

Agent	Indications	Dose
Verapamil (Isoptin, Calan)	Paroxysmal supraventricular tachycardia (PSVT) with narrow QRS complexes	1. IV bolus 5–10 mg repeated after 10 min, then 0.005 mg/kg/min if needed 2. IV infusion 1 mg/min to total of 10 mg 3. If myocardial disease, work up from 0.0001 mg/kg/min, titrating against heart rate
	Atrial flutter/fibrillation (control of ventricular rate)	IV infusion, if needed (3, above); or 80–120 mg 3x daily increasing to 80–120 mg 4x daily; beware of digitalis toxicity
	Prophylaxis of PSVT	Orally 80–120 mg 3x daily
	Angina of effort, unstable angina at rest, Prinzmetal's angina	Orally 240–480 mg daily in divided doses
	Hypertension, mild to moderate	Orally 240–360 mg daily in divided doses (or equivalent dose of slow-release tablets)
	Hypertrophic cardiomyopathy*	Orally 240–480 mg daily in divided doses
Diltiazem (Cardizem) (Herbesser) (Tildiem) (Tilazem)	Angina of effort, unstable angina at rest, Prinzmetal's angina	Orally 30–90 mg 3x daily increasing to 4x daily as indicated
	Non-Q-wave infarction*	Orally 60 mg 4x daily
	Hypertension	Orally 240–360 mg daily in divided doses
Nifedipine (Procardia) (Adalat) (Procardia XL)	Angina of effort	Orally 30–80 mg daily in 3 or 4 doses; Procardia XL 30-150 mg daily
	Prinzmetal's angina	Orally 10 mg 3x daily up to 20 mg every 4 hrs
	Hypertension, mild to moderate	Orally 10 mg 2–4x daily; Procardia XL 30-150 mg daily
	Severe urgent hypertension	10 mg sublingually or bite-and-swallow 6-hourly
	Acute LV failure (pulmonary edema) with hypertension	10 mg sublingually or bite-and-swallow 6-hourly
	Raynaud's phenomenon*	10 mg sublingually or bite-and-swallow at onset of attack

*Not FDA approved at present.
PSVT = paroxysmal supraventricular tachycardia.
IV   = intravenous.
LV   = left ventricular.

960 mg,[73] but such levels are rarely tolerated. During chronic oral dosing, the formation of norverapamil metabolites and altered rates of hepatic metabolism may mean that less frequent daily doses of verapamil are preferable;[55] for example, if verapamil has been given at a dose of 80 mg 3x daily, then 120 mg 2x daily would be as good, especially in the treatment of hypertension.[139] Lower doses are also required in elderly patients or those with advanced renal or hepatic disease.[60]

With **slow-release preparations**, the usual dose of verapamil is 1 to $1^1/_2$ tablets daily (240–360 mg); scored tablets allow 360 mg daily.

IV verapamil should be used only in monitored patients. For **supraventricular tachycardias**, when there is no myocardial depression, a bolus of 5 to 10 mg (0.1 to 0.15 mg/kg) can be given over 1 minute and repeated 10 minutes later if needed; the infusion rate after a successful bolus is 0.005 mg/kg/min for about 30 to 60 minutes, decreasing thereafter. When there is risk of hypotension (prior β-blockade, myocardial disease, disopyramide therapy), pretreatment with calcium gluconate (90 mg) should be tried before an infusion (1 mg/min for 10 minutes).[68] When used for uncontrolled **atrial fibrillation**, combined with myocardial disease, verapamil is infused at a very low dose (0.0001 mg/kg/min) and titrated against the ventricular response, especially if the patient has already received β-blockade or when digitalis toxicity is suspected. In the absence of these relative contraindications, verapamil may safely be given at a higher rate (0.005 mg/kg/min, increasing) or as an IV bolus of 5 mg (0.075 mg/kg) followed by double the dose if needed.[62]

Side-effects. Class side-effects are those of vasodilation, causing headaches, facial flushing, and dizziness. Constipation is specific and causes most trouble, especially in elderly patients.[48,61] Troublesome especially to female patients is ankle swelling not caused by overall fluid retention.

Rare Side-effects. Rare side-effects may include pain in the gums, facial pain, epigastric pain, hepatotoxicity, and transient mental confusion.

Severe Nodal Side-effects. When incorrectly given as a bolus to patients with pre-existing AV inhibition caused by disease or β-blockade, IV verapamil can be fatal. In patients with sick sinus syndrome, severe asystole may result after IV verapamil. With oral verapamil, lesser degrees of these side-effects are possible.

Myocardial Depressant Effects. A striking negative inotropic effect is seen with verapamil and other calcium antagonists in isolated preparations. Yet when correctly used, verapamil seldom causes serious cardiac depression. In supraventricular arrhythmias, the hemodynamic benefits of restoration of sinus rhythm usually outweigh any negative inotropic effect.[56]

Contraindications (Fig. 3–4, Table 3-4). Sick sinus syndrome; pre-existing AV nodal disease, excess therapy with β-adrenergic blockade, digitalis, quinidine, or disopyramide; or myocardial depression are all still contraindications that especially apply in the IV therapy of supraventricular tachycardias.[44,58] In the rarer type of Wolff-Parkinson-White (WPW) syndrome with anterograde conduction through the bypass tract, the risk is that the impulses of atrial fibrillation can be too rapidly conducted to the ventricles with danger of ventricular fibrillation (VF). Nonetheless, verapamil can safely be used in the vast majority of patients with supraventricular tachycardias and narrow QRS complexes.

Verapamil and β-Blockers: Interactions and Combination Therapy

Special care is required when verapamil is acutely added by IV injection in the presence of pre-existing β-adrenergic blockade.[66] Also, in patients with angina pectoris already receiving propranolol

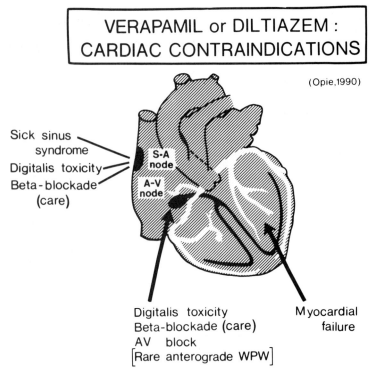

Sick sinus syndrome
Digitalis toxicity
Beta-blockade (care)

Digitalis toxicity
Beta-blockade (care)
AV block
[Rare anterograde WPW]

Myocardial failure

FIGURE 3–4. Contraindications to verapamil and diltiazem. For use of verapamil and diltiazem in patients already receiving β-blockers, see text.

or metoprolol, IV[31] or oral verapamil[46] can reduce contractility,[46] increase heart size,[28] and cause symptomatic sinus bradycardia.[72] There may be a hepatic pharmacokinetic interaction.[19] Depending on the dose, the combination β-blocker–verapamil may be well tolerated[28] or not.[23] Although Packer has recently drawn attention to the possible hazards of such combination therapy,[119] it remains true that, in practice, clinicians can safely combine verapamil with β-blocker in the therapy of angina pectoris or hypertension, provided that due care is taken and that the combination is avoided in elderly patients unless specific care is taken to exclude nodal disease. In angina, the combination improves myocardial function during exercise more than either agent does alone.[27] Verapamil–β-blocker works well for hypertension, although heart rate, AV conduction, and LV function may be adversely affected.[42] Similarly, with care, the combination verapamil-propranolol is used for the chronic prevention of supraventricular tachycardia.[74] To avoid any hepatic interactions, verapamil is best combined with a hydrophilic β-blocker such as atenolol rather than metoprolol or propranolol.[113]

In comparison, the combination of nifedipine–β-blocker is generally well tolerated.[45] The combination diltiazem–β-blocker may cause concern if bradycardia or hypotension develops.[23]

Other Drug Interactions with Verapamil

Digoxin. Verapamil can interact with digitalis to increase blood digoxin levels.[35] In digitalis toxicity, rapid IV verapamil is **absolutely contraindicated** because it can lethally exaggerate AV block. There is no reason why, in the absence of digitalis toxicity or AV block, oral verapamil and digitalis compounds should not be combined (checking the digoxin level), because digitalis does not inhibit the slow

TABLE 3–4 COMPARATIVE CONTRAINDICATIONS OF VERAPAMIL, DILTIAZEM, NIFEDIPINE AND OF β-ADRENERGIC BLOCKING AGENTS

Contraindications	Verapamil	Diltiazem	Nifedipine	β-blockade
Absolute:				
Sinus bradycardia	0/+	0/+	0	++
Sick sinus syndrome	++	+	0	++
AV conduction defects	++	++	0	+
Digitalis toxicity with AV block*	++	++	0	+
Asthma	0	0	0	+++
Bronchospasm	0	0	0	++
Heart failure	++	++	0/+	++
Hypotension	+	+	++	+
Coronary artery spasm	0	0	0	+
Raynaud's and active peripheral vascular disease	0	0	0	+
Severe mental depression	0	0	0	+
Severe aortic stenosis	+	+	++	+
Obstructive cardiomyopathy	0/+	0/+	++	Indicated
Relative:				
Adverse blood lipid profile	0	0	0	Care
Digitalis without toxicity	Care	Care	0	Care
β-blockade	Care	Care	Hypotension	0
Verapamil therapy	0	Avoid	Hypotension	Care
Quinidine therapy	Care/avoid[1]	Care[1]	Care**	Care
Disopyramide therapy	Care/avoid[1]	Care	0	Care
Unstable angina at rest	0/+	0	++	Indicated
Post-infarct protection	++(If LVF)	++(If LVF)	++	Indicated

"Indicated" means judged suitable for use by author, not necessarily FDA-approved.

+++ = absolutely contraindicated.
++ = strongly contraindicated.
+ = relative contraindication.
0 = not contraindicated.
LVF = left ventricular failure.
*Contraindication to rapid intravenous administration.
**Nifedipine depresses blood quinidine levels with rebound upon nifedipine-withdrawal.
[1]Exception: antiarrhythmic therapy.

inward calcium current. Experimentally, verapamil has proved effective against ventricular arrhythmias due to digitalis, but in practice IV verapamil should be given only with great caution to patients with digitalis poisoning.

Prazosin. Verapamil has also been used combined with prazosin in hypertension, with added and possibly synergistic effects;[10] the latter may be explained by pharmacokinetic interactions.[47]

Quinidine. Verapamil may adversely interact with quinidine, presumably due to the combined effect on peripheral α-receptors causing hypotension,[40] or due to increasing quinidine levels.

Disopyramide. Because the combined negative inotropic potential of verapamil and disopyramide is considerable the combination must be given with care.

Therapy of Verapamil Toxicity

There are few clinical reports on management of verapamil toxicity. Calcium gluconate (1 to 2 g IV) helps when heart failure or excess hypotension is induced. Calcium therapy, however, is not effective against excess AV block,[20] which apparently depends less on external calcium than does hypotension or the negative inotropic effect. To shorten AV conduction, atropine (1 mg IV) or isoproterenol should be effective.

Verapamil for Chronic Stable Angina, Unstable Angina, and Prinzmetal's Variant Angina

In **chronic stable effort angina**, verapamil acts by a combination of afterload reduction and a mild negative inotropic effect; there may also be an increase in the blood supply.[56] The heart rate usually stays the same as in controls. Thus verapamil can logically be combined with β-blockade (for precautions, see Fig. 3–7). In several recent studies, verapamil has been as effective as propranolol for effort angina, or more so, and there is less risk of serious side-effects. A daily dose of verapamil (about 360 mg) is the approximate equivalent of propranolol 300 mg daily,[38] metoprolol 200 mg 2x daily,[3] or nifedipine 60 mg daily.[8]

In **unstable angina at rest** with threat of infarction, verapamil has not been tested against placebo. Compared with propranolol, verapamil 480 mg daily was much better than propranolol 240 mg daily in preventing recurrent chest pain. However, 7 of the 20 patients had Prinzmetal's angina, a condition for which β-blockade is a relative contraindication.[84] IV verapamil 0.002 mg/kg/min, when added to nitroglycerin, improves ECG ischemic episodes.[111]

In **silent myocardial ischemia**, together with short-lived (<10 minutes) attacks of chest pain, verapamil in a mean dose of 400 mg is much better than propranolol, also in a mean dose of 300 mg.[121]

In **variant angina** (Prinzmetal's syndrome), verapamil (average daily dose 450 mg in 3 to 4 divided doses) and nifedipine (average daily dose 70 mg in 3 to 4 divided doses) were equally effective, with fewer dose-limiting side-effects with verapamil.[70] Combinations of verapamil or nifedipine with oral isosorbide dinitrate are more effective than isosorbide alone in reducing anginal frequency and ischemic ECG changes in variant angina.[71]

For **post-infarct protection**, the first trial failed to show any benefit of acute IV verapamil started at the onset of AMI followed by post-infarct oral verapamil. However, the design was flawed; in a second study (Danish Verapamil Infarct Trial, Second Trial [DAVIT II], soon to be published), verapamil 120 mg 3x daily started 7 to 15 days after the acute phase was more protective and decreased re-infarction and mortality by about 40% over 6 months.

Verapamil for Supraventricular Arrhythmias

In **paroxysmal supraventricular tachycardia (PSVT)**, an IV bolus of 5 to 10 mg restores sinus rhythm in 75% or more of cases.[57] Thereafter, oral prophylactic therapy against recurrent PSVT may use either verapamil[41] or verapamil-propranolol.[74] Verapamil by itself is about as effective as digoxin or propranolol.[71]

In rapid **atrial fibrillation**, whether or not previously treated with digitalis, IV verapamil reduces the ventricular rate with regularization in some cases and reduces conversion to sinus rhythm in a few, especially in those of recent onset. But the blood pressure may drop,[21] so that a slow infusion or oral treatment (taking only 2 hours to act) is preferred to bolus infusion unless reduction of ventricular rate is urgent (for example, in AMI when there are no facilities for cardioversion).

In **atrial flutter**, the block is increased; occasionally sinus rhythm is restored (especially in acute infarction), or atrial fibrillation ensues.[57]

In **recent onset atrial fibrillation or flutter**, verapamil, although effective, has a lower rate of conversion to sinus rhythm than the ultrashort-acting β-blocker, esmolol (see β-blocking section, p 21).

Verapamil for Hypertension

Verapamil is now approved for mild to moderate hypertension in the USA. Particularly, the slow-release preparation (240 mg tablet) is used and can be given 1 to 2x daily. Although monotherapy with verapamil is claimed to be effective in nearly 90% of patients by the manufacturers, in a long-term, double-blind comparative trial, hypertension was adequately controlled in only 45% of patients given verapamil 240 mg daily.[103] The corresponding figure for hydrochlorothiazide 25 mg daily was only 25%. Adding hydrochlorothiazide to verapamil, or vice versa, improved the response to about 60%. The response rate to verapamil in this study may be relatively low because the top dose was only 240 mg daily instead of the 360 to 480 mg used in some other studies.

Verapamil vs β-blockade for Hypertension

Verapamil compares well with β-blockade, with doses of 240 to 360 mg daily being the approximate equivalent of propranolol 160 to 240 mg daily, labetalol 400 mg daily, and atenolol 100 mg daily (for review, see Opie[140] Table 3-6). The combination of verapamil (360 mg) and propranolol (240 mg) gives better results than either agent alone, at the cost of more side-effects.[42]

In **black patients**, verapamil is probably better than propranolol.[88]

Other Uses for Verapamil

Verapamil for Hypertrophic Cardiomyopathy. In hypertrophic cardiomyopathy, of all the calcium antagonists verapamil has been best evaluated. It improves symptoms, reduces the outflow tract gradient, and improves exercise tolerance by 20 to 25%, at least when administered acutely.[51] Diastolic function is also improved by verapamil.[22] However, verapamil should not be given to patients with resting outflow tract obstruction,[69] when propranolol or disopyramide, with their stronger negative inotropic effects, may be better. At present there is no evidence of any protection by verapamil against ventricular arrhythmias associated with the disease, nor is it known whether verapamil produces a regression in the characteristic ventricular hypertrophy. A large number of patients on the drug develop significant side-effects with long-term verapamil, including sino-atrial and AV nodal dysfunction, and occasionally severe heart failure.[51] Although strict comparisons with β-blockade are lacking,[29] some patients respond better to verapamil, possibly because of improved diastolic mechanics.[22]

Verapamil for Ventricular Tachycardia. "For most patients with recurrent, sustained VT, verapamil is not effective and frequently deleterious."[4] In fact, verapamil can be lethal in wide complex VT. However, some patients with exercise-induced VT due to triggered automaticity may respond well,[73] as may young patients with idiopathic VT with right bundle branch block and left axis deviation.

New Derivatives of Verapamil

Gallopamil (investigational) has properties very similar to verapamil.

Anapamil (investigational) is long-acting and is being assessed for hypertension.

Summary: Verapamil

Among calcium antagonists, verapamil has the widest range of approved indications, including angina pectoris, supraventricular tachycardias, and hypertension. Compared with propranolol in the therapy of effort angina, it is at least as effective, has less risk of serious side-effects, and has fewer contraindications. Verapamil is now increasingly used as one of a number of early options in the therapy of hypertension. The combination verapamil-β-blockade can be more effective than either component in the therapy of angina or hypertension, but a number of cautions and contraindications must be observed.

DILTIAZEM

Diltiazem (Cardizem in the USA; Tildiem in the UK; Herbesser or Tilazem elsewhere), initially developed in Japan, is now available worldwide. Although modern opinion suggests that there are different binding sites for each of the three major calcium antagonists (nifedipine, diltiazem, and verapamil), in clinical practice, diltiazem and verapamil have somewhat similar therapeutic spectra and contraindications, so that these agents are combined in some classifications of calcium antagonists. Diltiazem seems more active on the sinus node, so that it is more likely to decrease the heart rate than is verapamil, whereas verapamil may be more active on the AV node. **Clinically, diltiazem is used for the same spectrum of disease as is verapamil: angina pectoris, hypertension, and arrhythmias (AV nodal inhibition).** Of these, angina and hypertension are usage approved in the USA. Diltiazem has a low side-effect profile, similar to that of verapamil, except that the incidence of constipation is much lower (Table 3-5). Like the other first-generation calcium antagonists, diltiazem must be given several times a day for optimal therapy unless slow-release preparations are used.

Pharmacologic Properties

Pharmacokinetics. Following oral administration, over 90% is absorbed, but bioavailability is about 45% (first-pass hepatic metabolism). The onset of action is within 15 to 30 minutes (oral), with a peak at 1 to 2 hours. The elimination half-life is 4 to 7 hours; hence, dosage every 6 to 8 hours is required for sustained therapeutic effect. The therapeutic plasma concentration range is 50 to 300 ng/ml. Protein binding is 80 to 86%. Diltiazem is acetylated in the liver to deacyldiltiazem (40% of the activity of the parent compound), which accumulates with chronic therapy. Unlike verapamil and nifedipine, only 35% of diltiazem is excreted by the kidneys (65% by the GI tract).

Dose. For all varieties of angina, the dose of diltiazem is 120 to 360 mg, usually in 4 daily doses. Strict 6-hour dosing may be needed for severe angina, yet a single 120-mg dose improves exercise tolerance for 8 hours, and 3x daily dosing may be effective even in unstable or variant angina.[6] Slow-release diltiazem-SR permits 2x daily doses. For hypertension and prophylaxis of supraventricular tachycardia, doses are similar. IV diltiazem, available in Japan, is given like verapamil with a dose of 0.15 to 0.25 mg/kg over 2 minutes with ECG and blood pressure control.

Side-effects. Normally side-effects are few and limited to headaches, dizziness, and ankle edema in about 6 to 10% of patients (see Table 3-5). With high-dose diltiazem (360 mg daily) one series reported no side-effects in the treatment of angina,[23] whereas leg edema, abdominal discomfort, and constipation limited the dose when used for atrial fibrillation.[127] Compared with nifedipine (120 mg daily), diltiazem 360 mg daily had fewer side-effects, the doses being equipotent for coronary artery spasm.[124] In the case of IV diltiazem, side-effects should resemble those of IV verapamil, including the possible risk of asystole and high-degree AV block when there is pre-existing nodal disease. In post-infarct patients with pre-existing poor

TABLE 3–5 SOME SIDE-EFFECTS OF THE THREE PROTOTYPICAL CALCIUM ANTAGONISTS COMPARED WITH LONG-ACTING COMPOUNDS

	Verapamil (%)	Diltiazem (%)	Nifedipine capsules (%)	Nifedipine XL (%)	Amlodipine (%)
Facial flushing	6–7	0–3	6–25	0	2
Headaches	6	4–9	7–34	16*	6+
Tachycardia	0	0	low–25	0	0
Lightheadedness, dizziness	7	6–7	3–12	4	5
Constipation	34	4	0	3	0
Ankle edema, swelling	6	6–10	1–8	10–30	10
Provocation of angina	0	0	low–14	0	0

DHP = dihydropyridine.

Data sources from Opie[140] (p 197). For nifedipine XL, see package insert. For amlodipine, mean values of 6 trials on 2573 patients calculated from Osterloh.[118]

N.B. Side-effects are dose-related; **no strict comparisons exist** except for nifedipine versus diltiazem.

* vs 10% in placebo.

+ vs 8% in placebo.

LV function, mortality is increased by diltiazem, not decreased.[114] Occasionally, severe skin rashes such as exfoliative dermatitis are found.

Contraindications. Contraindications resemble those of verapamil (see Fig. 3-4, Table 3-4)—pre-existing marked depression of the sinus or AV node and myocardial failure. Post-infarction, LV failure with an ejection fraction below 40%, is a clear contraindication.[114]

Drug Interactions

Like verapamil, diltiazem may increase the blood digoxin level, although the effect is often slight or negligible.[130]

Combination with β-Blockers and Other Drugs

Diltiazem plus propranolol may be used for angina with risk of excess bradycardia or hypotension;[19] however, the combination may be better tolerated than propranolol-nifedipine, which is hemodynamically sounder.[28] In some studies the combination was no more effective than diltiazem itself, presumably because of the bradycardia already induced by diltiazem.[23] When propranolol is ineffective in patients with coronary artery spasm, the combination of diltiazem-propranolol becomes effective, although without any obvious advantage over diltiazem alone.[65] Occasionally diltiazem-nifedipine is used for refractory coronary artery spasm.[124] **Diltiazem plus long-acting nitrates** may lead to excess hypotension.[5]

Diltiazem for Ischemic Syndromes

In **chronic stable effort angina**, the combination of vasodilatory and a mild bradycardic effect seems very desirable. The efficacy of diltiazem in chronic angina is at least as good as propranolol, and the doses required vary from 120 to 360 mg daily in 3 divided doses (Table 2-5, Opie[140]). The drug is generally safe with no effect on the PR-interval in the absence of pre-existing nodal disease, and severe subjective side-effects are unusual.

No studies compare diltiazem with placebo in **unstable angina at rest**. However, the properties of diltiazem should be ideal—coronary vasodilation and bradycardia, with only a relatively slight negative inotropic effect. In comparison with β-blockade (propranolol), diltiazem is at least as good,[64] or possibly even better.[1,65] Different results probably reflect different population groups, with varying degrees of coronary spasm as a cause of angina at rest. However, diltiazem has not been tested against placebo.

In **Prinzmetal's variant angina**, diltiazem 240 to 360 mg/day reduces the number of episodes of pain. At doses of 240 mg daily, 30% of patients become pain-free, and the frequency of angina is reduced in the remaining majority.[54]

In **AMI without Q waves**, diltiazem 360 mg daily may help to prevent early re-infarction, starting 24 to 72 hours after the onset[50] (the incorrect use of a one-tailed P-test brings statistical doubt).

Post-infarct diltiazem has no overall benefit; retrospective analysis suggests harm with previous LV failure and benefit in those without.[114]

Diltiazem for Hypertension

In an excellently designed multicenter trial on nearly 300 patients, monotherapy by diltiazem-SR (180 mg 2x daily) reduced the diastolic blood pressure <90 mm Hg in 57% of patients. BP started to fall after 1 week and a full effect was reached at 3 to 4 weeks. **Combination with hydrochlorothiazide** (12.5 mg daily) gave 68% response, and with 25 to 50 mg about 75%.[83] However, the combination increased blood sugar by 13 mg/dl and plasma cholesterol by 8 mg/dl, so that caution is required in diabetics, in whom diltiazem monotherapy should be much safer (blood sugar increase only 4 mg/dl).

Antiarrhythmic Properties of Diltiazem

The electrophysiologic properties of diltiazem closely resemble those of verapamil. The main effect is a depressant one on the AV node; the functional and effective refractory periods are prolonged by diltiazem. Diltiazem can be used for the elective as well as prophylactic control (90 mg 3x daily[75]) of most supraventricular tachyarrhythmias (not approved in the USA or UK). A particularly useful combination for termination of paroxysmal supraventricular tachycardia is single oral dose diltiazem (120 mg) and propranolol (160 mg), which usually works within 20 to 40 minutes.[76] Diltiazem is unlikely to be effective in ventricular arrhythmias except in those complicating coronary artery spasm or in those few in whom verapamil works. In chronic atrial fibrillation, diltiazem (usual dose 240 mg daily) added to digoxin improves control of ventricular rate.[130]

Summary: Diltiazem

Diltiazem, with its properties of peripheral vasodilation and a mild negative inotropic effect, is increasingly seen as having hemodynamic advantages in the therapy of angina pectoris. In the therapy of hypertension, it is well tolerated. Although effective, it is not approved for supraventricular tachycardias in the USA. The incidence of side-effects (usually low) will depend on the dose and the underlying state of the sinus or AV node and the myocardium, as well as any possible co-therapy with β-blockers.

NIFEDIPINE

The dihydropyridine calcium antagonists, of which nifedipine (Procardia, Adalat) is the prototype, inhibit the calcium channel by acting at a binding site different from verapamil and diltiazem. Nifedipine was first introduced in Europe (Adalat) and is now widely used in the USA (Procardia, Procardia XL). **Dihydropyridines are, in general, powerful arteriolar vasodilators with relatively scant effects on the AV node in clinical doses, and their direct negative inotropic effect is usually outweighed by arteriolar unloading effects in clinical practice** (Fig. 3–5).

Nifedipine, the most widely used dihydropyridine, is very successful in treating severe hypertension, Prinzmetal's variant angina, Raynaud's phenomenon, and other syndromes produced by arterial vasoconstriction. Nifedipine's action on isolated coronary smooth muscle is 10 or 12x more powerful than that of verapamil, although in clinical practice nifedipine is only marginally better for coronary spasm.[32]

Lacking a clinically significant effect against the AV node, nifedipine is ineffective against supraventricular arrhythmias, and the combination with β-blocking agents is theoretically less hazardous than with verapamil or diltiazem.

Pharmacologic Properties

Pharmacokinetics. Nifedipine (capsule form) is almost fully absorbed after an oral dose, reaching peak blood values within 20 to 45 minutes, with a half-life of 3 hours. Almost all circulating nifedipine is broken down by hepatic metabolism to inactive metabolites (high first-pass metabolism). The hypotensive effect starts within 20 min-

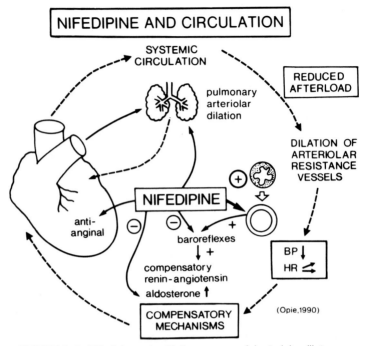

FIGURE 3–5. Nifedipine acts chiefly as a powerful arteriolar dilator. CHF = congestive heart failure.

utes of an oral dose and within 5 minutes of a sublingual or bite-and-swallow dose. The duration of action is 4 to 6 hours in some studies, and up to 8 hours in others, especially combined with other antihypertensives. With long-acting slow-release capsules (**Procardia XL**), 24-hour stable blood levels of about 20 to 30 ng/ml are achieved, which are within the therapeutic range (see Table 3-1). With nifedipine tablets (**Adalat Retard**), 20 mg, it is the slow rate of absorption rather than the decreased rate of breakdown that prolongs the half-life to 5 to 11 hours.

Dose. In **effort angina**, the usual total dose of nifedipine capsules is 30 to 90 mg daily (i.e., 1 to 3 capsules 3x daily) (Table 2-4, Opie[140]). Dose-titration is advisable to avoid precipitation of ischemic pain in some patients. In **cold-induced angina**, nifedipine capsules work at a dose of 10 mg 3x daily.[124] In **coronary artery spasm**, the usual dose is 80 to 120 mg in 3 or 4 doses.[124] In **severe hypertension**, 10 mg sublingually usually brings down the pressure within 20 to 60 minutes. In **mild to moderate hypertension**, the required dose as monotherapy is about 10 to 20 mg 3x daily (Table 3-7, Opie[140]). In **elderly patients**, it is prudent to avoid possible cerebral underperfusion as a result of abrupt vasodilation, so that the initial dose should be 5 mg (available in capsule form in many countries, or a 10 mg capsule cut in half).

Although sublingual administration is standard when rapid action is required, as in urgent hypertension, the bite-and-swallow method consistently gives the most rapid absorption and higher blood levels.[134]

The dose for extended-release capsules (Procardia XL) is about the same as the total daily dose of standard capsules.

Contraindications. Among the few side-effects (Table 3-4; Fig. 3–6) are aortic stenosis or obstructive hypertrophic cardiomyopathy (in both cases exaggeration of pressure gradient), severe myocardial depression (added negative inotropic effect), and unstable angina with threat of infarction (in the absence of concurrent β-blockade). Relative contraindications are subjective intolerance to nifedipine, previous adverse reactions, and pre-existing tachycardia.

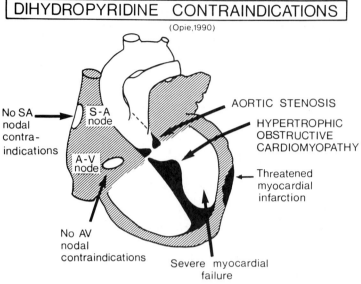

DIHYDROPYRIDINE CONTRAINDICATIONS

(Opie,1990)

No SA nodal contra-indications

S-A node

A-V node

No AV nodal contraindications

AORTIC STENOSIS

HYPERTROPHIC OBSTRUCTIVE CARDIOMYOPATHY

Threatened myocardial infarction

Severe myocardial failure

FIGURE 3–6. Contraindications to dihydropyridines (nifedipine-like agents) are chiefly obstructive lesions, such as aortic stenosis or hypertrophic obstructive cardiomyopathy. Unstable angina (threatened infarction) is a contraindication unless combined nifedipine-β-blockade therapy is used or unless (rarely) coronary spasm is suspected.

Minor Side-effects. Overall the drug is very safe when the above contraindications are observed. On the other hand, especially with the capsules, unpleasant subjective reactions are relatively common, resulting from peripheral vasodilation, including flushing, dizziness, headaches, and palpitations. Sometimes angina may be precipitated about 30 minutes after the dose,[24] the mechanism presumably being tachycardia or coronary underperfusion. Such side-effects may occur in nearly 40% of patients and are severe enough to require drug discontinuation in about 5%.[2] The bilateral ankle edema of nifedipine is distressing to patients but is not due to cardiac failure; the edema can usually be left alone but, if required, can be treated by conventional diuretics or captopril. Nifedipine itself has a mild diuretic effect. The incidence of subjective vasodilatory side-effects seems to be higher with nifedipine than with verapamil or diltiazem. With extended-release nifedipine capsules (Procardia XL), the manufacturers claim that side-effects are restricted to headache (nearly double that found in controls) and ankle edema (dose-dependent, 10% with 30 mg daily, 30% with 180 mg daily). These claims may be correct because the incidence of some vasodilatory side-effects is governed by the rate of rise of blood dihydropyridine levels.[135]

Severe Side-effects. Occasionally in very ill patients, the direct negative inotropic effect is a serious problem. Occasionally side-effects compatible with the effects of excess hypotension and organ underperfusion have been reported: myocardial ischemia, and even infarction, retinal and cerebral ischemia,[49] and renal failure.[9]

Rebound After Cessation of Nifedipine Therapy. In patients with vasospastic angina, abrupt cessation of nifedipine therapy may markedly increase the frequency and duration of attacks.[36,53] In effort angina, the evidence for rebound is less convincing. In previous unstable angina that has become stable on therapy, nifedipine may be withdrawn.[16]

Rare Side-effects. These include muscle cramps, myalgia, hypokalemia (via diuretic effect), gingival swelling, and precipitation of diabetes mellitus.

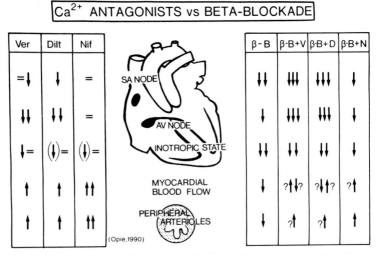

FIGURE 3–7. Proposed hemodynamic effects of calcium antagonists, singly or in combination with β-blockade. Some of these effects are based on animal data, and extrapolation to man should be made with caution. Ver = verapamil; Dilt = diltiazem; Nif = nifedipine; B = β-blockade.

Combination with β-Blockers and Other Drugs

In patients with reasonable LV function, nifedipine may be freely combined with β-blockers (Fig. 3–7), provided that excess hypotension is guarded against. In the therapy of angina pectoris, nifedipine-propranolol seems better than propranolol-isosorbide dinitrate (Chap. 2, p 37). For unstable angina at rest, nifedipine, if used, must be combined with a β-blocker (metoprolol was used in the HINT study[102]). In the therapy of angina caused by spasm, nifedipine may be combined with nitrates. In the therapy of hypertension, nifedipine may be combined with diuretics, β-blockers, methyldopa, or ACE inhibitors. Combination with prazosin may lead to adverse hypotensive interactions, so a test dose is required.[25] Occasionally nifedipine and diltiazem, however, have been combined with frequent side-effects.[124]

Nifedipine for Ischemic Syndromes

In **chronic stable angina**, nifedipine is consistently better than placebo. The initial baroreflex-mediated tachycardia can diminish the antianginal efficacy. Later the baroreflexes become blunted and the heart rate is unchanged. In a double-blind study on ambulatory patients where ST-segment shifts were monitored, propranolol (380 mg daily) was more effective than nifedipine 60 mg daily, although the combination was possibly most effective.[39] Likewise, nifedipine with metoprolol[67] or atenolol[13] is more effective in effort angina than either agent alone, while the β-blocker is marginally superior as monotherapy. Nifedipine causes a modest reflex increase in heart rate, which may be dose-dependent to limit the antianginal effect. Furthermore, the absence of any significant direct negative inotropic effect may also be a disadvantage in the therapy of angina of effort. **Combination with β-blockade is therefore logical therapy, giving better antianginal efficacy than nifedipine or β-blockade alone**[12,30,39,72] or propranolol-isosorbide dinitrate (see Chap. 2). When combined with nitrates, hypotension or syncope from excess peripheral vasodilation may become troublesome, even though nifedipine plus nitrates may give added vasodilator effects at the site of "dynamic stenosis."[37]

In **smokers with effort angina**, nifedipine is much less effective than in non-smokers,[90] a fact that might have obscured the benefit of nifedipine in some trials.

In **angina precipitated by cold**, nifedipine is preferable to propranolol,[123] presumably because it relieves reflex coronary vasoconstriction.

In **Prinzmetal's angina** (vasospastic angina), nifedipine 40 to 80 mg in 3 to 4 divided daily doses gives consistent relief[2,63] and is more effective combined with isosorbide dinitrate.[71] In some studies, up to 120 mg daily was needed.[124]

In **unstable angina at rest**, the closer the angina is to Prinzmetal's variety, the better is the effect of nifedipine.[59] In the **standard type of angina** at rest with threatened myocardial infarction, nifedipine by itself is contraindicated, as shown by the HINT study,[102] but achieves benefit when added to pre-existing β-blockade (see Chap. 1). Best results may be obtained by the combination β-blocker-nifedipine-nitrates,[17,43] taking care to avoid hypotension.

In **threatened and very early myocardial infarction**, nifedipine is contraindicated because of increased mortality.[43] Nonetheless, when unloading is required in early AMI, the hemodynamic benefit of sublingual nifedipine results from the first dose of 10 mg,[17] but routine prolonged therapy cannot be advised.[43]

Post-infarct, nifedipine "prophylaxis" carries no benefit.[100]

Other Uses of Nifedipine

In **hypertrophic cardiomyopathy,** nifedipine may have two opposing effects: peripheral vasodilation could exaggerate resting outflow tract obstruction (hence **hypertrophic obstructive cardiomyopathy** is a contraindication), whereas benefit presumably results from enhanced diastolic relaxation. The combination of nifedipine and propranolol reduces peak systolic and end-diastolic pressures, the peripheral resistance, and the outflow gradient.[34]

In **CHF**, nifedipine is being used less and less, unless hypertension is the basis.

In **chronic hypertensive heart failure** nifedipine (20 mg 4x daily) seems better than verapamil (160 mg 3x daily) in reducing symptoms and pulmonary wedge pressure.[18]

In **primary pulmonary hypertension**, nifedipine seems better than hydralazine,[14] yet must be used with care.

In **acute pulmonary edema** caused by hypertension, nifedipine 10 mg sublingually is effective.[11, 18]

PREVENTION OF NEW CORONARY LESIONS

In the INTACT study, nifedipine 20 mg 4x daily given for 3 years **decreased the development of new coronary atherosclerotic lesions** on angiography.[108] Overall non-cardiac mortality was increased in the nifedipine group, probably due to the small number of patients, so that larger trials are required to show any true patient benefit.

Nifedipine for Hypertension

In **systemic hypertension**, nifedipine and other DHPs are increasingly seen (together with other calcium antagonists) as standard third-line therapy (after diuretics and β-blockade). Many centers are using nifedipine as second-line therapy (in combination with β-blockade or ACE inhibitors) and occasionally as monotherapy when, like nicardipine, nifedipine capsules are likely to give variable control over 24 hours. In combination with methyldopa and (probably) β-blockers, nifedipine capsules have a more prolonged action, lasting up to 8 to 12 hours in mild to moderate hypertension. Because the standard capsules may act only for 4 to 6 hours, slow-release tablets are better for 1 to 2x daily dosage, and even better is the once-a-day extended release preparation (Procardia XL).

For **severe hypertension** (DBP>120 mm Hg), nifedipine 10 mg sublingually, which can be repeated once after 30 to 60 minutes, is now standard. It is quicker and cheaper than sodium nitroprusside infusion.[92] Although the first dose is often effective, a sustained hypotensive effect frequently requires additional treatment by a β-blocker, ACE inhibitor, or diuretic, or a combination of these agents. In **moderately severe hypertension**, the efficacy of nifedipine is apparently maintained during subsequent prolonged therapy without development of tolerance when combined with other agents.[26] In **malignant hypertension with papilledema**, slow-release nifedipine 40 mg 12-hourly caused a quicker fall in blood pressure than did atenolol, although both reached the same end-point.[104] In true **hypertensive crises**, however, it is not yet clear that such rapid reduction of blood pressure is safe or desirable.

In **systolic hypertension of the elderly**, nifedipine 10 mg often benefits when given acutely, in which case long-term therapy is warranted. Fear of abrupt peripheral vasodilation and absence of a corrective baroreflex response means that excessive hypotension with possible cerebral ischemia is a risk, so that the initial dose should be 5 mg.

Nifedipine Poisoning

In one case there was hypotension, SA and AV nodal block, and hyperglycemia.[101] Treatment was by infusions of calcium and dopamine.

Summary

Nifedipine is a widely used and powerful arterial vasodilator with few serious side-effects and is now part of the accepted therapy of effort- or cold-induced angina and of hypertension. However, in unstable angina at rest, nifedipine should not be used as monotherapy, although it is effective when added to pre-existing β-blockade. Nifedipine, like verapamil and diltiazem, is especially useful in patients with contraindications to β-blockade, such as bronchospasm, diabetes mellitus, or active peripheral vascular disease. Contraindications to nifedipine are few, and combination with β-blockade is usually simple. Vasodilatory side-effects are common and can seemingly be reduced by a prolonged release preparation, although headache remains a problem.

SECOND-GENERATION CALCIUM ANTAGONISTS

What Can be Predicted: Common Properties, Common Problems

Virtually all the second-generation calcium antagonists now being introduced are dihydropyridines (DHPs) and nifedipine-like in structure. Therefore, they will all by definition have certain common properties and contraindications and share certain side-effects with nifedipine. All DHPs interact with the dihydropyridine binding site (N site, Fig. 3–1) to modify the properties of the calcium channel so that the probability of the channel's being "opened" by voltage depolarization is lessened (i.e., the channel is "closed").

The **pharmacokinetics** of all DHPs can be predicted to have the following common features. First, they are all actively metabolized by the liver to inactive metabolites, which are excreted chiefly by the

**TABLE 3–6 PATIENT PROFILING FOR PREFERENTIAL
ANTIHYPERTENSIVE THERAPY WITH CALCIUM ANTAGONISTS,
INCLUDING DIHYDROPYRIDINES**

	Rationale
Patient Category	
Black	Low-renin or primary vasoconstriction
Elderly (controversial)	Low-renin or increased arterial wall stiffness
Physically active	Normal hemodynamics
Intense mental activity	Better hemodynamics than with conventional β-blockers
Associated Conditions	
Angina, cold-induced	Coronary vasodilation
Angina, β-blocker C/I (bronchospasm, diabetes)	Alternate antianginal mechanisms
Exercise-induced asthma	Bronchodilator (weak)
Renal disease	Renal plasma flow increased (evidence for GFR uncertain)
Raynaud's disease*	Peripheral vasodilation
Scleroderma (Raynaud's phenomenon*, coronary spasm)	Peripheral and coronary dilation
LV hypertrophy+	Regression of LV mass
LV diastolic dysfunction+	Improved relaxation

Abbreviations: C/I = contraindicated; LV = left ventricular; GFR = glomerular filtration rate.
* = Therapeutic effect not yet shown for verapamil.
+ = Beta-blockade is alternative therapy.
For data sources, see Opie.[140]

kidneys. A lower dosage of all DHPs can be anticipated in chronic liver disease (lower rate of metabolism). In chronic renal disease, the dose will be virtually unchanged. All DHPs will tend to accumulate in the elderly where the hepatic blood flow is decreased.

The **antihypertensive effects** of DHPs are well established. The success rate is not uniform and varies from about 45 to 70%, depending on the criteria chosen for success. There is little reason to believe that any one DHP should be more effective than any other, apart from the question of duration of action. All DHPs may be considered as potential first-line agents, particularly when there are certain specific co-existing conditions or states suggesting preferential use of these agents (Table 3-6). It is often thought that DHPs, like other calcium antagonists, are more effective in the elderly and in blacks. Data on the elderly tend to be contradictory, whereas more and more studies suggest that a vasodilatory rather than a β-blocking mode of antihypertensive action is better in black patients.

The **chief antihypertensive mechanism of DHPs** is on the systemic vascular resistance, where arteriolar dilation is of rapid onset, thereby causing the elevated blood pressure (BP) to fall. Some evidence suggests that the higher the level of the BP, the greater the fall induced by calcium antagonists. The peripheral vasodilation invokes a reflex activation of the baroreceptors, which results in adrenergic activation with an acute reflex tachycardia and release of renin with formation of angiotensin-II and a tendency to counterregulatory vasoconstriction. However, in severe hypertension the baroreflexes are blunted so that the BP falls with only a slight tachycardia. Furthermore, during chronic therapy the calcium antagonists directly inhibit the baroreflex response so that the tachycardia is less or non-existent.[115] Nonetheless, even during long-term therapy, most studies show a residual elevation of plasma norepinephrine. Although an increased aldosterone level could be expected, a direct inhibitory effect of calcium antagonists on the release of aldosterone probably explains the unchanged levels of aldosterone found during both acute and chronic therapy.[116]

The **acute hypotensive effect** of nifedipine and all rapidly acting DHPs (see time to peak blood level[117]) is one of the most useful properties in **severe hypertension** when baroreflex inhibition by the hypertensive process dampens the acute vasodilatory effects, so that there is no detectable tachycardia. It is precisely this use in severe and apparently refractory hypertension, where nifedipine is successful in the vast majority of cases, that has brought the antihypertensive qualities of these compounds to the forefront. However, long-acting preparations of slow onset (amlodipine, extended-release nifedipine) cannot be expected to induce acute hypotension.

Renal effects of DHPs include acute natriuresis, found consistently and in some studies persisting during chronic therapy. In the case of isradipine, there is repetitive post-dose natriuresis and diuresis even with chronic dosing.[105] MacGregor[110] proposes that a prolonged mild loss of sodium is part of the antihypertensive mechanism of DHPs, so that the combination with diuretics is likely to be less effective than expected. This issue is highly controversial. Although DHPs may acutely increase the glomerular filtration rate, there is no good evidence that this salutory change can be induced in patients with hypertension and impaired renal function.

Antianginal mechanisms of DHPs are complex and controversial and may include afterload reduction, coronary vasodilation to offset an exercise-induced coronary vasoconstriction, and improved diastolic compliance, which further increases ischemic blood flow. Although the acute tachycardia should diminish the antianginal effects of such agents and may be the cause of provocation of angina in certain studies, in time a direct inhibition of the baroreflexes results, so that, in most chronic studies, there is an unchanged heart rate or only a modest tachycardia.

Contraindications for all DHPs can be expected to be identical with those for nifedipine, including significant aortic stenosis, obstructive hypertrophic cardiomyopathy, threatened myocardial infarction, and unstable pre-infarction angina (contraindicated in the absence of β-blockade), as well as severe myocardial failure. Although some newer DHPs are relatively less cardiodepressant and more vascular selective, their safety and efficacy in severe congestive heart failure is not established.

Amlodipine (Norvasc; Istin in UK)

The major specific advantage compared with nifedipine is the slower onset of action and the much longer duration of activity (Fig. 3–8). It binds to the nifedipine (N) site, as do other DHPs. However, the binding is not entirely typical, and there is very slow association and dissociation[82] so that the channel block is slow in onset and offset.

Regarding **pharmacokinetics**, the absorption is also slow with peak blood levels being reached after 6 to 12 hours, followed by extensive hepatic metabolism to inactive metabolites. The plasma levels increase during chronic dosage probably because of the very long half-life. The elimination half-life is 35 to 48 hours, increasing slightly with chronic dosage.[78] In the **elderly**, the clearance is reduced and the dose may need reduction.[78]

Regarding **drug interactions**, no effect on digoxin levels has been found, nor is there any interaction with cimetidine.

In **hypertension**, as initial monotherapy, amlodipine 2.5 to 5 mg daily was effective in 56% of patients, where 73% responded to 5 to 10 mg daily.[93] Ambulatory monitoring has demonstrated 24-hour efficacy of 5 mg amlodipine. In comparative studies, amlodipine was equipotent to hydrochlorothiazide or atenolol. A mean dose of 9 mg of amlodipine is superior to verapamil in a mean dose of 320 mg.[109] In **angina pectoris**, amlodipine 10 mg was more effective than placebo,

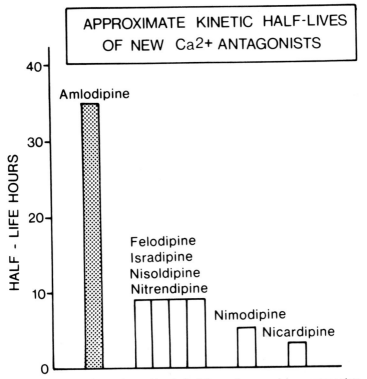

FIGURE 3–8. Approximate kinetic half-lives of new calcium antagonists. These half-lives (they are only approximate) separate the new calcium antagonists into one with a long half-life (amlodipine), those with moderately long half-lives (felodipine, isradipine, nisoldipine, and nitrendipine) and those with short half-lives (nimodipine and nicardipine). In every case the biological half-life, especially against hypertension, may be longer than the pharmacokinetic half-life.

and its antianginal effect persisted for 24 hours.[96] Amlodipine in a mean dose of 7.7 mg is at least as effective as nadolol 105 mg, judged by exercise parameters 24 hours after the last dose.[129]

The major **side-effect** is peripheral or facial edema, occurring in about 10% of patients (see Table 3-5). Next in significance are dizziness and flushing. Tachycardia has not been reported and headache seems less than with other DHPs, although there are no strict trials. Compared with verapamil, edema is more common but headache and constipation are less common.[118] Compared with diltiazem, fatigue is more common, with no other significant differences.[118]

In summary, the very long half-life of amlodipine makes it an effective once-a-day antihypertensive agent, setting it apart from many of the other agents, which are either 2x or 3x daily, or borderline once daily, in their dosages. Likewise, the antianginal effect is prolonged. These qualities distinguish amlodipine from other second-generation calcium antagonists. There may also be differences in the side-effect profile such as, possibly, fewer headaches.

Felodipine (Plendil, not approved in the USA)

This DHP has specifically been developed to be more vascular selective than nifedipine. For **hypertension**, the dose is 2.5 to 5 mg 2x daily; higher doses (10 mg b.d.) are more effective, but less well tolerated.[87] As monotherapy, it is approximately as effective as nifedipine.[77] Felodipine, like other DHPs, combines well with β-blockers. As a third-line agent after β-blockers and diuretics, felodipine is equal in effect to minoxidil[138] and better than hydralazine.[86] In **angina pectoris**, felodipine 5 to 10 mg given acutely can improve exercise time for 10 to 12 hours.[136]

The high vascular selectivity of felodipine has led to extensive testing in congestive heart failure, providing no proof of any sustained subjective benefit.[132]

Isradipine (DynaCirc)

This DHP has a medium-duration half-life (Fig. 3–8). Experimentally it is particularly well tested for antiatherogenic effects.

In **mild to moderate hypertension**, isradipine 2.5 to 5 mg 2x daily compares well with hydrochlorothiazide and diltiazem and is superior to propranolol and prazosin. An important finding relates to the antihypertensive mechanism of isradipine (up to 20 mg 2x daily), which may be (at least in part) explained by repetitive post-dose natriuresis and diuresis.[105] In **effort angina**, isradipine 2.5 to 7.5 mg 3x daily is similar to nifedipine 10 to 30 mg 3x daily.[133]

Side-effects of high doses used in the treatment of angina pectoris (dose 7.5 mg 3x daily) were ankle edema (25%), fatigue (22%), and facial flushing (6%). Unexpectedly, 14% of patients complained of arthralgia.[120] In contrast, for the lower doses used in hypertension, such as a mean dose of 3.4 mg 2x daily,[131] the incidence of edema was only 4%, although headache remained at 10% and flushing at 11%.

Interactions with digoxin are negligible.

Nicardipine (Cardene)

This DHP has many similarities to nifedipine, including the proposed indications and the short duration of action (Table 3-7). Claimed advantages over nifedipine are (1) less of a negative inotropic effect, so that nicardipine may be more vascular-specific with a relatively greater effect on arterial smooth muscle,[106] and (2) water-solubility without light-sensitivity, so that intravenous administration is easier. **Intracoronary nicardipine** gave less inhibition of systolic and diastolic function than did nifedipine in 12 patients with coronary artery disease, the doses of each being chosen to give an equal increase in coronary sinus outflow.[137]

In **angina pectoris**, nicardipine 30 to 40 mg 3x daily is well tested.[128] A lower starting dose (20 mg 3x daily) with upward titration to peak doses of 40 mg 3x daily is recommended in the USA and UK package inserts, and such titration should lessen the risk of precipitating angina.

In **silent ischemia** in patients who also had effort angina, nicardipine increased rather than decreased the number of episodes of ST-deviation, in contrast to the beneficial effects of verapamil.[126]

In **true vasospastic angina**, nicardipine gave benefit with a mean optimal dose of about 90 mg daily.[94] During percutaneous transluminal coronary angioplasty, pre-treatment with intracoronary nicardipine protected against ischemia.[99]

In **hypertension**, nicardipine 20 to 40 mg 3x daily is likely to be as effective as nifedipine without any compelling advantage for either agent. The package insert acknowledges the peak hypotensive effect at 1 to 2 hours post-dose is much more than at trough blood levels 6 to 8 hours post-dose, so that the BP should be checked at both times. After initial dose-titration (starting with 20 mg 3x daily), 2x daily therapy may be used according to the UK package insert. In comparative studies, nicardipine is similar in potency to verapamil, hydrochlorothiazide, and propranolol. Combination treatment in hypertension may be with atenolol, propranolol, or enalapril,[91] or with other agents such as diuretics or α-blockers. For treatment of severe hypertension (mean initial diastolic BP 127 mm Hg), IV nicardipine is undergoing evaluation.[85]

TABLE 3–7 SUMMARY OF SPECIFIC FEATURES OF NEW DIHYDROPYRIDINES (DHPs)

	Plasma Half-life	Possible Dose	Proposed Indications	Special Properties
Ultralong-Acting				
Amlodipine	36 hrs	2.5–10 mg 1x daily	Hypertension (angina)	Prolonged action. No digoxin interaction.
Medium Duration of Action				
Isradipine	8 hrs	5–10 mg 2x daily for hypertension; 5–7.5 mg 3x daily for angina	Hypertension (angina)	Vascular selective; no digoxin interaction
Felodipine	8 hrs	5–10 mg 2x daily for hypertension; 5–10 mg 3x daily for angina	Hypertension (angina)	Highly vascular selective
Nisoldipine	8–11 hrs	5–20 mg 1–2x daily For angina: 2x daily	(Hypertension) (angina)	Highly specific for calcium current; vascular selective
Nitrendipine	7–8 hrs	10–20 mg 1–2x daily	Hypertension (angina)	Doubles digoxin levels
Short Duration of Action				
Nicardipine	4–5 hrs or less	20–40 mg 3x daily	Hypertension, angina	Water-soluble, light-insensitive; vascular selective; registered for both angina and hypertension in USA
Nimodipine	5 hrs	0.35 mg/kg 4 hourly 30–40 mg 3–4 times daily	Cerebral spasm, subarachnoid hemorrhage (early stroke)	Best tested DHP in cerebral vascular disease. Truly selective.

For data sources, see Opie.[117]
( ) = possible indication, not yet registered in USA as far as could be ascertained.

In summary, a similar series of indications, contraindications, side-effects, and beneficial drug combinations can be anticipated with nicardipine as with nifedipine. The pharmacokinetics are similar. However, in contrast to nifedipine capsules, it is registered for use in both angina and hypertension in the USA. Unlike nifedipine, it is not light-sensitive, so that an intravenous form might come to be used in severe, urgent hypertension.

Nimodipine (Nimotop)

Nimodipine helps to prevent complications of **subarachnoid hemorrhage,**[79] for which it is licensed in the USA and UK. The dose in the USA is 60 mg (2 capsules) every 4 hours for 21 days, starting within 96 hours of aneurysmal subarachnoid hemorrhage, irrespective of evidence for coronary vascular spasm. In the UK, the dose is 1 to 2 mg/hr by central catheter starting as soon as possible and continuing for 5 days. It does not simply act as a vasodilator, rather the mechanism of benefit is still unknown.[107] The major side-effect is hypotension.[107] In **early ischemic stroke**, a dose of 120 mg daily in divided doses, added to standard therapy, reduced mortality at 4 weeks in male patients.[95]

Nisoldipine (Baymycard, not approved in USA)

This DHP is highly specific for the slow calcium current and therefore is one of the standard agents in experimental pharmacology. Nisoldipine is claimed to be 20x more specific as a vasodilator than is nifedipine. However, thus far it is not licensed for use in the USA or UK. In **hypertension**, 10 mg 1 to 2x daily was similar in benefit to hydrochlorothiazide,[89] and the combination achieved excellent control in 96% of patients, a figure which excludes 25% of the starting group who dropped out because of headache. When studied over 1 year at a mean dose of 25 mg daily, the BP reduction is maintained chiefly due to a reduced peripheral vascular resistance.[115] In **effort angina**, the dose is 5 to 20 mg 2x daily. When added to atenolol in the therapy of patients with **severe angina**, nifedipine 20 mg 3x daily was more effective than nisoldipine 20 mg once daily according to a preliminary communication.[122]

Nitrendipine (Baypress)

Because of its use as a reference standard in binding studies, nitrendipine has become well known to experimental pharmacologists. Nitrendipine is not a pure calcium channel antagonist; it also has some agonist properties. Clinically, it is of medium duration of action. In **hypertension**, the standard dose is 10 to 20 mg 1 to 2x daily. However, 10 to 30 mg once daily achieved satisfactory blood pressure reduction over 24 hours.[98] Regression of LV mass occurred within 3 months.[70] Nitrendipine is about as effective as amiloride, nifedipine, or hydralazine.[97] In black patients, it is better than atenolol.[112] Nitrendipine 20 mg daily almost doubles the **digoxin** level.

ADDITIONAL OR EXPERIMENTAL USES OF CALCIUM ANTAGONISTS

In **Raynaud's phenomenon**, nifedipine is well tested and can be taken either prophylactically or acutely (sublingual or bite-and-swallow) at the start of the attack. Diltiazem (but not verapamil) is also of documented benefit.

In **progressive systemic sclerosis** (scleroderma), nifedipine may relieve both the associated Raynaud's phenomenon and coronary artery spasm.

In **peripheral vascular disease**, calcium antagonists are poorly tested. Logically they should benefit most when spasm is the major component, as in severe disease associated with excess cigarette smoking or when intermittent claudication is precipitated by cold.

In **chronic renal failure**, nisoldipine (and by implication other DHPs) may prevent progression, acting by inhibition of renal calcinosis.

In **acute renal failure**, nifedipine given prophylactically may prolong the ischemic time, hence being of possible use in renal transplantation.

In **Conn's syndrome**, inhibition of release of aldosterone makes DHPs logical agents for the treatment of hypertension.

In **pulmonary hypertension of hypoxic origin**, nifedipine is best tested.

In **primary pulmonary hypertension**, high doses (nifedipine 240 mg or diltiazem 720 mg daily) may be tested cautiously after lower initial doses.

In **exercise-induced asthma**, nifedipine is a mild bronchodilator.

In **congestive heart failure**, calcium antagonists are being used less and less.

In **migraine**, verapamil (80 mg 4x daily) has been well studied, nifedipine and diltiazem are not. Nimodipine and **flunarizine** are also effective, the latter perhaps in part through antihistaminic mechanisms.

In **reperfusion "stunning"** in dogs, nifedipine or verapamil given 30 minutes after onset of reperfusion lessened "stunning."[125]

REFERENCES

References from Previous Editions

1. Andre-Fouet X, Usdin JP, Gayet C, et al: Eur Heart J 4:691–698, 1983
2. Antman E, Muller J, Goldberg S, et al: N Engl J Med 302:1269–1273, 1980
3. Arnman K, Ryden L: Am J Cardiol 49:821–827, 1982
4. Belhassen B, Horowitz LN: Am J Cardiol 54:1131–1133, 1984
5. Bruce RA, Hossack KF, Kusumi F, et al: Am Heart J 109:1020–1026, 1985
6. Chaitman BR, Wagniart P, Pasternac A, et al: Am J Cardiol 53:1–9, 1984
7. Chew CYC, Hecht HS, Collett JT, et al: Am J Cardiol 47:917–922, 1981
8. Dawson JR, Whitaker NHG, Sutton GC: Br Heart J 46:508–512, 1981
9. Diamond JR, Cheung JY, Fang LST: Am J Med 77:905–909, 1984
10. Elliott HL, Pasanisi F, Meredith PA, et al: Br Med J 288:238, 1984
11. Ellrodt AG, Ault MJ, Riedinger MS, et al: Am J Med 79(suppl 4A):19–25, 1985
12. Findlay IN, Dargie HJ: Postgrad Med J 59(suppl 2):70–73, 1983
13. Findlay IN, MacLeod K, Ford M, et al: Br Heart J 55:240–245, 1986
14. Fisher JF, Borer JS, Moses JW, et al: Am J Cardiol 54:646–650, 1984
15. Frishman W, Kirsten E, Klein M, et al: Am J Cardiol 50:1180–1184, 1982
16. Gottlieb SO, Ouyang P, Achuff SC, et al: J Am Coll Cardiol 4:382–388, 1984
17. Gottlieb SO, Weisfeldt M, Ouyang P, et al: Circulation 73:331–337, 1986
18. Guazzi MD, Cipolla C, Bella PD, et al: Am Heart J 108:116–123, 1984
19. Hamann SR, Kaltenborn KE, Vore M, et al: Am J Cardiol 56:147–156, 1985
20. Hariman RJ, Mangiardi LM, McAllister RG, et al: Circulation 59:797–804, 1979
21. Heng MK, Singh BN, Roche AHG, et al: Am Heart J 90:487–498, 1975
22. Hess O, Grimm J, Krayenbuehl HP: Eur Heart J 4(suppl F):47–56, 1983
23. Hung J, Lamb IH, Connolly SJ, et al: Circulation 68:560–567, 1983
24. Jariwalla AG, Anderson EG: Br Med J 1:1181–1182, 1978
25. Jee LD, Opie LH: Br Med J 287:1514–1516, 1983
26. Jennings AA, Jee LD, Smith JA, et al: Am Heart J 111:557–563, 1986
27. Johnston DL, Gebhardt VA, Donald A, et al: Circulation 68:1280–1289, 1983

28. Johnston DL, Lesoway R, Humen DP, et al: Am J Cardiol 55:680–687, 1985
29. Kaltenbach M, Hopf R: J Mol Cell Cardiol 17(suppl 2):59–68, 1985
30. Kenmure ACF, Scruton JH: Br J Clin Prac 33:49–51, 1979
31. Kieval J, Kirsten EB, Kessler KM, et al: Circulation 65:653–659, 1982
32. Kimura E, Kishida H: Circulation 63:844–848, 1981
33. Klein HO, Kaplinsky L: Am J Cardiol 50:894–902, 1982
34. Landmark K, Sire S, Thaulow E, et al: Br Heart J 48:19–26, 1982
35. Lessem J, Bellinetto A: Am J Cardiol 49:1025 (abstract), 1982
36. Lette J, Gagnon RM, Lemire JG, et al: Can Med Assoc J 130:1169–1171, 1984
37. Lichtlen PR, Engel H-J, Rafflenbeul W: In Opie LH (ed): Calcium Antagonists and Cardiovascular Disease. New York, Raven Press, 1984, pp 221–236
38. Livesley B, Catley PF, Campbell RC, et al: Br Med J 1:375–378, 1973
39. Lynch P, Dargie H, Krikler S, et al: Br Med J 2:184–187, 1980
40. Maisel AS, Motulsky HJ, Insel PA: N Engl J Med 312:167–171, 1985
41. Mauritson DR, Winniford MD, Walker WS, et al: Ann Intern Med 96:409–412, 1982
42. McInnes GT, Findlay IN, Murray G, et al: J Hypertens 3(suppl 3):S219–S221, 1985
43. Muller JE, Morrison J, Stone PH, et al: Circulation 69:740–747, 1984
44. Opie LH: Drugs and the Heart. London, Lancet, 1980, pp 27–38
45. Opie LH: Pharmacol Ther 25:271–295, 1984
46. Packer M, Meller J, Medina N, et al: Circulation 65:660–668, 1982
47. Pasanisi F, Elliott HL, Meredith PA, et al: Clin Pharmacol Ther 36:716–723, 1984
48. Pepine CJ, Feldman RL, Hill JA, et al: Am Heart J 106:1341–1347, 1983
49. Pitlik S, Manor RS, Lipshitz I, et al: Br Med J 287:1845–1846, 1983
50. Roberts R, Gibson RS, Boden WE, et al: J Am Coll Cardiol 7:68A (abstract), 1986
51. Rosing DR, Kent KM, Maron BJ, et al: Circulation 60:1208–1213, 1979
52. Schamroth L, Krikler DM, Garrett C: Br Med J 1:660–662, 1972
53. Schick EC, Heupler FA, Kerin NZ, et al: Am Heart J 104:690–697, 1982
54. Schroeder JS, Feldman RL, Giles TD, et al: Am J Med 72:227–232, 1982
55. Schwartz JB, Keefe DL, Kirsten E, et al: Am Heart J 104:198–203, 1982
56. Singh BN, Roche AHG: Am Heart J 94:593–599, 1977
57. Singh BN, Ellrodt G, Peter CT: Drugs 15:169–197, 1978
58. Singh BN, Opie LH: Drugs for the Heart. III. Calcium antagonists. Grune & Stratton, Orlando, 1984, pp 39–64
59. Stone PH, Muller JE, Turi ZG, et al: Am Heart J 106:644–652, 1983
60. Storstein L, Larsen A, Midtbo K, et al: Acta Med Scand (suppl 681):25–30, 1983
61. Subramanian VB: Calcium antagonists in chronic stable angina pectoris. Amsterdam, Excerpta Medica, 1983, pp 97–116, 217–229
62. Talano JV, Tommaso C: Prog Cardiovasc Dis 25:141–156, 1982
63. Theroux P, Waters DD, Affaki GS, et al: Circulation 60:504-510, 1979
64. Theroux P, Taeymans Y, Morissette D, et al: J Am Coll Cardiol 5:717-722, 1985
65. Tilmant PY, Lablanche JM, Thieuleux FA, et al: Am J Cardiol 52:230-233, 1983
66. Urthaler F, James TN: Am J Cardiol 44:651-656, 1979
67. Uusitalo A, Arstila M, Bae AE, et al: Am J Cardiol 57:733-737,1986
68. Weiss AT, Lewis BS, Halon DA, et al: Int J Cardiol 4:275–280, 1983
69. Wigle ED, Sasson Z, Henderson MA, et al: Prog Cardiovasc Dis 28:1–83, 1985
70. Winniford MD, Johnson SM, Mauritson DR, et al: Am J Cardiol 50:913–918, 1982
71. Winniford MD, Gabliani G, Johnson SM, et al: Am Heart J 108:1269–1273, 1984
72. Winniford MD, Fulton KL, Corbett JR, et al: Am J Cardiol 55: 281–285, 1985
73. Woelfel A, Foster JR, McAllister RG, et al: Am J Cardiol 56: 292-297, 1985
74. Yee R, Gulamhusein SS, Klein GJ: Am J Cardiol 53:757–763, 1984
75. Yeh S-J, Kou H-C, Lin F-C, et al: Am J Cardiol 52:271–278, 1983
76. Yeh S-J, Lin F-C, Chou Y-Y, et al: Circulation 71:104–109, 1985

New References

77. Aberg H, Lindsjo M, Morlin B: Comparative trial of felodipine and nifedipine in refractory hypertension. Drugs 29(suppl 2):117–123, 1985

78. Abernethy DR: The pharmacokinetic profile of amlodipine. Am Heart J 118:1100–1103, 1989
79. Allen GS, Ahn HS, Preziosi TJ, et al: Cerebral arterial spasm: A controlled trial of nimodipine in patients with subarachnoid hemorrhage. N Engl J Med 308:619–624, 1983
80. Bender VF: Die Behandlung der tachycarden arrhythmien und der arteriellen hypertonie mit verapamil. Drug Res 20:1310–1316, 1970
81. Betocchi S, Bonow RO, Cannon RO, et al: Relation between serum nifedipine concentration and hemodynamic effects in non-obstructive hypertrophic cardiomyopathy. Am J Cardiol 61:830–835, 1988
82. Burges RA, Dodd MG, Gardiner DG: Pharmacologic profile of amlodipine. Am J Cardiol 64:10 I–20 I, 1989
83. Burris JF, Weir MR, Oparil S, et al: An assessment of diltiazem and hydrochlorothiazide in hypertension: Application of factorial trial design to a multicenter clinical trial of combination therapy. JAMA 263:1507–1512, 1990
84. Capucci A, Bassein L, Bracchetti D, et al: Propranolol v. verapamil in the treatment of unstable angina: A double-blind cross-over study. Eur Heart J 4:148–154, 1983
85. Clifton GG, Cook E, Bienvenu GS, Wallin JD: Intravenous nicardipine in severe systemic hypertension. Am J Cardiol 64:16H–18H, 1989
86. Co-operative Study Group: Felodipine vs hydralazine: A controlled trial as third line therapy in hypertension. Br J Clin Pharmacol 21:621–626, 1986
87. Co-operative Study Group: Felodipine, a new calcium antagonist, as monotherapy in mild or moderate hypertension. Drugs 34(suppl 3):139–148, 1987
88. Cubeddu LX, Aranda J, Singh B, et al: A comparison of verapamil and propranolol for the initial treatment of hypertension: Racial differences in response. JAMA 256:2214–2221, 1986
89. Daniels AR, Opie LH: Monotherapy with the calcium channel antagonist nisoldipine for systemic hypertension and comparison with diuretic drugs. Am J Cardiol 60:703–707, 1987
90. Deanfield J, Wright C, Krikler S, et al: Cigarette smoking and the treatment of angina with propranolol, atenolol and nifedipine. N Engl J Med 310:951–954, 1984
91. Donnelly R, Elliott HL, Meredith PA, Reid JL: Enalapril in essential hypertension: The comparative effects of additional placebo, nicardipine and chlorthalidone. Br J Clin Pharmacol 24:842–845, 1987
92. Franklin C, Nightingale S, Mamdani B: A randomized comparison of nifedipine and sodium nitroprusside in severe hypertension. Chest 90:500–503, 1986
93. Frick MH, McGibney D, Tyler HM, et al: Amlodipine: A double-blind evaluation of the dose-response relationship in mild to moderate hypertension. J Cardiovasc Pharmacol 12(suppl 7):S76–S78, 1988
94. Gelman JS, Feldman RL, Scott E, et al: Nicardipine for angina pectoris at rest and coronary arterial spasm. Am J Cardiol 56:232–236, 1985
95. Gelmers HJ, Gorter K, de Weerdt CJ, Wiezer HJA: A controlled trial of nimodipine in acute ischemic stroke. N Engl J Med 318:203–207, 1988
96. Glasser SP, West TW: Clinical safety and efficacy of once-a-day amlodipine for chronic stable angina pectoris. Am J Cardiol 62:518–522, 1988
97. Goa KL, Sorkin EM: Nitrendipine: A review of its pharmacodynamic and pharmacokinetic properties, and therapeutic efficacy in the treatment of hypertension. Drugs 33:123–155, 1987
98. Grossman E, Oren S, Garavaglia GE, et al: Systemic and regional hemodynamic and humoral effects of nitrendipine in essential hypertension. Circulation 78:1394–1400, 1988
99. Hanet C, Rousseau MF, Vincent M-F, et al: Myocardial protection by intracoronary nicardipine administration during percutaneous transluminal coronary angioplasty. Am J Cardiol 59:1035–1040, 1987
100. Held PH, Yusuf S, Furberg CD: Calcium channel blockers in acute myocardial infarction and unstable angina: An overview. Br Med J 299:1187–1192, 1989
101. Herrington DM, Insley BM, Weinmann GG: Nifedipine overdose. Am J Med 81:344–346, 1986
102. HINT Research Group (Holland Interuniversity Nifedipine/Metoprolol Trial): Early treatment of unstable angina in the coronary care unit: A randomised double-blind placebo-controlled comparison of recurrent ischaemia in patients treated with nifedipine or metoprolol or both. Br Heart J 56:400–413, 1986

103. Holzgreve H, Distler A, Michaelis J, et al: Verapamil versus hydrochlorothiazide in the treatment of hypertension: Results of long-term double-blind comparative trial. Br Med J 299:881–886, 1989
104. Isles CG, Johnson OC, Milne FJ: Slow-release nifedipine and atenolol as initial treatment in blacks with malignant hypertension. Br J Clin Pharmacol 21:377–383, 1986
105. Krusell LR, Jespersen LT, Schmitz A, et al: Repetitive natriuresis and blood pressure: Long-term calcium entry blockade with isradipine. Hypertension 10:577–581, 1987
106. Lambert CR, Pepine CJ: Effects of intravenous and intracoronary nicardipine. Am J Cardiol 64:8H–15H, 1989
107. Langley MS, Sorkin EM: Nimodipine: A review of its pharmacodynamic and pharmacokinetic properties, and therapeutic potential in cerebro-vascular disease. Drugs 37:669–699, 1989
108. Lichtlen PR, Hugenholtz P, Rafflenbeul W, INTACT group: Retardation of the angiographic progression of coronary artery disease in man by the calcium channel blocker nifedipine: Results of the international nifedipine trial on antiatherosclerotic therapy (INTACT). Lancet, 1990
109. Lorimer AR, Smedsrud T, Walker P, Tyler HM: Comparison of amlodipine and verapamil in the treatment of mild to moderate hypertension. J Cardiovasc Pharmacol 12(suppl 7):S89–S93, 1988
110. MacGregor GA: Nifedipine and hypertension: Roles of vasodilation and sodium diuresis. Cardiovasc Drugs Ther 3:295–301, 1989
111. Mauri F, Mafrici A, Biraghi P, et al: Effectiveness of calcium antagonist drugs in patients with unstable angina and proven coronary artery disease. Eur Heart J 9(suppl N):158–163, 1988
112. M'Buyamba-Kabangu J-R, Lepira B, Lijnen P, et al: Intracellular sodium and the response to nitrendipine or atenolol in African blacks. Hypertension 11:100–105, 1988
113. McLean AJ, Knight R, Harrison PM, et al: Clearance based oral drug interaction between verapamil and metoprolol and comparison with atenolol. Am J Cardiol 55:1628–1629, 1985
114. Multicenter Diltiazem Postinfarction Trial Research Group: The effect of diltiazem on mortality and reinfarction after myocardial infarction. N Engl J Med 319:385–392, 1988
115. Omvik P, Lund-Johansen P, Haugland H: Nisoldipine: Central haemodynamics at rest and during exercise in essential hypertension: Acute and chronic studies. J Hypertens 6:95–103, 1988
116. Opie LH: Calcium channel antagonists: A Review. Part I: Fundamental properties: Mechanisms, classification, sites of action. Cardiovasc Drugs Ther 1:411–430, 1987
117. Opie LH: Calcium channel antagonists. Part V: Second generation agents. Cardiovasc Drugs Ther 2:191–203, 1988
118. Osterloh I: The safety of amlodipine. Am Heart J 118:1114–1120, 1989
119. Packer M: Combined β-adrenergic and calcium entry blockade in angina pectoris. N Engl J Med 320:709–718, 1989
120. Parker JO, Enjalbert M, Bernstein V: Efficacy of the calcium antagonist isradipine in angina pectoris. Cardiovasc Drugs Ther 1:661–664, 1988
121. Parodi O, Simonetti I, Michelassi C, et al: Comparison of verapamil and propranolol therapy for angina pectoris at rest: A randomized, multiple crossover, controlled trial in the coronary care unit. Am J Cardiol 57:899–906, 1986
122. Pedersen TR, Kantor M: Nifedipine three times daily versus nisoldipine once daily in patients with severe effort angina pectoris pretreated with atenolol (abstract). Cardiovasc Drugs Ther 1:275, 1987
123. Peart I, Bullock RE, Albers C, Hall RJC: Cold intolerance in patients with angina pectoris: Effect of nifedipine and propranolol. Br Heart J 61:521–528, 1989
124. Prida XE, Gelman JS, Feldman RL, et al: Comparison of diltiazem and nifedipine alone and in combination in patients with coronary artery spasm. J Am Coll Cardiol 9:412–419, 1987
125. Przyklenk K, Ghafari GB, Eitzman DT, Kloner RA: Nifedipine adminis-tered after reperfusion ablates systolic contractile dysfunction of post-ischemic "stunned" myocardium. J Am Coll Cardiol 13:1176–1183, 1989
126. Rodrigues EA, Kohli RS, Hains ADB, et al: Comparison of nicardipine and verapamil in the management of chronic stable angina. Int J Cardiol 18:357–369, 1988
127. Roth A, Harrison E, Mitani G, et al: Efficacy and safety of medium- and high-dose diltiazem alone and in combination with digoxin for control of heart rate at rest and during exercise in patients with chronic atrial fibrillation. Circulation 73:316–324, 1986

128. Scheidt S, LeWinter MM, Hermanovich J, et al: Efficacy and safety of nicardipine for chronic, stable angina pectoris: A multicenter randomized trial. Am J Cardiol 58:715–721, 1986

129. Singh S, Doherty J, Udhoji V, et al: Amlodipine versus nadolol in patients with stable angina pectoris. Am Heart J 118:1137–1138, 1989

130. Steinberg JS, Katz RJ, Bren GB, et al: Efficacy of oral diltiazem to control ventricular response in chronic atrial fibrillation at rest and during exercise. J Am Coll Cardiol 9:405–411, 1987

131. Sundstedt C-D, Ruegg PC, Keller A, Waite R: A multicenter evaluation of the safety, tolerability, and efficacy of isradipine in the treatment of essential hypertension. Am J Med 86(suppl 4A):98–102, 1989

132. Tan LB, Murray RG, Littler WA: Felodipine in patients with chronic heart failure: Discrepant haemodynamic and clinical effects. Br Heart J 58:122–128, 1987

133. Taylor SH, Jackson NC, Allen J, et al: Efficacy of a new calcium antagonist PN 200-110 (Isradipine) in angina pectoris. Am J Cardiol 59:123B–129B, 1987

134. Van Harten J, Burggraaf K, Danhof M, et al: Negligible sublingual absorption of nifedipine. Lancet 2:1363–1365, 1987

135. Van Harten J, Van Brummelen P, Zeegers RRECM, et al: The influence of infusion rate on the pharmacokinetics and haemodynamic effects of nisoldipine in man. Br J Clin Pharmacol 25:709–717, 1988

136. Verdecchia P, Gatteschi C, Benemio G, et al: Increased exercise tolerance and reduced electrocardiographic ischaemia 3 and 12 hours after oral felodipine in effort angina. Eur Heart J 10:70–76, 1989

137. Visser CA, Koolen JJ, Van Wezel H, et al: Hemodynamics of nicardipine in coronary artery disease. Am J Cardiol 59:9J–12J, 1987

138. Wathan CG, MacLeod D, Tucker L, Muir AL: Felodipine as a replacement for minoxidil in the treatment of severe hypertension. Eur Heart J 7:893–897, 1986

139. Wicker P, Roudaut R, Gosse P, Dallocchio M: Short- and long-term treatment of mild to moderate hypertension with verapamil. Am J Cardiol 57:83D–86D, 1986

Book

140. Opie LH: Clinical Use of Calcium Antagonist Drugs. Boston, Kluwer Academic Publishers, 1990

L.H. Opie
N.M. Kaplan

4

Diuretics

By definition a diuretic induces a diuresis of water and solutes. Loss of sodium is essential for the anti-edema effect, and for at least one major component of the antihypertensive effect. However, loss of sodium is inevitably accompanied by loss of other ions—potassium is most frequently emphasized (Table 4-1). Magnesium and calcium may also be lost, especially during a vigorous diuresis, depending on the diuretic used.

When used as antihypertensive agents, diuretics act at least in part by volume and sodium depletion.[22] In addition, diuretics might be effective by non-diuretic mechanisms,[2,32] at least in doses low enough to avoid the subjective feeling of a diuresis. In subdiuretic doses, diuretics may act as vascular dilators, or in a more subtle way by altering the sodium balance. Whatever the exact mechanisms, diuretics given to treat hypertension are used in doses lower than when a major diuretic effect is required.

Despite the potentially serious side-effects of diuretic therapy when used on a long-term basis, such agents remain valuable in treatment of congestive heart failure (CHF) because of the high ratio of efficacy to serious side-effects. In other words, **the benefit-risk ratio of diuretics is very high in CHF. In contrast, the benefit-risk ratio of diuretics in the therapy of mild hypertension is increasingly questioned**, especially because of the "wrong-way" blood biochemical changes. Therefore, the time-honored role of diuretics as first-line therapy in hypertension is increasingly challenged though these agents still have an important place in the therapy of certain groups of hypertensive patients—the elderly, the obese, and blacks—and those already receiving ACE inhibitors. In those with renal impairment, loop diuretics are used.

For practical purposes, the three major groups of diuretics are the loop diuretics, the thiazides, and the potassium-sparing diuretics. Each type of diuretic acts at a different site of the nephron (Fig. 4–1) leading to the concept of **sequential nephron blockade**.

LOOP DIURETICS

In the therapy of CHF, a loop diuretic is often chosen as initial therapy, especially when the CHF is severe. A particular advantage of loop diuretics (Table 4-2), such as furosemide, is that increasing doses exert an increasing diuresis before the ceiling is reached (**high-ceiling diuretics**).

TABLE 4–1 URINARY ELECTROLYTE COMPOSITION DURING DIURESIS

	Volume (ml/min)	pH	Na⁺ (mM/l)	K⁺ (mM/l)	Cl⁻	HCO₃⁻	Ca²⁺
Control	1	6.0	50	15	60	1	Variable
Thiazides	3	7.4	150	25	150	25	0
Furosemide	8	6.0	140	10	155	1	+
Triamterene	3	7.2	130	5	120	15	0
Amiloride	2	7.2	130	5	110	15	0

Modified from Mudge,[50] with permission. 0 = decreased, + = increased.

Furosemide

Furosemide (= frusemide; Lasix, Dryptal, Frusetic, Frusid) is one of the standard loop diuretics for CHF. Furosemide is initial therapy in acute pulmonary edema and in left-sided failure of acute myocardial infarction (AMI). Relief of dyspnea even before diuresis results from venodilation and preload reduction.[7] Furosemide is also widely used for maintenance therapy in CHF. Increasingly it is being appreciated that subdiuretic doses of furosemide are also antihypertensive.

Pharmacologic Effects and Pharmacokinetics. Loop diuretics, including furosemide (see Fig. 4–1), inhibit the Na⁺/K⁺/Cl⁻ cotransporter concerned with the transport of chloride across the lining cells of the ascending limb of the loop of Henle (site 2). This site of action is reached intraluminally, after the drug has been excreted by the proximal tubule. The effect of the cotransport inhibition is that chloride, sodium, potassium, and hydrogen ions all remain intraluminally and are lost in the urine with the possible side-effects of hyponatremia, hypochloremia, hypokalemia, and alkalosis. The plasma half-life of furosemide is 1.5 hours; the duration of action is 4 to 6 hours. Diuresis starts within 10 to 20 minutes of an IV dose and peaks 1 to 1.5 hours after an oral dose.[8]

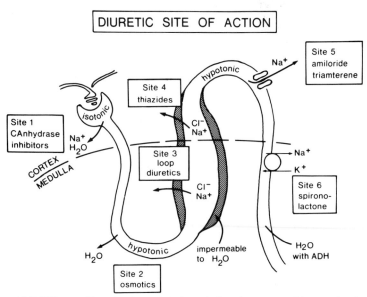

FIGURE 4–1. The six sites of action of diuretic agents. CA = carbonic anhydrase inhibitors. A common maximal combination is a loop diuretic plus a thiazide plus a K⁺-sparing agent (sequential nephron sites). (Figure copyright L.H. Opie.)

TABLE 4-2 LOOP DIURETICS: DOSES AND KINETICS

Drug	Dose	Pharmacokinetics
Furosemide (USA) Frusemide (UK) = Lasix	10–40 mg oral, once daily for BP 20–80 mg 1–2x for CHF 250–2000 mg oral or IV for refractory CHF, oliguria	Diuresis starts within 10–20 min of IV dose, reaches peak at 1.5 hr Total duration of action 4–5 hr Renal excretion
Bumetanide = Bumex (USA) = Burinex (UK)	0.5–2 mg oral 1–2x daily for CHF 5 mg oral or IV for oliguria	Peak diuresis 75–90 min Total duration of action 4–5 hr Renal excretion

Modified from Opie LH, Commerford PJ, Swanepoel CR: Diuretic Therapy. In Wenger N, Julian D (eds): Management of Heart Failure. London, Butterworths, 1986, pp 119–142, with permission.

BP = Blood pressure.

CHF = Use for congestive heart failure.

IV = Intravenous.

Dose. **IV furosemide** is usually started as a slow 40-mg injection (give 80 mg slow IV 1 hour later if needed); surprisingly, higher doses are required in elderly patients,[3] and much higher doses are required in renal failure and severe CHF. **Oral furosemide** also has a wide dose range (20–250 mg/day or even more; 20, 40, and 80 mg tablets in the USA; in Europe, also scored 500 mg tablets). A short duration of action (4–5 hours) means that frequent doses are needed when sustained diuresis is required. When 2 daily doses are required, they should be given in the early morning and mid-afternoon to obviate nocturia and to protect against volume depletion. Once acute relief has been obtained, however, twice daily dosage, reducing to once daily, is usually given to rest the kidneys and the patients (at night). Because of variable responses, such as a brisk initial diuresis with a residual resistant component, the dose regime must be individualized. For **hypertension**, doses are usually lower (20–40 mg 1–2x daily). Subdiuretic doses of furosemide can be antihypertensive. For **hypertension with renal impairment**, the initial dose becomes 80 mg daily, which can be titrated upward. A retard preparation (Lasix Retard) available in Europe is given once daily (30–60 mg); the longer duration of action may not be an advantage, as less time is allowed for interval self-correction of electrolyte deficits. In the presence of **oliguria**, as the GFR drops below 20 ml/min, up to 250–2000 mg of furosemide may be required because the site of action in the loop is reached from the lumen only after excretion of furosemide from the proximal tubule (the latter process is reduced as the renal blood flow falls). Similar arguments lead to similar doses of furosemide in **severe refractory heart failure**.

Indications. Furosemide is frequently the diuretic of choice for **severe heart failure** for four reasons. First, it is more powerful than the thiazides; second, it is effective (in high doses) in promoting diuresis even in the presence of a low glomerular filtration rate (GFR); third, furosemide promotes venodilation and preload reduction;[7,11] and fourth, it acts rapidly. Similar reasons make it the initial drug of choice in **acute pulmonary edema. After initial IV use, oral furosemide is usually continued as standard diuretic therapy, to be replaced by thiazides as the heart failure ameliorates.** In **AMI**, prophylactic furosemide in the absence of LVF only causes disadvantageous hemodynamic changes resulting from excess reduction of preload.[84] **Post-infarct**, a low ejection fraction is better treated by captopril than by furosemide.[90] In **hypertension**, low-dose furosemide can be effective even as monotherapy,[40] or combined with other agents such as ß-blockers[67] and ACE inhibitors. However, if thiazides do not work for hypertension, furosemide probably will not work either unless the problem is a very low GFR. In **severe renal failure**, it is widely believed that furosemide increases the GFR, yet the subject is poorly understood. In **severe hypertension**, IV furosemide is sometimes used, especially if fluid overload is present.

Contraindications. Anuria, although listed as a contraindication to use of furosemide, may be treated (as is oliguria) by furosemide in the hope of evoking a diuresis); first exclude dehydration, a history of hypersensitivity to furosemide, or sulfonamides. Furosemide (like other sulfonamides) may precipitate or exaggerate lupus erythematosus or photosensitive skin eruptions or may cause blood dyscrasias. Furosemide also should not be used intravenously when electrolytes cannot be monitored, to treat AMI in the absence of LV failure,[39,84] when optimal diuresis has already been achieved by other agents, or to treat patent ductus arteriosus in the neonate (see below).

Side-effects. The risk of **hypokalemia** is greatest with high-dose furosemide, especially when given intravenously, and at the start of myocardial infarction when hypokalemia is in any case common even in the absence of diuretic therapy. Any lowering of plasma potassium can dangerously precipitate arrhythmias in early myocardial infarction.[31] Carefully regulated IV potassium supplements may be required in these circumstances. In acute heart failure, too, digitalis toxicity may be precipitated by over-diuresis and hypokalemia. Standard oral doses of furosemide (40–80 mg daily), as used for the chronic therapy of heart failure and hypertension, probably cause less hypokalemia than do some thiazides (Table 4-1).[13,40,49] Clearly, much depends on the doses chosen and the degree of diuresis achieved. A lesser degree of hypokalemia than expected occurs because (1) the actual potassium concentration lost per unit volume during the diuresis is less (see Table 4-1), and (2) the short action of loop diuretics allows for post-diuresis correction of potassium and magnesium balance. Addition of potassium supplements to furosemide therapy is neither needed nor very effective;[41,77] addition of potassium-sparing diuretics is probably better.[44,49]

Other Side-effects. In 2580 patients, the chief side-effects, in addition to hypokalemia, were hypovolemia and hyperuricemia.[41] Hypovolemia can be lessened by a low initial dose (20–40 mg); if hypovolemia occurs, prerenal azotemia may develop (monitor blood urea).

Despite such fears of hemoconcentration, hemodilution is more likely, as shown by measurements of blood viscosity and hematocrit in patients with acute cardiogenic pulmonary edema treated by IV furosemide.[30] A few patients on high-dose furosemide have developed severe hyperosmolar non-ketotic **hyperglycemic states**.[16] **Atherogenic blood lipid changes**, similar to those found with thiazides, have recently been reported for loop diuretics.[70] Occasionally, gout or diabetes may be precipitated; it is not clear whether furosemide causes fewer metabolic side-effects than conventional thiazides.

Reversible dose-related **ototoxicity** (electrolyte disturbances of the endolymphatic system) can be avoided by infusing furosemide at rates not greater than 4 mg/min and keeping the oral dose below 1000 mg daily.

In **patent ductus arteriosus**, furosemide inhibits the degradation of prostaglandin E_2, which is a potent dilator of the ductus arteriosus so that the incidence of patent ductus arteriosus is increased.[23]

Drug Combinations and Interactions. Additional diuresis may be achieved by a combination of furosemide with hydrochlorothiazide or metolazone. Furosemide-hydrochlorothiazide-amiloride (low-dose Lasix plus Moduretic) is a combination that usually avoids the traditional requirement for potassium supplements with furosemide; nonetheless, the plasma potassium level requires checking, especially in the presence of renal failure.

Probenecid may interfere with the effects of thiazides or loop diuretics by blocking their secretion into the urine of the proximal tubule.[50,61] **Indomethacin** and other nonsteroidal anti-inflammatory drugs (**NSAIDs**) cause loss of response of the kidney to loop diuretics, presumably by interfering with formation of vasodilatory prostaglandins.[53,69] High doses of furosemide may competitively inhibit the excretion of salicylates to predispose to salicylate poisoning with tinnitus. Steroid or ACTH therapy may predispose to hypokalemia. Loop diuretics do not alter blood digoxin levels, nor do they interact with warfarin.

Bumetanide

The site of action of bumetanide (Bumex, Burinex) and its effects (and side-effects) are very similar to that of furosemide. The onset of diuresis is within 30 minutes, with a peak at 75 to 90 minutes, and a total duration of action of 270 minutes.[4,8] Although it has been claimed that potassium loss may be less than that caused by furosemide while achieving a comparable loss of sodium,[16] other studies show a powerful potassium losing capacity.[9] Ototoxicity may be less with bumetanide than with furosemide, but renal toxicity more. **The really striking differences between these two agents are the much greater**

bioavailability and potency of bumetanide, so that smaller (but not less frequent) doses are needed.[8] In practice, as with furosemide, low-dose therapy need not occasion undue concern regarding hypokalemia as a possible side-effect, whereas higher doses can cause considerable electrolyte disturbances including hypokalemia. Again, as in the case of furosemide, a combined diuretic effect is obtained by addition of a thiazide diuretic.

Dose and Clinical Uses. In CHF, bumetanide is claimed to be effective in patients with edema resistant to furosemide, but additional studies are required to prove this point. The usual oral dose is 0.5 to 2 mg (0.5- and 1-mg tablets) with 1 mg bumetanide being equal to 40 mg furosemide;[4] other estimates are that bumetanide is 70x more powerful than furosemide.[8] In renal failure, the comparative potency of bumetanide might be much less than 40.[16] In acute pulmonary edema, a single dose of 1 to 3 mg can be effective; usually it is given intravenously over 1 to 2 minutes, and the dose can be repeated at 2 to 3 hourly intervals to a maximum of 10 mg daily. In renal edema, the effects of bumetanide are similar to those of furosemide. In the USA, bumetanide is not approved for hypertension.

Side-effects. These are rather similar to those of furosemide; ototoxicity may be less[16] and renal toxicity more, so that the combination with other potentially nephrotoxic drugs, such as aminoglycosides, should be avoided. In patients with renal failure, high doses have caused myalgia, so that the dose should not exceed 4 mg/day when the GFR is below 5 ml/min.[29] Patients allergic to sulfonamides may also be hypersensitive to bumetanide; however, the package insert suggests that bumetanide might be safe when allergy to furosemide develops. Glucose tolerance may be well preserved.[20]

Summary

Until more careful studies are available on the comparison between bumetanide and furosemide, most clinicians will continue to use the agent they know best (i.e., furosemide) unless there is a specific reason for not giving furosemide (allergic reaction, ototoxicity). As furosemide is widely available in generic form, its cost is likely to be less than that of bumetanide. Nonetheless, the use of bumetanide is increasing.

Ethacrynic Acid

Ethacrynic acid (Edecrin) closely resembles furosemide in dose (50-mg tablet), duration of diuresis, and side-effects (except for more ototoxicity). Furosemide is much more widely used because it has a broader dose-response curve than ethacrynic acid, which allows easier definition of the optimal dose for a given patient.[50]

Piretanide

This agent is a new loop diuretic (Arlix, dose 6–24 mg), is claimed to have little effect on potassium homeostasis despite its potency,[51] and is being promoted for hypertension.

THIAZIDE DIURETICS

Thiazide diuretics (Table 4-3) **remain the most widely used first-line therapy for hypertension**, although increasingly other first-liners such as β-blockade, α-blockade, calcium antagonists, and ACE inhibitors are being chosen. Thiazides are also standard therapy for chronic CHF, when edema is modest, either alone or in combination with loop diuretics.

TABLE 4-3 THIAZIDE DIURETICS: DOSES AND DURATION OF ACTION

Drug	Dose		Duration of Action (hr)	Trade Name (UK, Europe)	Trade Name (USA)
1. Hydrochlorothiazide	12.5–25 mg 25–100 mg	(BP) (CHF)	6–12	Esidrex HydroSaluric	HydroDiuril Esidrix Thiuretic
2. Hydroflumethazide	12.5–25 mg 25–200 mg	(BP) (CHF)	6–12	Hydrenox	Saluron Diucardin
3. Chlorthalidone	12.5–50 mg		48–72	Hygroton	Hygroton Thalitone
4. Metolazone	1–5 mg 5–20 mg	(BP) (CHF)	18–25	Metenix Microx Diulo	Zaroxolyn Diulo
5. Bendrofluazide[+] = bendroflumethiazide	1.25–2.5 mg 10 mg	(BP) (CHF)	6–12	Aprinox Centyl Urizide	Naturetin
6. Polythiazide	1–2 mg	(BP)	24–48	–	Renese

7. Chlorothiazide	250–1000 mg	6–12	Saluric	Diuril
8. Cyclothiazide	1–2 mg	6–12	–	Anhydron
9. Trichlormethiazide	1–4 mg	About 24	Fluitran (not in UK)	Metahydrin Naqua
10. Cyclopenthiazide	0.125–0.25 mg*	6–12	Navidrex	–
11. Indapamide	2.5 mg (BP)	16–36	Natrilix	Lozol
12. Xipamide	20–40 mg (BP)	6–12	Diurexan	–

Modified from Opie LH, Commerford PJ, Swanepoel CR: Diuretic Therapy. In Wenger N, Julian D (eds): Management of Heart Failure. London, Butterworths, 1986, pp 119–142, with permission.

+See Carlsen, et al: Br Med J 300:975, 1990.

*Combination agents.

BP = Use for blood-pressure lowering.

CHF = Use for congestive heart failure.

NB: The doses given for antihypertensive therapy are generally **LOWER** than those recommended by the manufacturers. In our view high doses of diuretics are **contraindicated** for hypertension. See Carlsen, et al: Br Med J 300:975, 1990.

**TABLE 4-4 SIDE-EFFECTS OF PROLONGED THERAPY OF MILD
HYPERTENSION WITH HIGH-DOSE THIAZIDE***

Causing withdrawal of therapy

   Impaired glucose tolerance[+]
   Gout
   Impotence
   Lethargy
   Nausea, dizziness, or headache

Blood biochemical changes

   Glucose
   Uric acid
   Urea
   Potassium
   Cholesterol

*Bendroflumethiazide 10 mg daily.[46]
[+]Lower doses of bendroflumethiazide (2.5–5.0 mg) have been given over 6
years without any detectable glucose intolerance or changes in uric acid or
cholesterol, and with only a minimal fall of potassium.[6]

Pharmacologic Action and Pharmacokinetics. Thiazide diuretics act to inhibit the reabsorption of sodium and chloride in the more distal part of the nephron (site 3). This cotransporter is insensitive to the loop diuretics. More sodium reaches the distal tubules where more is exchanged with potassium, particularly in the presence of an activated renin-angiotensin-aldosterone system. Thiazides may also increase the active excretion of potassium in the distal renal tubule.[61]

Thiazides are rapidly absorbed from the GI tract to produce a diuresis within 1 to 2 hours, which lasts for 6 to 12 hours in the case of the prototype thiazide, hydrochlorothiazide. Some major differences from the loop diuretics are (1) the longer duration of action; (2) the different site of action (see Fig. 4–1); (3) the relatively low "ceiling" of thiazide diuretics (i.e., the maximal response is reached at a relatively low dosage); and (4) the much decreased capacity of thiazides to work in the presence of renal failure (serum creatinine >2.0 mg/dl; GFR below 15 to 20 ml/min.[59] The fact that thiazides and loop diuretics act at different sites explains the additive effects of these agents. The fact that thiazides, loop diuretics, and potassium-sparing agents act at different sites explains the additive effects of these agents (**sequential nephron block**).

Dose and Indications. In **hypertension**, thiazide doses have generally been too high, and high doses continue to be recommended by the manufacturers. Although long-term prospective studies are lacking, indirect evidence suggests a dose of 25 mg hydrochlorothiazide daily[5,40] or even lower doses (12.5 mg), especially in combination therapy.[42] In the case of cyclopenthiazide, widely used in the UK, only 0.125 mg (the approximate equivalent of hydrochlorothiazide 8 mg) gives as much antihypertensive effect as 0.5 mg with fewer metabolic side-effects.[85] Higher doses are marginally more effective, with greater risks of undesirable metabolic and subjective side-effects (Table 4-4: hypokalemia[25,27,40]), glucose intolerance, hyperuricemia, and atherogenic lipid changes. In combination with β-blockade, even lower doses (12.5 mg hydrochlorothiazide daily) appear to be effective.[42] **With hydrochlorothiazide, the full antihypertensive effect may take up to 12 weeks,[60] and a common error is "premature step therapy" (i.e., going on to the next step too soon).** Diuretics may be the initial agent of choice in the elderly, in blacks, and in obese[58] patients. Chlorthalidone 25 to 50 mg daily has been used in systolic hypertension in the elderly;[28] the long duration of action and tendency to hypokalemia[25] may not be advantages. High-dose diuretic (bendrofluazide 10 mg daily) was used in the giant British MRC trial[46] and, compared with propranolol up to 320 mg daily, had different side-effects, with (surprisingly) fatigue and impotence more common in the diuretic group, as were arrhythmias. A lower dose of bendrofluazide (2.5–5 mg) was used in Denmark over a 6-year period, however, with fewer metabolic side-effects.[6]

The **response rate in hypertension** to thiazide monotherapy may be disappointing, being only about 45% in one recent trial with 12.5 to 25 mg hydrochlorothiazide daily, although the rate increased to about 90% by the addition of verapamil.[81]

In **CHF**, higher doses are justified (50–100 mg hydrochlorothiazide daily are probably ceiling doses), while watching the plasma potassium. In **renal edema**, thiazides are not used if the GFR is low.[59]

Choice of Thiazide. It seems to matter little which of the various thiazide preparations is chosen; the majority, including hydrochlorothiazide, have an intermediate duration of action (6–12 hours). However, an ultra-long-acting compound such as chlorthalidone (24–72 hours; dose same as hydrochlorothiazide) has the potential disadvantages of nocturia and greater risk of electrolyte disturbances.

Contraindications. Contraindications include renal edema, hypokalemia, ventricular arrhythmias, and co-therapy with pro-arrhythmic drugs (Class IA and III drugs, including sotalol) (see Chap. 8). In hypokalemia (including early AMI), thiazide diuretics may precipitate arrhythmias. Relative contraindications include pregnancy hypertension, because of the risk of a decreased blood volume; moreover, thiazides can cross the placental barrier with risk of neonatal jaundice. In renal impairment, the GFR may fall as thiazides decrease the blood volume.

Side-effects. Besides the increasingly emphasized "wrong way" metabolic side-effects, such as hypokalemia, hyponatremia, and increased blood triglyceride and cholesterol levels, thiazide diuretics rarely cause sulfonamide-type immune side-effects including intrahepatic jaundice, pancreatitis, blood dyscrasias, angiitis, pneumonitis, and interstitial nephritis. Impotence can occur with high doses.[46]

Drug Interactions. Prior treatment with nifedipine-type calcium antagonists may diminish the response to diuretics in hypertension, presumably because of the pre-existing mild diuretic effect of these agents. Steroids and estrogens (e.g., the contraceptive pill) may cause salt retention to antagonize the action of thiazide diuretics. **Indomethacin** and NSAIDs blunt the response to thiazide diuretics[69] and may worsen CHF.[19] **Captopril** or **enalapril**, when combined with a potassium-retaining diuretic, may cause hyperkalemia, so this combination should be avoided. Hypokalemia induced by diuretics may predispose to torsades de pointes when there is additional therapy with agents that prolong the QT-interval, such as sotalol[45] or ketanserin (an antihypertensive available in Europe). The nephrotoxic effects of certain antibiotics such as the aminoglycosides may be potentiated by diuretics. **Probenecid** (for the therapy of gout) and **lithium** (for mania) may block thiazide effects by interfering with thiazide excretion into the urine. **Lithium** interacts with diuretics by impairing their renal clearance and by possible additive effects of lithium toxicity.

Combination Therapy. Combination with amiloride, triamterene, or spironolactone is commonly used in the therapy of hypertension and CHF.

OTHER THIAZIDES AND THIAZIDE-LIKE AGENTS

Metolazone—in a Class of its Own

Metolazone (Zaroxolyn, Diulo, Metenix) belongs to the category of thiazide diuretics. An important additional property is that **metolazone**

appears to be effective even in patients with reduced renal function,[12] thus resembling furosemide. The duration of action is up to 24 hours, so a single daily dose is recommended. In combination with furosemide, metolazone may provoke a profound diuresis, with the risk of excessive volume and potassium depletion.[34] Therefore, patients should be carefully observed and probably hospitalized when the combination is started, especially in elderly patients. Alternatively, once-a-day low-dose (2.5 or 5 mg) metolazone may be used instead of 2 to 3 daily doses of furosemide. If added diuresis is needed, metolazone may be added to furosemide with care, especially in patients with renal as well as cardiac failure. The side-effect profile of metolazone closely resembles that of the ordinary thiazides.

In 17 patients with severe CHF, almost all of whom are already on furosemide, captopril, and digoxin, metolazone 1.25–10 mg daily was given in titrated doses; most responded by a brisk diuresis within 48–72 hours.[82]

Indapamide

Indapamide (Lozol, Natrilix) is a thiazide-like diuretic (albeit with a different molecular structure) that lowers the blood pressure in a dose of 2.5 mg/day, with a terminal half-life of 14 to 16 hours; in higher doses, a vigorous diuresis can be achieved.[10] Part of the antihypertensive action might be peripheral vasodilation.[36] In hypertension, indapamide can evoke a rapid hypotensive response, more so than the thiazides, so that in elderly patients reduced organ perfusion is a theoretical risk.[60] Although originally thought not to have metabolic side-effects, indapamide 2.5 mg daily has a **metabolic side-effect profile similar to hydrochlorothiazide 50 mg daily,**[36] with particular reference to changes in the serum potassium, serum uric acid, and blood cholesterol (strict comparisons of glucose tolerance were not made). Another study[91] suggests that indapamide is more lipid-neutral than is hydrochlorothiazide; however, the dose of hydrochlorothiazide chosen for that comparison was 100 mg daily. In cardiac edema the drug has little advantage over other well-tried diuretics.[43] As a third-line antihypertensive agent, after β-blocker with calcium antagonist, adding indapamide 2.5 mg was as effective as adding hydrochlorothiazide 25 mg plus amiloride 2.5 mg ($^{1}/_{2}$ Moduretic tablet). Hypokalemia was somewhat more common with indapamide and hyperuricemia equally frequent in both regimens.[86]

Xipamide

This compound, not available in the USA, structurally resembles chlorthalidone and also causes a prolonged diuresis that may be disturbing to elderly patients, for whom it is otherwise recommended.[43] In doses recommended for hypertension (10–20 mg), prolonged diuresis is no problem.[88] Hypokalemia remains a risk. The true place of this agent is not yet known.

MINOR DIURETICS

Carbonic anhydrase inhibitors such as acetazolamide (Diamox) are weak diuretics. They decrease the secretion of hydrogen ions by the proximal renal tubule (site 1), with increased loss of bicarbonate and hence of sodium. These agents, seldom used as primary diuretics, have found a place in the therapy of glaucoma because carbonic anhydrase plays a role in the secretion of aqueous humor in the ciliary processes of the eye. In salicylate poisoning, the alkalinizing effect of carbonic anhydrase inhibitors increases the renal excretion of lipid-soluble weak organic acids.[50]

Calcium antagonists have a direct diuretic effect that contributes to the long-term antihypertensive effect.[38,83] For example, nifedipine increases urine volume and sodium excretion[35] and may inhibit aldosterone release by angiotensin.[48] Diuresis explains the occasional tendency to hypokalemia with high-dose nifedipine. The diuretic action is quite independent of any change in renal blood flow or glomerular filtration.

METABOLIC SIDE-EFFECTS OF THIAZIDES

Many side-effects of thiazides are similar to those of the loop diuretics: electrolyte disturbances, including hypokalemia, hyponatremia, hyperuricemia, the precipitation of gout and diabetes, a decreased blood volume, and alkalosis. **Atherogenic** blood lipid changes and impotence have recently been described. **Hyponatremia** may sometimes occur in the elderly, even with low diuretic doses.

Hypokalemia

As in the case of loop diuretics, hypokalemia is probably an overfeared complication, especially when low doses of thiazides are used.[40] Yet many physicians remain impressed by the average fall in plasma potassium of about 0.7 mM/L, which will lower the K^+ level to below 3.5 mM/L in about one-third of hypertensives with impairment of control of blood pressure.[33] Hence the frequent choice of combination potassium-retaining diuretics with triamterene or amiloride. This choice in turn brings about the alternative but lesser risk that some patients will develop **hyperkalemia**, especially in the presence of renal impairment or during the concomitant use of potassium supplements or converting enzyme inhibitors.

ARRHYTHMIAS

A detailed retrospective analysis highlights the complexity of assessing the relationship between hypokalemia and arrhythmias in patients with mild hypertension treated by diuretics.[47] Only one fact emerged clearly: in patients chronically treated by bendrofluazide (daily dose, 10 mg), there were more malignant or premalignant arrhythmias. It seemed that diuretic therapy itself rather than a low plasma potassium was associated with arrhythmias; perhaps magnesium depletion played a role. Other trials have also shown the problems of trying to relate **potassium levels** to arrhythmias. In 13 patients with torsades de pointes receiving sotalol,[45] only 6 had potassium values of less than 3.4 mM/L. Correction of diuretic-induced hypokalemia was not linked to a decreased incidence of extrasystoles in patients with uncomplicated systemic hypertension.[55] The problem with some of the above studies may be that the analyses were retrospective. For reviews with conflicting conclusions, see Helfant[25] and Papademetriou.[54]

In a prospective trial in patients with mild hypertension and typical effort angina, amiloride 10 mg 2x daily (potassium-retaining) was used as a sole agent in comparison with chlorthalidone 25 mg daily (potassium-losing[63]). Equal control of blood pressure was achieved. The potassium-losing phase brought down plasma K^+ from 4.3 to 3.3 mEq/L and gave a higher incidence of ventricular arrhythmias both during ambulatory monitoring and during programmed stimulation. Plasma magnesium was unchanged throughout. This study proves that even mild hypokalemia must be avoided in patients with angina pectoris.

In **AMI**, initial hypokalemia is linked to ventricular arrhythmias including ventricular fibrillation (VF).[17,52] The hypokalemia could be caused both by diuretic therapy and by adrenergic discharge.[64] β-adrenergic blockade (especially by non-selective agents) appears to inhibit the stress-induced hypokalemia with lessening of ventricular arrhythmias.[31]

THERAPEUTIC STRATEGIES FOR HYPOKALEMIA.

Although the arrhythmogenic dangers of thiazide-induced hypokalemia are not convincingly established, common sense says that in patients with a higher risk of arrhythmias, as in ischemic heart disease, heart failure on digitalis, or hypertension with LV hypertrophy, a potassium- and magnesium-sparing diuretic should be part of the therapy unless contraindicated by renal failure or by co-therapy with captopril or enalapril. Such a diuretic may be better than potassium supplementation,[44] especially because the supplements do not avoid hypomagnesemia; yet these issues are not completely resolved. For heart failure, a standard combination daily therapy might be 1 to 2 tablets of Moduretic (hydrochlorothiazide 50 mg, amiloride 5 mg), 2 to 4 tablets of Dyazide (hydrochlorothiazide 25 mg, triamterene 50 mg), or 1 to 2 tablets of Maxzide (hydrochlorothiazide 50 mg, triamterene 75 mg). For **hypertension**, the doses are approximately halved, bearing in mind the requirement for the ideal thiazide dose of no more than and probably less than 25 mg/day as in 1 tablet of Dyazide. In some countries, a new mini-Moduretic (Moduret 25), with half-strength hydrochlorothiazide (25 mg) and amiloride 2.5 mg, is now available. K+-containing supplements such as Slow-K or K-Lyte (both with KCel) should not be given unless there is still proven hypokalemia despite the combination therapy. **When ACE inhibitors are part of the therapy, potassium supplements must be avoided and potassium-sparing diuretics should be replaced by simple hydrochlorothiazide.** It must be stressed that the above proposals are based on extrapolation, albeit reasonable, so that revision may be needed as new data arrive.

When **cost is important**, a generic thiazide may be cheaper than a potassium-sparing thiazide combination; and when hypokalemia is suspected or detected, oral K-supplementation with a salt substitute is less expensive than KCel supplements.

Hypomagnesemia

Hypomagnesemia,[27] like hypokalemia, is blamed for arrhythmias during diuretic therapy, although the facts are few. Even in the case of some digitalis-induced arrhythmias, there is no clear case for a role for hypomagnesemia. Recently, magnesium infusions have been recommended for patients with early myocardial infarction (Chap. 8), but more trials are required. Animal data suggest that hypomagnesemia can be prevented by the addition of a potassium-retaining component such as amiloride to the thiazide diuretic.[14,15] Despite the marketing of an oral magnesium preparation (**Slow Mag**), there is no good evidence that such supplements avoid arrhythmias or improve blood-pressure control even during prolonged diuretic therapy.[79] The only sure effect of magnesium supplementation is to restore body potassium depletion more rapidly.[80]

Diabetogenic Effects

The thiazides are sulfonamide derivatives which explains their potential pancreatic toxicity and provocation of diabetes in a minority of patients. The mechanism may act indirectly, via hypokalemia with decreased insulin secretion.[57] Patients with a familial tendency to diabetes are probably prone to the diabetogenic side-effects and should be excluded whenever possible. Even a hydrochlorothiazide dose of only 25 mg daily for 4 months increased fasting glucose by 11% and fasting plasma insulin by 31%.[87]

Urate Excretion

Most diuretics decrease urate excretion with the risk of increasing blood uric acid and causing gout in those predisposed; thus a personal or family history of gout should lead to therapy with non-thiazide diuretics. When **allopurinol** is given for associated gout, or when the blood urate is high in association with a family history of gout, it must be remembered that the normal dose of 300 mg daily is for a normal creatinine clearance. With a clearance of only 40 ml/min, the dose drops to 150 mg daily and, for 10 ml/min down, to 100 mg every 2 days.[78] **Dose reduction is essential** to avoid serious skin reactions, which are dose-related and can even be fatal.

Atherogenic Changes in Blood Lipids

Thiazides may increase the total blood cholesterol by an average of 15 to 20 mg/dl[87] in a dose-related fashion.[74] Also the LDL-cholesterol (LDL = low density lipoprotein) and triglycerides increase even after 4 months with low-dose hydrochlorothiazide (25 mg daily)[87] (see Table 10-2). **During prolonged thiazide therapy a lipid-lowering diet is advisable.**

Hypercalcemia

Thiazide diuretics tend to retain calcium by an unknown mechanism. Especially in hyperparathyroid patients, hypercalcemia can be precipitated.[75]

Prevention of Metabolic Side-effects

Reduction in the dose of diuretic, restriction of dietary sodium, and additional dietary potassium will reduce the frequency of hypokalemia. Combination of a thiazide with a potassium-sparer lessens hypokalemia. Addition of potassium supplements seems ineffective.[77] Combination therapy of hydrochlorothiazide (about 50 mg daily) with captopril (25–50 mg 2–3x daily) reduces the incidence of hypokalemia and hyperuricemia, and possibly also of hyperglycemia. Hence, combination therapy with hydrochlorothiazide and potassium-sparing or potassium-retaining diuretics is frequently used. In the treatment of hypertension, diuretics should not be combined, if possible, with other drugs with unfavorable effects on blood lipids, such as the β-blockers, but rather ACE inhibitors or calcium antagonists should be selected (see Table 10-2).

POTASSIUM-SPARING OR -RETAINING DIURETICS

Agents such as amiloride and triamterene inhibit sodium reabsorption distally, thereby indirectly sparing potassium. Spironolactone inhibits sodium-potassium exchange and therefore retains potassium. Sodium-potassium exchange in the collecting tubules only accounts for a small part of the sodium re-uptake into the renal cells, so that a powerful diuresis cannot be obtained by distally acting potassium-retaining agents acting alone (Table 4-5).

TABLE 4-5 POTASSIUM-SPARING DIURETICS (GENERALLY ALSO SPARE MAGNESIUM)

Drug	Dose	Duration of Action	Trade Name (UK, Europe)	Trade Name (USA)
Spironolactone	25–200 mg	3–5 days	Aldactone	Aldactone
Amiloride	2.5–20 mg	4–5 days	Midamor	Midamor
Triamterene	25–200 mg	8–12 hr	Dytac	Dyrenium

Modified from Opie LH, Commerford PJ, Swanepoel CR: Diuretic Therapy. In Wenger N, Julian D (eds): Management of Heart Failure. London, Butterworths, 1986, pp 119–142, with permission.

Amiloride and Triamterene

Amiloride inhibits the sodium channel, which is concerned with sodium reabsorption in the distal tubules and collecting tubules. This specific action means that there is no direct loss of potassium or of magnesium. Despite the relatively weak diuretic action (see Table 4-1), these agents are frequently used in combination with thiazide diuretics. Advantages are that (1) the loss of sodium is achieved without a major loss of potassium or magnesium, and (2) there is an action independent of the activity of aldosterone. As sole agents they are too weak for diuresis in CHF; they may be antihypertensive in their own right,[63,66] but the data are incomplete. Side-effects are few: hyperkalemia (a contraindication) and acidosis may rarely occur, and then mostly in those with renal disease. In particular the thiazide-related risks of diabetes mellitus and gout have not been reported. There is a suggestion that amiloride may be preferable to triamterene (the latter is excreted by the kidneys with risks of renal casts on standard doses and occasional renal dysfunction[37]). In practice, compounds with triamterene have been widely and extensively used without many detectable risks. (For combination with thiazides, see p 90.)

Spironolactone

Spironolactone acts on the distal tubule to inhibit Na^+/K^+ exchange at the site of aldosterone action. It is logical therapy in those few patients who develop heart failure or hypertension in the presence of high mineralocorticoid levels, as during prednisone therapy or as part of Conn's syndrome. **This diuretic is the agent of choice when diabetes or gout may be present or when there is fear of their precipitation, or when it is important to retain potassium.** Spironolactone is a more powerful diuretic than amiloride or triamterene in the presence of hyperaldosteronism and is probably more effective as a sole agent in hypertension (strict trials are lacking). Spironolactone can be more effective than amiloride in remedying thiazide-induced hypokalemia. One daily dose of spironolactone is usually adequate for diuresis (25–100 mg); in contrast, for therapy of Conn's syndrome 100 mg or more 3x daily with meals may be needed (food enhances bioavailability of canrenone). Side-effects include antitestosterone effects such as gynecomastia and impotence, particularly when large doses (>100 mg daily) and long-term treatment are used, or in liver disease or alcoholism. Spironolactone may benefit hirsuties in females.

Canrenone

Spironolactone becomes active by hepatic transformation to canrenone. Canrenoate potassium 200 mg can be given IV for severe cardiac or hepatic edema.

ACE Inhibitors

Because captopril and enalapril ultimately exert an anti-aldosterone effect, they too act as mild potassium-retaining diuretics. Combination therapy with other potassium retainers should be avoided.

Hyperkalemia—A Specific Risk

Amiloride, triamterene, and spironolactone may all cause hyperkalemia (serum potassium equal to or exceeds 5.5 mEq/L) especially in the presence of pre-existing renal disease, diabetes, in elderly patients during co-therapy with ACE inhibitors, or in patients receiving possible nephrotoxic agents without careful monitoring of the serum potassium. Hyperkalemia is treated by drug withdrawal, infusions of glucose-insulin, and cation-exchange resins such as sodium, polystyrene sulfonate, and sometimes dialysis. IV calcium chloride may be required to avoid VF. The risk of hyperkalemia is also there with most diuretic combinations.

COMBINATION DIURETICS

Besides addition of one class of diuretic to another, the fear of hypokalemia has increased the use of potassium-retaining diuretic combinations (Table 4-6), such as **Dyazide**, **Moduretic**, **Maxzide** and **Aldactazide**. **When used for hypertension, special attention must be given to the thiazide dose** (25 mg hydrochlorothiazide in Dyazide; 50 mg in Moduretic and Maxzide), where the lower dose is preferable. On the other hand, amiloride (in Moduretic) is marginally preferable to triamterene (in Dyazide and Maxzide), as judged by renal side-effects.[37] Of interest is the new mini-Moduretic (Moduret, 25 mg hydrochlorothiazide, 2.5 mg amiloride) available in Europe. **Maxzide** (see Table 4-6) appears to have few metabolic side-effects, especially when given as half-tablet daily (= 25 mg hydrochloro-thiazide, 37.5 mg triamterene).[26] A potassium-retaining furosemide combination (**Frumil** in Europe) is another reasonable alternative.

Another combination is that of **capozide** and **Vaseretic** (see Table 4-6). Thiazide diuretics increase renin levels, and captopril decreases metabolic side-effects of thiazides. Hence the combination is logical.

POTASSIUM SUPPLEMENTS

The routine practice in many centers of giving potassium supplements with loop diuretics is usually unnecessary (Table 4-1) and leads to extra cost and loss of compliance. Addition of low-dose potassium-retaining diuretics is usually better if really required. Even high doses of furosemide may not automatically require potassium replacement because such doses are usually given in the presence of renal impairment or severe CHF when renal potassium handling may be abnormal. Clearly potassium levels need periodic checking during therapy with all diuretics. To avoid hypokalemia, low-dose diuretics are preferred. A high-potassium, low-salt diet is advised and can be simply and cheaply achieved by the use of salt substitutes. Sometimes, despite all reasonable care, problematic hypokalemia develops, especially after prolonged diuretic therapy or in the presence of diarrhea or alkalosis. Then potassium supplements may become necessary.

Potassium chloride (KCel) in liquid form is theoretically best because (1) co-administration of chloride is required to correct fully potassium deficiency in hypokalemic hypochloremic alkalosis;[62] (2) slow-release tablets may cause GI ulceration, which liquid KCel does not.[56] The dose is variable. About 20 mEq daily are required to avoid potassium depletion and 40 to 100 mEq are required to treat potassium depletion. Absorption is rapid and bioavailability good. To help avoid the frequent GI irritation, liquid KCel needs dilution in water or another liquid and titration against the patient's acceptability. KCel may also be given in some effervescent preparations. **Slow-release potassium chloride wax-matrix tablets** (Slow-K, each with 8 mEq or 600 mg KCel; Klotrix, K-Tab, and Ten-K each contain 10 mEq KCel; Kaon-CL, 6.7 or 10 mEq KCel) although widely used and well tolerated, should not be given (according to the package insert in the USA) unless liquid or effervescent potassium preparations are not tolerated. The chloride salt, although able to correct co-existing chloride deficiency, carries the risk of GI ulceration or bleeding, especially when

TABLE 4–6 SOME COMBINATION DIURETIC AGENTS

Drug	Dose		Trade Name (UK, Europe)	Trade Name (USA)
Hydrochlorothiazide + triamterene	25 mg	1–2 tablets/day (up to 4 in CHF)	Dyazide	Dyazide
	50 mg			
Hydrochlorothiazide + amiloride	50 mg	1/2–1 tablet/day (up to 2 in CHF)	Moduretic*	Moduretic
	5 mg			
Hydrochlorothiazide + triamterene	50 mg	1/2–1 tablet/day (limited clinical experience with higher dose)	–	Maxzide
	75 mg			
Spironolactone + hydrochlorothiazide	25 mg	1–4 tablets/day	Aldactazide	Aldactazide
	25 mg			
Cyclopenthiazide + potassium chloride	0.25 mg	1/2–1 tablet/day	Navidrex-K	–
	600 mg			
Furosemide + amiloride	40 mg	1–2 tablets/day	Frumil	–
	5 mg			
Captopril + hydrochlorothiazide	25–50 mg	1 tablet 2x/day	Capozide+	Capozide+
	15–25 mg			
Enalapril + hydrochlorothiazide	10 mg	1–2 tablets daily	–	Vaseretic
	25 mg			

Modified from Opie LH, Commerford PJ, Swanepoel CR: Diuretic Therapy. In Wenger N, Julian D (eds): Management of Heart Failure. London, Butterworths, 1986, pp 119–142, with permission.

CHF = congestive heart failure.

For hypertension, see text — low doses generally preferred and high doses are **contraindicated**.

*Available in half-strength in Europe as Moduret 25 mg.

+Captopril 50 mg, hydrochlorothiazide 25 mg in UK; captopril 50 or 25 mg, hydrochlorothiazide 25 or 15 mg in USA.

GI motility is impaired (as in elderly, immobile, or diabetic patients, or in the presence of scleroderma), esophageal stricture, massive left atrial enlargement, or co-therapy with anticholinergic drugs including disopyramide. To avoid esophageal ulceration, tablets should be taken with the patient upright or sitting, and with a meal or beverage, and anticholinergic therapy should be avoided. **Microencapsulated KCel** (Micro-K, 8 mEq KCel or 10 mEq KCel) may reduce GI ulceration to only 1 per 100,000 patient years, but the package insert still carries the same warning as for wax-matrix tablets. High doses of Micro-K cause GI ulcers, especially during anticholinergic therapy.[56]

Effervescent preparations lessen the risk of GI ulceration and those with KCel include Klorvess (20 mEq), K-Lor (20 mEq KCel per packet), K-Lyte/Cl (25 mEq per tablet), and K-Lyte/Cl 50 (50 mEq tablet). K-Lyte contains potassium bicarbonate and citrate, 25 mEq. GI intolerance frequently limits the use of these agents, which are best given with liquid meals and in relatively small doses. **Potassium gluconate** (with citrate), Bi-K 20 mEq, or Twin K tends to minimize the GI irritative effects of the effervescent preparations but lacks chloride.

The simplest is a high-potassium, low-sodium diet achieved by salt substitutes. When K^+ supplements become essential, KCel is preferred. The best preparation will be one well tolerated by the patient and inexpensive. "No comprehensive adequately controlled studies of the relative efficacy of the various KCel preparations in clinical settings are available."[65]

SPECIAL DIURETIC PROBLEMS

Over-diuresis

During therapy of **edematous states**, over-vigorous diuresis may reduce venous pressure and ventricular filling so that the cardiac output drops and tissues become underperfused. The renin-angiotensin axis is further activated. Probably many patients are protected against the extremely effective potent diuretics by poor compliance. Over-diuresis is most frequently seen during hospital admissions when a rigid policy of regular administration of diuretics is carried out.

Fixed diuretic regimens are largely unsatisfactory in edematous patients. Often, responsible patients can manage their therapy well by tailoring a flexible diuretic schedule to their own needs, using a simple bathroom scale, knowing how to recognize pedal edema and the time course of maximal effect of their diuretic often allows a patient to adjust his own diuretic dose and administration schedule to fit in with daily activities.

Patients who may experience **adverse effects** due to over-diuresis include (1) those with mild chronic heart failure overtreated with potent diuretics; (2) patients requiring a high filling pressure particularly those with a "restrictive" pathophysiology as in restrictive cardiomyopathy or hypertrophic cardiomyopathy; and (3) patients in early phase AMI,[21] when the problem of excessive diuresis is most commonly encountered when using potent IV diuretics for acute heart failure. It may be necessary cautiously to administer a "**fluid challenge**" with saline solution or a colloid preparation while checking the patient's cardiovascular status. If the resting heart rate falls, renal function improves, and blood pressure stabilizes, the ventricular filling pressure has been inadequate.[71]

Diuretic Resistance

Repetitive diuretic administration leads to a levelling off of the effect, because (in the face of a shrunken intravascular volume) the

SOME CAUSES OF DIURETIC RESISTANCE

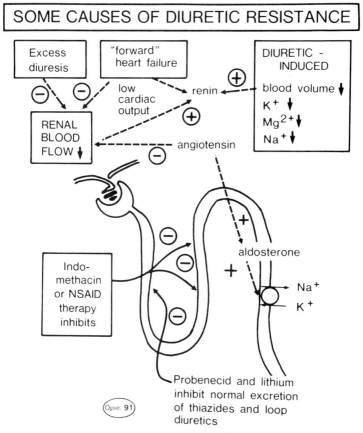

FIGURE 4–2. The causes of resistance to diuretics.

part of the tubular system not affected reacts by reabsorbing more sodium. Additional mechanisms are an abnormally low cardiac output in patients with heart failure; prominent activation of the angiotensin-renin axis; or an electrolyte-induced resistance (Fig. 4–2, Table 4-7). Apparent resistance can also develop when there is concomitant therapy with indomethacin or with other NSAIDs (exception: sulindac;[69,73]) or with probenecid. The thiazide diuretics (exception: metolazone) will not work well if the GFR is below 15 to 20 ml/min.[59] When potassium depletion is severe, diuretics will not work well for complex reasons.

Is there compliance with dietary salt restriction? Is complete bed rest required? Is the optimal agent being used, avoiding thiazide diuretics (except metolazone), when the GFR is low? Is the optimal dose being used? Are there interfering drugs or severe electrolyte or volume imbalances that can be remedied? Has the general cardiovascular status been made optimal by judicious use of unloading or inotropic drugs? **To achieve diuresis, an ACE inhibitor may have to be added to thiazide or loop diuretics, or metolazone may have to be combined with loop diuretics. In out-patients, compliance and dietary salt restriction must be carefully checked, while all unnecessary drugs are eliminated. Sometimes fewer drugs work better than more (here the prime sinners are potassium supplements, requiring many daily tablets frequently not taken).**

Renal Failure

In patients with mild chronic renal failure, treated without success with high-dose furosemide (up to 480–500 mg/day), the addition of

TABLE 4–7   SOME CAUSES OF APPARENT RESISTANCE TO DIURETICS IN THERAPY OF CARDIAC FAILURE

Incorrect use of diuretic agent
- combination of 2 thiazides or 2 loop diuretics instead of 1 of each type
- use of thiazides when GFR is low* (exception: metolazone)
- excessive diuretic dose (see 2 and 3)
- poor compliance, especially caused by multiple tablets of oral K^+ supplements

Electrolyte volume imbalance
- hyponatremia, hypokalemia, hypovolemia
- hypomagnesemia may need correction to correct hypokalemia

Poor renal perfusion diuretic-induced hypovolemia
- cardiac output too low
- excess hypotension (vasodilators including ACE inhibitors)

Excess circulating catecholamines
(frequent in severe congestive heart failure; causes vasoconstriction and limits renal blood flow)
- correct by increased inotropic support if possible, or by appropriate unloading agents

Activation of renin-angiotensin-aldosterone system
(frequent in severe congestive heart failure)
- correct by angiotensin converting enzyme inhibition (captopril, enalapril)

Interfering drugs
- indomethacin and other nonsteroidal anti-inflammatories inhibit diuresis (prostaglandins inhibit action of vasopressin)
- probenecid and lithium inhibit tubular excretion of thiazides and loop diuretics

*GFR = glomerular filtration rate below 15–20 ml/min.

hydrochlorothiazide 25 to 50 mg 2x daily may produce a marked diuresis, so that the combination may be effective when either agent singly fails.[72] Metolazone and furosemide may likewise be combined (see section on metolazone), especially when the GFR is low. Whether the latter combination is truly more powerful than hydrochlorothiazide-furosemide (as some anecdotal observations suggest) remains to be rigorously tested.[24]

Hyponatremia

In patients severely ill with CHF, despite overall sodium retention, a hyponatremic state may develop from predominant water retention. Recent studies point to (1) the inappropriate release of arginine vasopressin–antidiuretic hormone;[65] and (2) increased activity of angiotensin-II.[19] The best treatment seems to be the combination of furosemide and an ACE inhibitor;[18] restriction of water intake is also important.

Adverse Drug Interactions

Indomethacin and other NSAIDs may cause serious deterioration of cardiovascular status in some patients with severe heart failure[19] because the vasoconstrictor response to angiotensin may evoke the release of vasodilatory prostaglandins to exert a compensatory effect on the circulation. Most NSAIDs impair control of blood pressure by thiazides and other agents (exception: sulindac = Clinoril).[73] Probenecid and lithium decrease the normal renal excretion of thiazide and loop diuretics, so that the diuretic effect is decreased.

LESS COMMON USES OF DIURETICS

Less common indications are (1) **hypernatremia** when not due to fluid depletion; (2) IV furosemide in **malignant or premalignant hypertension,** especially if there is associated CHF and fluid retention; (3) high-dose furosemide for **acute or chronic renal failure** when it is hoped that the drug may initiate diuresis; (4) in **hypercalcemia,** high-dose loop diuretics increase urinary excretion of calcium; IV furosemide is used in the emergency treatment of severe hypercalcemia; (5) thiazides for the **nephrogenic form of diabetes insipidus**—the mechanism of action is not clear, but there is a diminution in "free water" clearance; and (6) thiazide diuretics decrease the urinary calcium output through a mechanism that is not well understood, so that they are used in **idiopathic hypercalciuria** to decrease the formation of renal stones (in contrast, loop diuretics increase urinary excretion of calcium). **The inhibitory effect of thiazides on urinary calcium loss may explain why these agents may increase bone mineralization**[68] and decrease the incidence of hip fractures,[89] hence suggesting a possible **new therapeutic use for thiazides in osteoporosis.** The latter benefit is another argument for first-line (low-dose) diuretic therapy in elderly hypertensives.

An additional use, entirely unrelated, is in **mania** when **lithium** therapy is insufficient (thiazides sensitize to lithium effects).

STEP-CARE THERAPY OF CHF

Diuretics

In **mild to moderate CHF,** diuretics are standard first-line therapy, although no good placebo-controlled studies have been published. The usual step-care therapy has been (1) dietary sodium restriction and the use of thiazide diuretics; (2) increasing doses of thiazides to the ceiling, which is rapidly reached, and monitoring plasma potassium (and sometimes magnesium); (3) low-dose furosemide; and (4) high-dose furosemide or other loop diuretics. However, the current trend is to add ACE inhibitors when the dose of furosemide exceeds 120 mg daily,[76] which helps to avoid metabolic side-effects of high-dose diuretics. When the patient is only receiving a low dose of furosemide, such as 40 mg daily, it is better to increase the dose of furosemide up to 120 mg daily than to add captopril.[76]

For **severe CHF,** when congestion and edema are prominent symptoms, initial therapy is usually with furosemide, especially when renal perfusion may be impaired. Complete bed rest helps to promote an early diuresis.[1] The dose of furosemide required may be very high (500–1500 mg daily).

Digitalis

In the USA, digitalis is usually introduced when diuresis by itself seems inadequate—probably at the stage of low-dose or high-dose furosemide unless there is atrial fibrillation, in which case digitalis will be introduced earlier. In the USA and in Germany, digitalis is still sometimes given as the primary agent. In the UK, digitalis is usually given after the combination of diuretics with an ACE inhibitor. (For use of digitalis in heart failure, see Chap. 6).

ACE Inhibitors

ACE inhibitors are increasingly used in heart failure (Chap. 5, p 109), especially in preference to high-dose diuretics or other vasodilators. However, there is no case for the use of ACE inhibitors without diuretics. In CHF, the action of diuretics may be inhibited by poor renal perfusion and vasoconstrictive formation of renin, with a low GFR, lessening sodium excretion. Hence ACE inhibitors are logical additions to diuretics. Relatively little tolerance to these agents has been found. They also have an indirect diuretic effect ultimately by inhibiting aldosterone release. Unfortunately the use of all ACE inhibitors may be limited by hypotension, especially in CHF. Therefore a low initial test dose is essential.

Vasodilators Other Than ACE Inhibitors

The problem with vasodilators other than the ACE inhibitors is, in general, the frequent development of tolerance, so that classical vasodilators are now being replaced by ACE inhibitors. Nonetheless, nitrates have a specific role in reducing the preload and relieving dyspnea. They can, for example, be given intermittently (to avoid tolerance) in anticipation of exertional dyspnea or at bedtime to avoid nocturnal dyspnea.

Short-term Inotropic Support

In a number of seriously ill patients, short-term support by agents such as amrinone, milrinone, or the sympathomimetics may give dramatic relief. This is essentially a rescue operation.

General Measures

Especially in the presence of poor renal perfusion, water restriction is required (the patient being told to restrict both water and salt). Physically, the patient should be kept active as much as is possible, and recent trials suggest a beneficial effect of mild exercise training within limits.

Special Problems

In unusual patients who have heart failure and severe restriction of the GFR (such as 15–20 ml/min), high doses of furosemide alone or combined with metolazone are used. In patients with borderline diabetes, mild diabetes, increasing glucose intolerance, or gout, neither thiazides nor furosemide can be used with impunity; now spironolactone becomes the agent of choice, yet it is unfortunately only of low diuretic potency.

SUMMARY

Diuretics are powerful therapeutic agents with the potential for major and serious side-effects. Thus the benefit-risk ratio in the therapy of mild hypertension is increasingly questioned except in three groups of patients: the elderly, black patients, and the obese. Patients with renal impairment also require a diuretic (loop or metolazone). For most hypertensives, low-dose thiazide diuretic, probably with a potassium-retaining component (amiloride or triamterene) might be the answer. An alternative is a subdiuretic dose of a loop diuretic which, by the nature of its short duration of action allows a corrective period of gain of K^+ and magnesium. Another alternative for hypertension is low-dose spironolactone. Thiazide diuretics combine well with ACE inhibitors, in which case a K^+-sparing component is not advisable. The benefit-risk ratio of diuretics is high in the therapy of heart failure, and their use remains standard.

Yet not all patients require vigorous diuresis; rather each patient needs careful clinical evaluation with a specific cardiological diagnosis so that surgically correctable defects are appropriately handled. First choice of therapy is a thiazide (for mild heart failure) or a loop diuretic (for severe heart failure). With intermediate severities of failure, increasing doses of thiazide or metolazone may be used before switching to a loop diuretic such as furosemide. We stress that automatic addition of oral potassium supplements is far from ideal practice. Rather, the combination of a loop diuretic plus low-dose thiazide plus potassium-retaining diuretic is reasonable, except in the presence of renal failure, when loop diuretics with metolazone seem better.

The next step is variable. High-dose furosemide used to be the next choice and can still be used; the dangers of volume depletion, electrolyte imbalance, and activation of the renin-angiotensin axis are very real. Therefore additional therapy with an ACE inhibitor seems preferable unless limited by side-effects such as hypotension. Potassium-retaining diuretics (amiloride, triamterene, spironolactone) must be avoided with ACE inhibitors, as should oral potassium supplements, unless there is still proven hypokalemia.

REFERENCES

References from Previous Editions

1. Abildgaard U, Aldershvile J, Ring-Larsen H, et al: Eur Heart J 6:1040–1046, 1985
2. Acchiardo SR, Skoutakis VA: Am Heart J 106:237–244, 1983
3. Andreasen F, Hansen U, Husted SE: Br J Clin Pharmacol 18:65–74, 1984
4. Asbury MJ, Gatenby PBB, O'Sullivan S, et al: Br Med J 1:211–213, 1972
5. Beermann B, Groschinsky-Grind M: Eur J Clin Pharmacol 13:195–201, 1978
6. Berglund G, Andersson O: Lancet 1:744–747, 1981
7. Biddle TL, Yu PN: Am J Cardiol 43:86–90, 1979
8. Brater DC, Chennavasin P, Day B, et al: Clin Pharmacol Ther 34:207–213, 1983
9. Carriere S, Dandavino R: Clin Pharmacol Ther 20:424–438, 1976
10. Caruso FS, Szabadi RR, Vukovich RA: Am Heart J 106:212–220, 1983
11. Chatterjee K, Parmley WW: J Am Coll Cardiol 1:133–153, 1983
12. Dargie HJ, Allison MEM, Kennedy AC, et al: Br Med J 4:196–198, 1972
13. Davidov ME, McNight JE, Osborne JL: Curr Ther Res 25:1–9, 1979
14. Devane J, Ryan MP: Br J Pharmacol 72:285–289, 1981
15. Devane J, Ryan MP: Br J Pharmacol 79:891–896, 1983
16. Drug and Therapeutics Bulletin: Drug Ther Bull 17:47–48, 1979
17. Dyckner T, Helmers C, Lundman T, et al: Acta Med Scand 197:207–210, 1975
18. Dzau VJ, Hollenberg NK: Ann Intern Med 100:777–782, 1984
19. Dzau VJ, Packer M, Lilly LS, et al: N Engl J Med 310:347–352, 1984
20. Flamenbaum W, Friedman R: Pharmacotherapy 2:213–222, 1982
21. Forrester JS, Diamond G, Chatterjee K, et al: N Engl J Med 295:1356–1362; 1404–1413, 1976
22. Freis ED: Am Heart J 106:185–187, 1983
23. Green TP, Thompson TR, Johnson DE, et al: N Engl J Med 308:743–748, 1983
24. Greenberg A, Walia R, Puschett JB: First International Conference on Diuretics, 1984, p 36
25. Helfant RH: Am J Med 80(suppl 4A):13–22, 1986
26. Hollenberg NK, Bannon JA: Am J Med 80(suppl 4A):30–36, 1986
27. Hollifield JW: Am J Med 80(suppl 4A):8–12, 1986
28. Hulley SB, Furberg CD, Gurland B, et al: Am J Cardiol 1985; 56:913–920.
29. Huston G: In Hamer J (ed): Drugs for Heart Disease. London, Chapman & Hall, 1979, pp 513–547
30. Jahnsen T, Skovborg F, Hansen F, et al: Scand J Clin Lab Invest 43:297–300, 1983
31. Johansson BW, Dziamski R: Drugs 28(suppl 1):77–85, 1984
32. Jones B, Nanra RS: Lancet 1979; 2: 1258–1260.

33. Kaplan NM, Carnegie A, Raskin P, et al: N Engl J Med 312:746–749, 1985
34. Kehoe WA, Guslielmo BJ: Clin Pharmac 2:304–305, 1983
35. Klutsch K, Schmidt P, Grosswendt J: Arzneim-Forschung (Drug Res) 22:377–380, 1972
36. Kreeft JH, Langlois S, Ogilvie RI: J Cardiovasc Pharmacol 6:622–626, 1984
37. Lancet review: Lancet 1:424, 1986
38. Landmark K: J Cardiovasc Pharmacol 7:12–17, 1985
39. Larsen FF, Mogensen L: Eur Heart J 7:210–216, 1986
40. Licht JH, Haley RJ, Pugh B, et al: Arch Intern Med 143:1694–1699, 1983
41. Lowe J, Gray J, Henry DA, et al: Br Med J 2:360–362, 1979
42. MacGregor GA, Banks RA, Markandu ND, et al: Br Med J 286:1535–1538, 1983
43. Maclean D, Tudhope GR: Br Med J 286:1419–1422, 1983
44. Maronde RF, Milgrom M, Vlachakis ND, et al: JAMA 249:237–241, 1983
45. McKibbin JK, Pocock WA, Barlow JB, et al: Br Heart J 51:157-162, 1984
46. Medical Research Council Working Party on Mild to Moderate Hypertension: Lancet 2:539–543, 1981
47. Medical Research Council Working Party on Mild to Moderate Hypertension: Br Med J 287:1249–1253, 1983
48. Millar JA, McLean K, Reid JL: Clin Sci 61:65S–68S, 1981
49. Morgan DB, Davidson C: Br Med J 280:905–908, 1980
50. Mudge GH: In Gilman AG, Goodman LS, Gilman AG (eds): The Pharmacological Basis of Therapeutics, 6th ed. New York, MacMillan, 1980, pp 892–915
51. Muller FO, Meyer BH, de Waal A, et al: Clin Pharmacol Ther 31:339–342, 1982
52. Nordrehaug JE, von der Lippe G: Br Heart J 50:525–529, 1983
53. Oliw E, Kover G, Larsson C, et al: Eur J Pharmacol 38:95–100, 1976
54. Papademetriou V: Am Heart J 111:1217–1224, 1986
55. Papademetriou V, Fletcher R, Khatri I, et al: Am J Cardiol 52:1017–1022, 1983
56. Patterson DJ, Weinstein GS, Jeffries GH: Lancet 2:1077–1078, 1983
57. Perez-Stable E, Caralis PV: Am Heart J 106:245–251, 1983
58. Raison J, Achimastos A, Asmar R, et al: Am J Cardiol 57:223–226, 1986
59. Reubi FC, Cottier PT: Circulation 23:200–210, 1961
60. Reyes AJ, Leary WP: S Afr Med J 64(suppl):1–5, 1983
61. Smith TW, Braunwald E: In Braunwald E (ed): Heart Disease, 2nd ed. Philadelphia, WB Saunders, 1984, pp 527–534
62. Stanaszek WF, Romankiewicz JA: Drug Intell Clin Pharm 19:176–183, 1985
63. Stewart DE, Ikram H, Espiner EA, et al: Br Heart J 54:290–297, 1985
64. Struthers AD, Whitesmith R, Reid JL: Lancet 1:1358–1361, 1983
65. Szatalowicz VL, Arnold PE, Chaimovitz C, et al: N Engl J Med 305:263–266, 1981
66. Thomas JP, Thompson WH: Br Med J 286:2015–2018, 1983
67. Van der Elst E, Dombey SL, Lawrence J: Am Heart J 102:734–740, 1981
68. Wasnich RD, Benfante RJ, Yano K, et al: N Engl J Med 309:344–347, 1983
69. Webster J: Drugs 30:32–41, 1985
70. Weidmann P, Uehlinger DE, Gerber A: J Hypertens 3:297–306, 1985
71. Williams ES, Fisch C: In Rosen MR, Hoffman BF (eds): Cardiac Therapy. Boston, Martinus Nijhoff, 1983, pp 453–479
72. Wollam GL, Tarazi RC, Bravo EL, et al: Am J Med 72:929–938, 1982
73. Wong DG, Spence JD, Lamki L, et al: Lancet 1:997–1001, 1986

New References

74. Burris JF, Weir MR, Oparil S, et al: An assessment of diltiazem and hydrochlorothiazide in hypertension: Application of factorial trial design to a Multicenter clinical trial of combination therapy. JAMA 263:1507–1512, 1990
75. Christensson T, Hellstrom K, Wengle B: Hypercalcemia and primary hyperparathyroidism. Arch Intern Med 137:1138–1142, 1977
76. Cowley AJ, Stainer K, Wynne RD, et al: Symptomatic assessment of patients with heart failure: Double-blind comparison of increasing doses of diuretics and captopril in moderate heart failure. Lancet 2:770–772, 1986
77. Dorup I, Skajaa K, Clausen T, Kjeldsen K: Reduced concentrations of potassium, magnesium, and sodium-potassium pumps in human skeletal muscle during treatment with diuretics. Br Med J 296:455–458, 1988

78. Hande KR, Noone RM, Stone WJ. Severe allopurinol toxicity: Description and guidelines for prevention in patients with renal insufficiency. Am J Med 76:47–56, 1984

79. Henderson DG, Schierup J, Schodt T: Effect of magnesium supplementation on blood pressure and electrolyte concentrations in hypertensive patients receiving long-term diuretic treatment. Br Med J 293:664–665, 1986

80. Hollifield JW: Thiazide treatment of systemic hypertension: Effects on serum magnesium and ventricular ectopic activity. Am J Cardiol 63:22G–25G, 1989

81. Holzgreve H, Distler A, Michaelis J, et al: Verapamil versus hydrochlorothiazide in the treatment of hypertension: Results of long-term double-blind comparative trial. Br Med J 299:881–886, 1989

82. Kiyingi A, Field MJ, Pawsey CC, Yiannikas J, et al: Metolazone in treatment of severe refractory congestive cardiac failure. Lancet 335:29–31, 1990

83. Krusell LR, Jespersen LT, Schmitz A, et al: Repetitive natriuresis and blood pressure: Long-term calcium entry blockade with isradipine. Hypertension 10:577–581, 1987

84. Larsen FF: Haemodynamic effects of high or low doses of furosemide in acute myocardial infarction. Eur Heart J 9:125–131, 1988

85. McVeigh G, Galloway D, Johnston D: The case for low dose diuretics in hypertension: Comparison of low and conventional doses of cyclopenthiazide. Br Med J 297:95–98, 1988

86. Poulsen L, Friberg M, Noer I, Kruskell K, Pedersen OL: Comparison of indapamide and hydrochlorothiazide plus amiloride as a third drug in the treatment of arterial hypertension. Cardiovasc Drugs Ther 3:141–144, 1989

87. Pollare T, Lithell H, Berne C: A comparison of the effects of hydrochlorothiazide and captopril on glucose and lipid metabolism in patients with hypertension. N Engl J Med 321:868–873, 1989

88. Prichard BNC, Brogden RN: Xipamide: A review of its pharmacodynamic and pharmacokinetic properties and therapeutic efficacy. Drugs 30:313–332, 1985

89. Ray WA, Griffin MR, Downey W, Melton LJ III: Long-term use of thiazide diuretics and risk of hip fractures. Lancet 1:687–690, 1989

90. Sharpe N, Murphy J, Smith H, Hannan S: Treatment of patients with symptomless left ventricular dysfunction after myocardial infarction. Lancet 1:255–259, 1988

91. Shaw KM: Hypertension in diabetes: Effect of indapamide on glucose tolerance in diabetic hypertensive patients. S Afr Med J (suppl):18–21, 1989

L.H. Opie
K. Chatterjee
P.A. Poole-Wilson
E. Sonnenblick

5

Angiotensin Converting Enzyme Inhibitors and Conventional Vasodilators

PRINCIPLES OF VASODILATION

Vasodilation, once a specialized procedure, is now commonplace in the therapy of congestive heart failure (CHF) and hypertension, as the peripheral circulation has become one of the prime sites of cardiac drug action (Table 5-1). **There are two major classifications for vasodilators.** First, according to the site of action in the circulation, preload reducers may be separated from those reducing primarily the afterload, while mixed agents act on both pre- and afterload (Fig. 5–1). Reduction of the preload is chiefly required in "backward" CHF or in acute pulmonary edema, whereas reduction of the afterload is required in "forward" CHF or in other low-output states (not resulting from obstructive valvular disease), or in systemic hypertension. Second, vasodilators may be classified according to their cellular site of action on vasoconstrictive vascular receptors or on cell signal systems (Fig. 5–2). **Angiotensin converting enzyme (ACE) inhibitors** diminish the formation of angiotensin-II, which lessens the "opening" of receptor-operated calcium channels and decreases the permissive effect of angiotensin-II on norepinephrine (NE) release from terminal neurons (see Fig. 5–2). Prazosin and other α_1-**receptor blockers** inhibit the action of NE on vasoconstrictor α_1-receptors. **Calcium channel blockers** inhibit both receptor-operated channels (α_2-receptor activity in response to NE stimulation) and voltage-operated channels, which respond to depolarization. Conversely, vasodilatory stimuli (not shown in Fig. 5–2) are mediated by β_2-receptor stimulation, for example, as a result of the administration of dobutamine. Other agents act on intracellular signal pathways (Fig. 5–2, panel *B*) to stimulate formation of vasodilatory cyclic GMP by guanylate cyclase. This is the mode of action of **nitrates and nitroprusside**.

Other "direct" vasodilators such as **hydralazine** also act ultimately by a decrease of vascular smooth muscle calcium, but the mechanism involved is not yet known. An important physiologic vasodilatory effect is exerted by EDRF (**endothelium derived relaxation factor**), now known to be nitric oxide, which is liberated from the vascular endothelium, for example, by acetylcholine. EDRF promotes vasodilation (see Fig. 2–2), so that as the vasoconstrictive effect of NE is opposed, the vessel diameter enlarges. β_2-Agonists and phosphodiesterase inhibitors such as **amrinone** and **milrinone** stimulate the formation of **vasodilatory cyclic AMP**, which inhibits the kinase essential for myosin light chain phosphorylation and, ultimately, for myocyte contraction (Fig. 5–2, panel *B*). **Adenosine** indirectly decreases cell calcium by hyperpolarization as a result of potassium

TABLE 5–1 TYPES OF VASODILATORS

Category	Proposed Mechanism	Examples
Angiotensin converting enzyme inhibitors	Decrease formation of vaso-constrictory angiotensin-II; inhibit secretion of aldosterone	Captopril Enalapril Lisinopril
Nitrate-like agents	Stimulate guanylate cyclase with formation of cyclic GMP	Nitrates Nitroprusside
Direct vasodilators	Unknown	Hydralazine Diazoxide
Potassium channel "openers"	Hyperpolarization	Minoxidil Pinacidil Cromakalim
α_1-Antagonists	Inhibition of α_1 mediated calcium ingress	Prazosin Labetalol (Indoramin)*
α_1-α_2-Antagonists	Inhibition of α_1-α_2 mediated calcium ingress	Phentolamine Phenoxybenzamine
Calcium antagonists	Inhibit calcium ingress	Nifedipine Verapamil Diltiazem New dihydropyridines
β_2-agonists	Inhibit formation of cyclic AMP to decrease myosin light chain kinase activity in vessel wall	Isoproterenol Dobutamine Salbutamol = albuterol
Dopamine agonists	Inhibition of release of NE from terminal neurons	Dopamine (Ibopamine, Dopexamine)*
Central α_2-agonists	Central inhibition of adrenergic outflow	Clonidine Methyldopa
Serotonin antagonists	Inhibition of vasoconstriction	(Ketanserin)*
Under development	Prostacyclin-like agents Atrial natriuretic peptide	– –

*Not in the USA.
Compiled by LH Opie.

channel "opening," thereby shifting the resting membrane potential away from the zone required for calcium channel "opening." Another example of a potassium opener is **minoxidil**, and new ones such as cromakalim and pinacidil that will constitute a new generation of antihypertensives.

Neurohumoral Effects of Severe Heart Failure. A crucial problem in CHF is the inability of the failing LV to maintain a normal blood pressure.[61] The result is a baroreflex-mediated reflex increase in sympathetic adrenergic discharge, which stimulates the myocardium to beat faster and stronger, yet increases peripheral vasoconstriction so that the afterload rises and the load on the failing myocardium augments (Fig. 5–3). Enhanced activity of the renin-angiotensin system, another result of excess adrenergic activity, further increases peripheral vascular resistance and contributes to fluid retention (edema) by stimulation of the secretion of aldosterone (**renin-angiotensin-aldosterone activation**). Furthermore, angiotensin promotes the release of vasopressin to contribute to abnormal volume regulation and hyponatremia in severe CHF.[11] Thus the compensatory processes set in motion by hypotension and increased baroreceptor activity are accompanied by neurohumoral overcompensation and further overloading of the left ventricle.

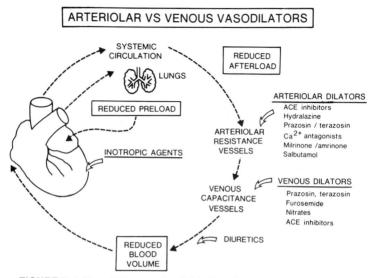

FIGURE 5–1. Vasodilators can be divided into those acting on the afterload, or the arteriolar dilators; those acting on the preload, or the venodilators; and those acting on both sites, such as the ACE inhibitors. The diagram also shows the action of positively inotropic agents and diuretics in CHF. (Figure copyright L.H. Opie.)

Increased Systemic Vascular Resistance. It follows that there is an "afterload mismatch" between the level of vascular resistance and the heart's ability to deliver enough blood to meet the body's demands, especially during exertion, when systolic wall stress has become too high for the depressed contractility of the failing myocardium. The result is exertional fatigue. Systemic vasoconstriction reduces renal plasma flow, which detrimentally affects salt excretion and further promotes renin formation. The inability of the left ventricle to empty itself during systole increases the preload with exertional dyspnea (Fig. 5–4). The combination of increased pre- and afterload, so common in CHF, leads to **progressive ventricular dilation with wall remodeling** (cell hypertrophy and slippage), so that the ejection fraction declines progressively with time. Load reduction may help to stop or retard this detrimental process. Today, vasodilators and especially the ACE inhibitors are widely used as a crucial component of the therapy of CHF. There are also other agents that act selectively on pre- or afterload (Fig. 5–2).

Preload Reduction. Normally as the preload (the LV filling pressure) increases, so also does the peak LV systolic pressure, and the cardiac output rises (ascending limb of the Frank-Starling curve, Fig. 5–4). In diseased hearts the increase in cardiac output is much less than normal, and the output fails to rise and may even fall as the filling pressure rises (the apparent descending limb of Frank-Starling curve). However, the optimal filling pressure for the diseased heart is variable, not always being higher than normal so that reduction of the preload is generally useful, but not always. Clinically, the major drugs reducing the preload in CHF are (1) furosemide, by its diuretic effect (see Fig. 4–1), and (2) the nitrates that dilate the systemic veins to reduce the venous return and thus the filling pressure in both the right and left heart chambers (Table 5-2).

Afterload Reduction. The therapeutic aim is reduction of the peripheral vascular resistance to lessen the load on the heart, improved renal function, and improved skeletal muscle perfusion. Reduction of the systemic vascular resistance is not the same as blood pressure reduction, because in CHF a compensatory increase in the cardiac output

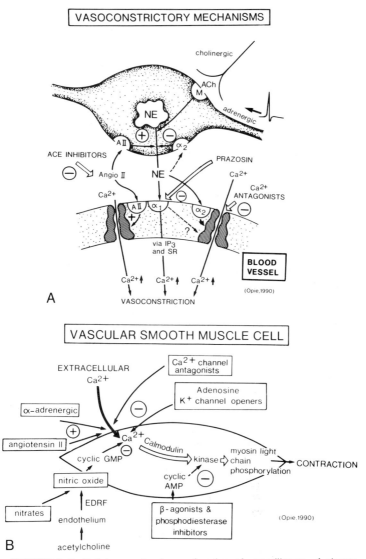

FIGURE 5–2. Cellular mechanisms of action of vasodilators. *A* shows agents modifying the release and effects of NE (norepinephrine) and angiotensin-II, the major neurohumoral vasoconstrictors. *B* shows the effects of agents modifying the intracellular regulation of calcium by cyclic GMP (nitrates) or cyclic AMP (β–stimulants). M=muscarinic receptor; EDRF=endothelial-derived relaxation factor.

tends to maintain the arterial pressure. According to the Laplace law, the tension on the walls of a thin-walled sphere equals the intraluminal pressure times the radius. Wall tension is one of the major determinants of the myocardial oxygen uptake. Afterload reduction hence implies a decrease in the myocardial oxygen demand. In contrast, positive inotropes, such as digitalis, increase the work of the heart and the oxygen demand unless they reduce the heart size, which will reduce wall tension and tend to reduce oxygen demand. **Thus, as in ischemic heart disease, one of the aims in chronic heart failure is to reduce preload and afterload and thus to enhance ventricular emptying and to improve the myocardial oxygen balance.**

Specific afterload reducers are few and limited in practice to two: hydralazine, a non-specific agent whose cellular mode of action is still

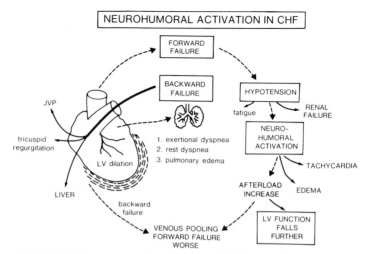

FIGURE 5–3. Neurohumoral adaptation in CHF. The crucial consequence of LV failure is the inability to maintain a normal BP, which elicits a baroreflex-mediated increase in sympathetic adrenergic activity, including a tachycardia, thereby increasing the cardiac output and the degree of vasoconstriction, the latter restoring the BP to normal. Such compensation places even greater demands on the failing LV, however, as the increased SVR causes increased LV failure because the myocardium is afterload-dependent. Furthermore, increased adrenergic β-stimulation leads to increased release of renin with increased vasoconstrictive angiotensin-II (see Fig. 5–2) and more release of aldosterone (see Fig. 5–5). Thus, compensation is accompanied by over-compensation. (Figure copyright L.H. Opie.)

unknown; and the calcium antagonists, which, unfortunately, also have a negative inotropic effect, thereby restricting their use in CHF.

Differing Effects of Vasodilators in Heart Failure and Hypertension

In **heart failure**, the filling pressure is high and the cardiac output is decreased because of myocardial inadequacy. The ventricle performs along the flattened portion of the ventricular function curve (Fig. 5–4), so that a decreased preload due to venodilation, for example by nitrate therapy, relieves symptoms of pulmonary congestion with-out necessarily changing the stroke volume. In contrast to the situation in hypertension, in CHF the failing myocardium is afterload-dependent. Thus, when the systemic vascular resistance (SVR, also known as PVR, peripheral vascular resistance) is therapeutically reduced, the ventricular function curve moves upwards and to the left so that stroke volume and cardiac output rise. In heart failure, the higher the systemic vascular resistance, the greater the increase in cardiac output achieved by peripheral arteriolar vasodilation, as, for example, by nitroprusside, hydralazine, or ACE inhibitors.

In **hypertension**, vasodilation is an important principle of therapy, with hemodynamics as follows. A raised peripheral vascular resistance is an important perpetuating and/or initiating mechanism, because BP = CO x SVR (CO = cardiac output, SVR = systemic vascular resistance). As the SVR rises, the BP must rise since the cardiac output remains normal. The LV filling pressure is normal and the patient is on the steep portion of the function curve, so that a dominant venodilator effect, as with nitrates, may not increase but rather may decrease the stroke volume. When a predominant arteriolar vasodilator is used, such as a calcium antagonist, the reduction in aortic impedance causes little change in the cardiac output (Fig. 5–4), because the well-compensated ventricle is not afterload-dependent, and peripheral

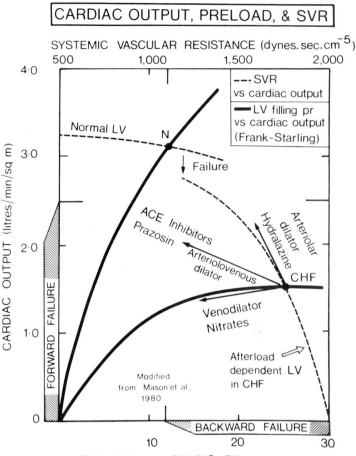

FIGURE 5-4. A high left ventricular (LV) end-diastolic pressure causes congestive symptoms (e.g., dyspnea). A low cardiac output causes symptoms of forward failure (e.g., fatigue). Two basic therapies are vasodilators reducing the LV end-diastolic pressure and agents increasing contractile activity of the heart, such as digitalis. In normal heart (point N), cardiac output (CO) is principally regulated by changes in preload and heart rate; alterations in impedance are of less importance. In contrast, in CHF, CO is principally regulated by minor changes in impedance (afterload-dependent); alterations in preload are of less importance. In CHF, the pure arteriodilator, hydralazine, raises lowered CO markedly with mild decline of elevated left ventricular end-diastolic pressure (LVEDP); the angiotensin converting enzyme inhibitors and prazosin act on both venous and arterial systems to raise the lowered CO and to decrease elevated LVEDP. The pure venodilator, sublingual nitroglycerin, decreases elevated LVEDP markedly, with little or no improvement of lowered CO. Modified from Mason, et al. Arch Intern Med 140:1577–1581, 1980, with permission.

autoregulation keeps the same cardiac output. In response to vasodilation, circulatory reflexes may produce tachycardia. Sometimes, as with hydralazine, tachycardia may be excessive due to unopposed sympathetic stimulation. In contrast, the same vasodilators usually do not produce any change in heart rate in patients with heart failure, presumably due to blunted baroreceptor activity. **The advent of a new generation of vasodilators with relatively few side-effects, including the calcium antagonists and ACE inhibitors, means that vasodilation is increasingly seen as first-line therapy in hypertension.**

**TABLE 5–2 HEMODYNAMICS OF VASODILATORS
IN CHRONIC HEART FAILURE**

Vasodilator	BP	CO	SVR	RAP
Nitrates	0/–	0/–	0/–	—
Hydralazine Minoxidil	0/–	++	—	0
Prazosin Trimazosin	–	+	—	—
ACE inhibitors	–	+	—	–
Salbutamol	0/–	+	–	0/–

BP = blood pressure; CO = cardiac output; SVR = systemic vascular resistance; RAP = right atrial pressure; 0 = no effect; + = moderate increase; ++ = marked increase; – = moderate decrease; — = marked decrease.

Heart rate effects are as follows: Nitrates, hydralazine, minoxidil, and salbutamol tend to increase the heart rate; prazosin, trimazosin, and ACE inhibitors tend to decrease the heart rate.

Modified from Chatterjee K: Vasodilators, in Weatherall DJ, Ledingham JCG (eds): Oxford Textbook of Medicine. Oxford, Oxford University Press, 1968.

ANGIOTENSIN CONVERTING ENZYME (ACE) INHIBITORS

The ACE inhibitors have major roles as vasodilators in both hypertension and CHF. Furthermore, in CHF, ACE inhibitors are able to inhibit the deleterious neurohumoral vicious circle involving angiotensin-renin-aldosterone.

ACE inhibitors (= converting enzyme inhibitors = CEI) act on the angiotensin-renin-aldosterone system by inhibition of the ACE. The ACE inhibitors, captopril, enalapril, and lisinopril (and many others, including ramipril, perindopril, quinapril, and cilazapril, which have already appeared in Europe), act as mixed arteriolar and venous vasodilators. **Theoretically, ACE inhibitors should be of most benefit when CHF is accompanied by high plasma renin activity, or when hypertension is caused by a high renin state as in renal artery stenosis. Yet these agents frequently are of benefit in ordinary essential hypertension and mild degrees of CHF.** In CHF, ACE inhibitors are increasingly seen as the vasodilators of choice because of their added neurohumoral benefit, and are therefore being used earlier and earlier, though there is no evidence that they are effective in the absence of co-therapy with diuretics. The "permissive" role of angiotensin in the release of NE from the terminal adrenergic neurons and elsewhere (Fig. 5–5) leads to the proposal that angiotensin inhibitors may be tested in various other "hyperadrenergic" states, such as acute myocardial infarction (AMI) and some ventricular arrhythmias.

Possible Sites of Angiotensin Inhibition. Angiotensin-II is an octapeptide, and its formation from its precursor, decapeptide (angiotensin-I) requires the converting enzyme (Fig. 5–6). Renin is the rate-limiting enzyme required to form angiotensin-I from the substrate angiotensinogen, which comes from the liver (Fig. 5–7). The synthesis of angiotensin-II can be decreased by ACE inhibitors. The synthesis of both angiotensin-I and -II can be prevented by blocking the formation of renin, normally synthesized and released by the juxtaglomerular cells of the kidney, by experimental renin-inhibiting peptides. Finally, angiotensin-II can undergo competitive antagonism at its receptor sites by the investigational agent saralasin.

Tissue ACE Inhibition. Recently local renin-angiotensin systems (autocrine-paracine) have been identified in many tissues, including blood vessels, heart, adrenals, kidney, and brain. For example, vaso-constriction may be precipitated either by circulating angiotensin or by angiotensin formed locally at or near the receptor site. Interaction

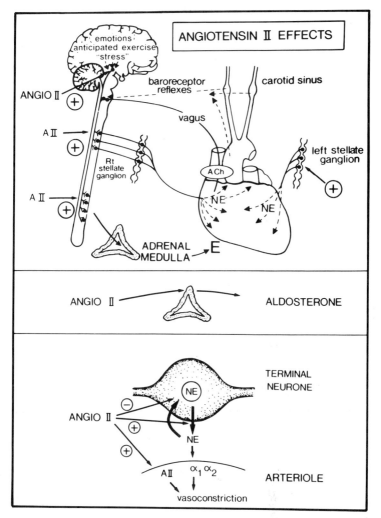

FIGURE 5–5. Multiple sites of action of angiotensin-II (= angio-II), including central adrenergic activation, facilitation of ganglionic transmission, release of aldosterone from the adrenal medulla, release of norepinephrine (NE) from terminal sympathetic varicosities with inhibition of re-uptake, and direct stimulation of vascular angiotensin-II receptors. The major net effect is powerful vasoconstriction. Modified from Opie LH: The Heart: Physiology, Metabolism, Pharmacology and Therapy. Grune & Stratton, Orlando & London, 1984, with permission.

with adrenergic terminal neurons and endothelial synthesis of prostacyclin are other sites of regulation of vascular tone. In the myocardium, local angiotensin has a small positive inotropic effect. Thus the overall hemodynamic effects of ACE inhibitors result from inhibition of circulating and local angiotensin-renin systems.

Bradykinin. Another function of the converting enzyme is to degrade the potent vasodilator kinin peptide (bradykinin) to inactive metabolites (Fig. 5–7). ACE inhibition therefore increases bradykinin to contribute to peripheral vasodilation by stimulating the synthesis and release of vasodilator prostaglandins. This sequence explains why indomethacin attenuates the effects of the ACE inhibitor captopril.[49] Increased formation of bradykinin may explain the relatively high incidence of cough as a side-effect of the ACE inhibitors, and the rare yet serious angioedema.[56]

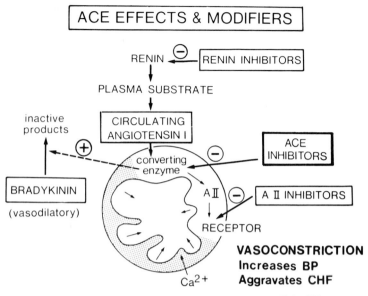

FIGURE 5–6. Site of action of angiotensin-converting enzyme (ACE) and its modifiers. ACE is found especially in the pulmonary vascular bed. ACE inhibitors reduce formation of angiotensin-II (AII), and also decrease breakdown of the vasodilator bradykinin. The latter mechanism is thought to account for an effect of captopril detected even in anephric patients. Angiotensin-II receptor antagonists (e.g., saralasin, not in clinical use) interact with the same vascular binding site as does angiotensin-II, thereby causing vasodilation. Anti-renin agents are under development. Modified from Opie LH: The Heart: Physiology, Metabolism, Pharmacology and Therapy. Grune & Stratton, Orlando & London, 1984.

ACE Inhibitors for Hypertension

In hypertension, increased activity of the renin-angiotensin-aldosterone system is most obvious in cases of unilateral renal artery stenosis, when the decreased perfusion pressure to the renal arteries results in increased release of renin from the juxtaglomerular apparatus. However, the renin-angiotensin system also helps to maintain blood pressure both in normal people and in essential hypertension, especially when sodium intake is restricted. Therefore, although ACE inhibition leads to the most dramatic falls of blood pressure in the presence of an underlying renal mechanism, ACE inhibition also may be an effective antihypertensive therapy in mild to moderate hypertension, possibly acting by indirect adrenergic modulation (Fig. 5–5). As ACE inhibitors do not alter glucose tolerance, blood uric acid, or cholesterol levels,[71] and as these agents seldom cause subjective side-effects other than cough, their use in hypertension is rapidly increasing.

ACE inhibitors appear to lower blood pressure by five mechanisms. First, they inhibit the normal conversion of circulating angiotensin-I to the powerful vasoconstrictor angiotensin-II. Second, they reduce the secretion of aldosterone to induce a natriuresis. Third, specific renal vasodilation may enhance natriuresis. Fourth, the inactivation of vasodilatory bradykinins is reduced. Fifth, they inhibit local formation of angiotensin-II in vascular tissue and in myocardium.[81]

Quality of Life in Hypertension. Although it is claimed that ACE inhibitors produce a good quality of life, the classic study[12] used as comparison not placebo but two agents already known to have central and sexual side-effects, namely methyldopa and propranolol. When

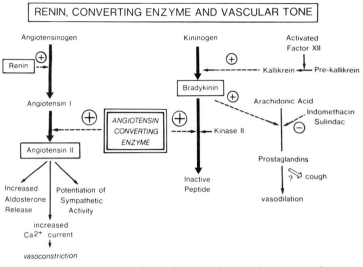

FIGURE 5–7. Interacting effects of renin and converting enzyme that contribute to alterations in vascular tone. The effects of inhibitors at various sites are (1) renin blockers, (2) ACE inhibitors, and (3) competitive inhibitors.

compared with a cardioselective β-blocker such as atenolol, differences in the quality of life become trivial, except for a mild memory impairment with atenolol.[64] Likewise, the quality of life with ACE inhibitors does not differ much from that with the calcium-antagonist agents, although the irritating side-effects may differ. For example, with ACE-inhibitor therapy, cough may cause discontinuation, whereas in the case of calcium antagonists, ankle edema or headache may do likewise.

ACE Inhibitors for CHF

In the therapy of severe CHF, **captopril** (usual dose 25–50 mg 3x daily with lower initial doses to avoid hypotension) is well tested, and gives sustained benefit during prolonged double-blind randomized trials.[4] Because of the rapid onset of action of captopril, reactive hypotension may be a problem; hence, a test dose of 6.25 mg is usually given first, while vigorous diuretic doses are avoided and the circulating volume is maintained. **Enalapril** (5 mg 2x daily after test dose of 2.5 mg, range 2.5–20 mg 2x daily) is equally effective. Although 5 mg was given twice daily in the Consensus study,[53] a single 5-mg dose may be used.[51] In a crucial study, enalapril added to diuretics and digitalis decreased mortality rate in severe CHF.[53] The slower onset of action means that reactive hypotension may be less of a problem, yet first-dose reactions can occur with doses as low as 2.5 mg,[13] and hypotension will be prolonged. Lisinopril and other ACE inhibitors are probably equally effective in CHF. **Hypotension with any ACE inhibitor carries with it the risk of renal failure and anuria**.[13] In CHF with severe liver dysfunction, captopril would appear to be preferable to enalapril because of the requirement of the latter for activation by the liver; otherwise lisinopril (no liver metabolism) is a logical choice. Patients with CHF may constitute a high-risk group for serious **ventricular arrhythmias** (risk factors: myocardial disease, therapy with digoxin and thiazide diuretics, excess circulating catecholamines). ACE inhibitors, by relieving heart failure, increasing plasma potassium, and decreasing circulating NE levels,[13] can be expected to have an indirect antiarrhythmic effect;[7] specific studies are required.

Selection of Patients with CHF for ACE-Inhibitor Therapy. Mostly the efficacy of these agents has been shown in patients not responding well to diuretics and digitalis.[80] Nonetheless, ACE inhibitors are now widely used as second-line agents after diuretics. They seem not to work in the absence of diuretic therapy;[74] therefore, by implication they are not appropriate for use as first-line agents. Certain conditions are particularly suitable for ACE inhibitor therapy: (1) hypertension and CHF; (2) angina plus CHF when ACE inhibitors may improve coronary blood flow; and (3) CHF with an elevated plasma renin activity (however, as with hypertension, captopril also works when the renin level is normal).[27] Plasma sodium concentrations of 130 mEq/L or less are more frequently associated with increased plasma renin activity and may warn of a brisk response to ACE inhibitors.[32] In patients with high plasma renin levels, ACE inhibitors may be less effective than anticipated because of persistent pulmonary vasoconstriction.[33]

Precautions. **Hypotension** may occur in many patients with CHF with pre-existing normal or low blood pressures treated by ACE inhibitors. Transient hypotension has the risk of precipitating symptomatic orthostasis or arrhythmias or prerenal azotemia. Hypotension may be avoided by decreasing the diuretic dose, maintaining circulating blood volume and using low initial doses. Otherwise, therapy of CHF with ACE inhibition is relatively straightforward, provided that the precautions outlined under captopril are followed. Readjustment of the diuretic dose is frequently required. **Hyperkalemia** is a risk in patients treated with potassium-retaining diuretics or with potassium supplements, especially if renal function is impaired. **Aortic stenosis** is a contraindication to all vasodilator therapy. **Renal failure** is also a contraindication, because of the risk of prolonged deterioration in renal function following excess hypotension.

ACE Inhibitors for Post-Infarct Remodeling

Experimental[72] and clinical[70,78] studies support the use of ACE inhibitors in presenting an increase in decreasing LV size post-infarction. By unloading the left ventricle and decreasing LV chamber size, they may improve LV ejection fraction and do so better than furosemide in patients without overt heart failure.[78] This leads to the logical but untested suggestion that ACE inhibitors, tending to decrease LV cavity size post-infarct, should combine well with β-blockers, which tend to increase cavity size. In the presence of early overt post-infarct LV failure, which is an important cause of an increased LV volume,[59] it makes sense to combine ACE inhibitor and diuretic therapy.

ACE Inhibitor Therapy in Patients with Renal Impairment

ACE inhibitors may have a specific renal vasodilatory effect, acting to dilate the efferent arterioles and thereby relieving intraglomerular pressure.

In **diabetic nephropathy**, captopril (37.5 mg 3x daily) improved proteinuria without changing serum creatinine, possibly by reduction of intrarenal hypertension.[44] In a comparative study, captopril decreased filtration fraction, whereas nifedipine increased it; correspondingly, captopril reduced albuminuria, whereas nifedipine increased it.[66]

In **early renal failure** of hypertension, ACE inhibitors are being tested for a possible beneficial reduction of intrarenal hypertension.[10]

In **ischemic renal failure**, ACE inhibitors should theoretically relieve angiotensin-induced vasoconstriction.[28]

In **severe CHF and impaired creatinine clearance**, ACE inhibitors (especially captopril) may maintain renal function (renal vasodilator effect), but there is risk of exaggeration of the renal defect.[34]

Class Side-effects of ACE Inhibitors

Cough. Of the various side-effects, some serious and some not, cough has emerged as one of the most troublesome and common. This side-effect took a long time to be discovered. Patients with CHF cough in any case, and in patients with hypertension, side-effects are generally discovered only if volunteered. Cough was ignored in the famous "quality of life" study.[12] In some centers, the incidence of cough is thought to be as high as 10 to 15%, whereas others report a much lower incidence. Disabling cough is probably the most limiting factor in the use of ACE inhibitors for hypertension. The cough is due to an increased sensitivity of the cough reflex, resulting in a dry, irritating non-productive cough, quite different from bronchospasm. Increased formation of bradykinin and prostaglandins may play a role (Fig. 5–7). Preliminary data suggest relief of the cough by added **sulindac**, a non-steroidal anti-inflammatory drug.[65] However, use of nonsteroidal anti-inflammatories will greatly diminish the vasodilator effects of ACE inhibition.[67]

Hypotension. Particularly in CHF, where the BP tends to be low, added pre- and afterload reduction can give rise to excess hypotension (Fig. 5–8), sometimes necessitating dose reduction or even cessation of ACE inhibitor therapy. The major threat of hypotension lies in tissue underperfusion, especially renal failure.

Renal Side-effects. Hypotension can precipitate renal failure, usually temporary; predisposing conditions include severe CHF and underlying renal disease, such as renal artery stenosis. Occasionally, irreversible renal failure has been precipitated in patients with bilateral renal artery stenosis, which is therefore a contraindication to the use of ACE inhibitors. In unilateral renal artery disease, with high circulating renin values, ACE inhibitors may also cause excessive hypotensive responses with oliguria or azotemia. To obviate and minimize such problems, a low first test dose (6.25 mg captopril) should always be given to patients with CHF and to hypertensive patients in whom a renal artery stenosis has not been excluded.

Angioedema. Although rare (about 0.1%), this condition is life-threatening. There is no known method of prediction. The mechanism may be by formation of bradykinin, and steroid treatment may be required.

Hyperkalemia. When ACE inhibitors are given with potassium-sparing diuretics or in the presence of renal failure, the mild potassium retention induced by ACE inhibition may precipitate hyperkalemia.

ACE Inhibitors: Drug Combinations and Interactions

ACE Inhibitors Plus Diuretics. ACE inhibitors may be combined with other antihypertensive or antifailure regimens. In **hypertension**, captopril may be combined with thiazide diuretics[1] to enhance its hypotensive effects, but with some diuretic-related loss of quality of life.[12] ACE inhibitors also tend to decrease the metabolic and hypovolemic side-effects of diuretic therapy.[1] When combined with potassium-retaining thiazide diuretics (Dyazide, Moduretic, Maxzide), and especially spironolactone,[40] there is a **risk of hyperkalemia** because captopril/enalapril decreases aldosterone secretion.

In **CHF**, additive effects of ACE inhibitors on the preload may lead to syncope or hypotension, so that the diuretic dose is usually halved before starting ACE inhibitors. The result may be a true diuretic-sparing effect in about half of patients with mild CHF upon addition of the ACE inhibitor, yet in severe CHF the full diuretic dose usually must be reinstituted.[68] A low serum sodium is an indirect indicator of a high renin state, because high aldosterone levels retain the sodium

PRECAUTIONS :ACE INHIBITORS IN HEART FAILURE

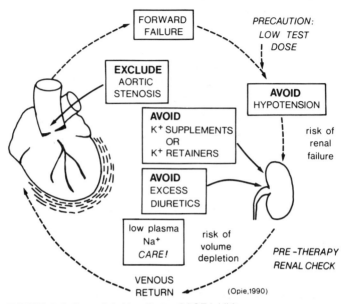

FIGURE 5–8. Potential side-effects of ACE inhibitors.

that stimulates vasopressin secretion. In such hyponatremic patients therapy by furosemide alone is ineffective and the addition of ACE inhibition is required.[54]

ACE Inhibitors Plus Digoxin for CHF. In the specific case of CHF, ACE inhibitors are frequently combined with diuretics and digoxin, as in the Consensus Trial Study Group.[53] Logically, digoxin decreases heart size and rate, whereas ACE inhibitors decrease the load, so that the combination should be better than either agent alone.[60] However, captopril increases blood digoxin levels (see Table 6-4).

ACE Inhibitors Plus β-Blockade. This combination has been widely used in hypertension, although theoretically it is not the combination of choice because both agents have an ultimate antirenin effect. Although the overall antihypertensive response to ACE inhibition–β-blockade is usually held to be less than additive, more recent data suggest that there is after all an additive effect.[50]

ACE Inhibitors Plus Calcium Antagonists. This combination, now increasingly used in the therapy of hypertension, appears logical because of the two different modalities of attack—first on the renin-angiotensin system, and second on the increased peripheral vascular resistance found especially in moderate and severe hypertension. Furthermore, both agents should be free of CNS side-effects.

ACE Inhibitors Plus Other Vasodilators. As different vasodilators have different supplementary qualities, each patient has to be managed on a pragmatic basis. Combination of ACE inhibitors with other vasodilators, such as nitrates, nifedipine, or hydralazine, should be undertaken with care because of the added risk of hypotension. In the therapy of CHF, milrinone may be added to captopril without excess hypotensive effect and yet increase the stroke volume.[26] Combination hydralazine-captopril may have an added risk of altered immune function, so that careful monitoring of neutrophils is mandatory.

ACE Inhibitors and Nonsteroidal Anti-inflammatories. Formation of bradykinin and prostaglandins is thought to be part of the mechanism of cough production by ACE inhibitors, as well as playing an important role in peripheral vasodilation.[65,67] Hence, nonsteroidal anti-inflammatories should lessen cough and also lessen the effectiveness of ACE inhibitors in CHF.

Possible New Uses of ACE Inhibitors

Insulin Resistance. Recently it has been proposed that insulin resistance is an important component of hypertension and that ACE inhibitors have a more beneficial effect on the insulin-mediated disposal of glucose and on the insulin response to glucose than a diuretic.[71] Hence, everything else being equal, to maintain metabolic normality in hypertensives, the ACE inhibitor would be better than the diuretic.

Arteriosclerosis. Preliminary work suggests that ACE inhibitors can slow the rate of intimal hyperplasia, an important component of atherogenesis.[58]

SPECIFIC ACE INHIBITORS

Captopril

Captopril (Capoten; Lopril in France; Lopirin in Germany; Captopril in Japan), the first widely available ACE inhibitor, was originally seen to be an agent with significant and serious side-effects, such as loss of taste, renal impairment, and neutropenia. Now it is recognized that these are rare side-effects than can be avoided largely by reducing the daily dose and by appropriate monitoring. The result is that captopril is now widely used for both CHF and hypertension. Whether captopril and other ACE inhibitors actually improve the quality of life in hypertension needs proof.

Pharmacokinetics. After absorption from the stomach, captopril is metabolized by the liver and kidney, with an elimination half-life of approximately 2 to 3 hours. A dose of 20 mg given orally to normal volunteers blocks the pressor response to exogenous angiotensin-I within 15 minutes and for over 2 hours.[15] In hypertension its biological half-life is long enough to allow 2x daily dosage.

Dose and Indications. In **hypertension**, captopril is given in an average daily dose of 25 to 50 mg orally, 2x daily (instead) of much higher 3x daily doses previously prescribed). For maximum bioavailability, captopril should be taken on an empty stomach, yet food has little influence on the overall antihypertensive effect.[37] In hypertension, although 2x daily doses are conventional, a single daily dose of 50 to 100 mg may be used with dietary salt restriction.[36] The risk of excess hypotension is highest in patients with high renin states (renal artery stenosis, pre-existing vigorous diuretic therapy, or severe sodium restriction) when the initial dose should be low (6.25–12.5 mg). When given sublingually (25 mg, chewed), captopril may relieve severe hypertension,[46] but renal contraindications must first be excluded.

In **CHF**, the usual maintenance dose is 75 to 150 mg daily in three divided doses; 2x daily therapy seems logical.[57] Captopril may cause excessive hypotension, especially in vigorously diuresed patients, so that a **test dose** of 6.25 mg is required (if given sublingually the safety can be assessed within 1 hour, followed by 12.5 mg 3x daily).

In **renal disease**, when captopril is not contraindicated (next section), the dose is reduced.

In **diabetic nephropathy**, captopril improves proteinuria.

In **rheumatoid arthritis**, captopril appears to work by virtue of the sulfhydryl (SH) group.[20]

In **nitrate tolerance**, preliminary data suggest amelioration of tolerance by captopril.[62]

Contraindications. These include bilateral renal artery stenosis;

renal artery stenosis in a single kidney; immune-based renal disease; severe renal failure (serum creatinine >1.6 mg/dl or >150 μmol/L); pre-existing neutropenia; and systemic hypotension. **Relative contraindications include** co-administration of other drugs likely to alter immune function, such as procainamide, tocainide, hydralazine, probenecid, and possibly acebutolol.

Side-effects. In general, the side-effects are seldom serious provided that the total daily dose is 150 mg daily or less.[19] Cough is the most common and frequently troublesome side-effect. Other class side-effects include renal failure, angioedema, and hyperkalemia. Immune-based side-effects are probably specific to captopril, such as taste disturbances, skin rashes, and (in a subgroup of patients) neutropenia.

Neutropenia (<1000/mm³) may occur with captopril, extremely rarely in hypertensive patients with normal renal function (1/8600 according to the package insert), more commonly (1/500) with pre-existing impaired renal function with a serum creatinine of 1.6 mg/dl or more, and as a serious risk (4/100) in patients with both collagen vascular disease and renal impairment. When captopril is discontinued, recovery from neutropenia is usual except when there is associated serious disease, such as severe renal or heart failure or collagen vascular disease.

Proteinuria occurs in about 1% of patients receiving captopril, especially in the presence of pre-existing renal disease or with high doses of captopril (>150 mg/day[22]). There appears to be a double mechanism for renal damage induced by captopril: first, an altered immune response, and second, excess hypotension, as shared with enalapril.[3] Paradoxically, captopril may be used in the therapy of diabetic nephropathy with proteinuria.[44]

Other side-effects include hypotension (frequent in the treatment of CHF); impaired taste (2–7%); skin rashes (4–10%), sometimes with eosinophilia; and, rarely (1/100 to 1/1000), serious angioedema. Hepatic damage is also very rare. Renal failure in patients with CHF may be exacerbated by captopril.

Pre-treatment Precautions. Bilateral renal artery stenosis must be excluded as far as possible. Patients with renal impairment caused by collagen disease, or patients receiving immunosuppressives or immune system modifiers such as steroids and hydralazine, should be excluded, as should patients with a history of hematological disease or pre-treatment depression of neutrophils or platelets. Pre-treatment hypotension excludes therapy.

Precautions at the Start of Therapy. First-dose hypotension may occur, especially in patients with high-renin states, including those over-diuresed, on severe salt restriction, or with severe hyponatremia or renal artery stenosis. Hypotension is a common risk in patients with CHF. Hypotension may be avoided by (1) using an **initial test dose** with captopril (6.25 mg in heart failure, 6.25–12.5 mg in patients with hypertension or high-renin states), and (2) decreasing the dose of the diuretic with attention to volume repletion in CHF. In all cases, therapy should be started under close medical supervision (emphasized in the package insert). A sublingual test dose of captopril may be tried in out-patient practice when the patient does not require hospital admission.

Precautions During Treatment. Regular monitoring of neutrophil counts is required in patients with pre-existing serious renal impairment (pre-treatment count, then 2 weekly counts for 3 months). Captopril should not be given to patients with collagen vascular disease. The risk of renal damage from captopril may be reduced by keeping total daily doses below 150 mg/day.[22]

Enalapril

Enalapril (Vasotec in the US; Innovace in the UK; Xanef, Renitec or Pres in Europe; Renivace in Japan) is now available throughout the world. In many ways enalapril is similar to captopril with, however, (1) a longer half-life; (2) a slower onset of effect because of the requirement of hydrolysis of the pro-drug to the active form, enalaprilat, in the liver so that the therapeutic effect depends on hepatic metabolism; and (3) the absence of the SH group from the structure, thus theoretically lessening or removing the risk of immune-based side-effects.

Pharmacokinetics. About 60% of the oral dose is absorbed[43] with no influence of meals. Enalapril is de-esterified in the liver and kidney to the active form enalaprilat, which, however, is poorly absorbed when given orally. Time to peak serum concentration is about 2 hours for enalapril, and about 5 hours for enalaprilat,[38] with some delay in CHF. Excretion is 95% renal as enalapril or enalaprilat (hence the lower doses in renal failure). The elimination half-life of enalaprilat is about 4 to 5 hours in hypertension and 7 to 8 hours in CHF.[38] Following multiple doses, the effective elimination half-life of enalaprilat is 11 hours (package insert). One oral 10 mg-dose of enalapril yields sufficient enalaprilat to cause significant ACE inhibition for 19 hours.[43] The peak hypotensive response to enalapril occurs about 4 to 6 hours after the oral dose, both in hypertension and in CHF,[38] which may account for the marked depression of renal function that may occur at that time.[3] Peak effects on cardiac index and other hemodynamic parameters occur earlier, after about 1 to 2 hours, and are sustained for at least 12 hours.[13] In severe liver disease, the dose may have to be increased.

Dose. In hypertension, the dose is 2.5 to 20 mg given as 1 or 2 daily doses. Doses higher than 10 to 20 mg daily give no added benefit.[76,77] A low initial dose (2.5 mg) is a wise precaution, especially when enalapril is added to a diuretic or the patient is salt-depleted,[48] in the elderly, or when high-renin hypertension is suspected. In CHF, enalapril is started under close supervision in hospital with an initial dose of 2.5 mg (risk of hypotension and renal failure) and a usual maintenance dose of 10 to 20 mg 2x daily. When added to digoxin and diuretics, a low dose of only 5 mg daily also achieves good results.[51] In renal failure (glomerular filtration rate [GFR] below 30 ml/min), the dose of enalapril must be reduced.

Side-effects. Cough is most common, as for all ACE inhibitors. In animals, very high doses of enalapril may cause renal tubular damage, probably the result of excess prolonged hypotension. Rarely neutropenia has been reported, and the relationship to enalapril has not been proven. Taste disturbances have not occurred, and enalapril can be safe when captopril has induced a skin rash.[29] **Angioedema is a risk highlighted in the package insert.**

Precautions. As in the case of captopril, (1) the major risk is excess hypotension (use low initial dose); and (2) pre-treatment evaluation of renal function and of drug co-therapy is essential. In hypertensives, bilateral renal artery stenosis or stenosis in a single kidney should be excluded. It is presumed that enalapril, without the SH group found in captopril, does not produce the same immune-based toxic effects, and regular monitoring of the neutrophil count or proteinuria is not required. If ACE inhibition is required for patients with collagen vascular disease, or during co-therapy with other drugs altering the immune status, enalapril seems preferable to captopril; yet the white cell count would still need periodic monitoring (package insert).

Lisinopril

This relatively new ACE inhibitor (Zestril, Prinivil), approved for hypertension in the USA and also effective in CHF, differs from the other two available in the USA in its unusual pharmacokinetic properties (Table 5-3). It is not a pro-drug, it is not metabolized by the liver, it is water soluble, and it is excreted unchanged by the kidneys (reminiscent of the kinetic patterns of water-soluble β-blockers). The

TABLE 5–3 SALIENT FEATURES OF CAPTOPRIL, ENALAPRIL, AND LISINOPRIL

	Captopril	Enalapril	Lisinopril
Trade name in USA	Capoten	Vasotec	Zestril, Prinivil
Pro-drug	No	Yes	No
Onset time,	0.5	2–4	2–4
Plasma T$\frac{1}{2}$	2–3	4–11	12–14
Duration of action	6–12	12–24	24–36
Metabolism	L,K	L	None
SH-group	Yes	No	No
Immune side-effects	Yes	No	No
Hypotension risk	Yes	Yes	Yes
Angioedema risk	Yes	Yes	Yes
Hypertension license*	Yes	Yes	Yes
CHF license*	Yes	Yes	No
Total oral dose (mg/day)	25–150	5–20	5–20
Frequency of dose	2–3x	1–2x	1x
Test dose (mg)	6.25	2.5	2.5
Sublingual dose	25 mg	None	None

L = liver; K = kidney; CHF = congestive heart failure.
*In USA.

half-life (12–14 hours) is longer than that of the other two agents approved in the USA, with a duration of action exceeding 24 hours. Effects start 2 hours after ingestion and peak at 4 to 8 hours. Lisinopril does not contain an SH-group and therefore should not be prone to immune-related side-effects. The initial dose is 2.5 to 5 mg with a maintenance dose of 10 to 20 mg, which is similar to enalapril. In the USA, it is licensed only for hypertension, although well tested for CHF.[52]

New ACE and Renin Inhibitors

An increasingly large number of new ACE inhibitors are being promoted in the hope of capturing a segment of the increasing market. From the practical point of view, it seems doubtful that these agents have anything to add to captopril or its immediate successors, enalapril and lisinopril. **Ramipril** is long-acting and hypotensive in a 5- to 10-mg dose once daily and is proposed to be a more tissue-specific ACE inhibitor without that claim being translated into any definite clinical differences from the others. **Perindopril** (Coversyl in UK, 2–8 mg once daily) is long-acting and is claimed to improve vascular structure and function in hypertension. **Cilazapril**, like enalapril, is a pro-drug with similar kinetics. Like many of the other agents, it needs conversion to the active form in the liver (cilazaprilat), the half-life of which appears to be nearly 40 hours. **Quinapril** (Accupro in UK) also has a long half-life and in the UK is licensed for once daily therapy in hypertension (5–40 mg daily) and twice daily therapy in CHF (2.5 mg upwards). **Benzapril** has an optimal dose of 10 mg twice daily in hypertension. **Zofenopril** is 5 times more potent than captopril, longer-acting, and, with the SH-group, complexed to a ring structure.

Specific **renin-inhibition** acts on the renin-angiotensin-aldosterone axis at a different site from the ACE inhibitors; no renin inhibitors are yet beyond the investigational stage.

Choice of ACE Inhibitor

In general, we see little advantage for one agent compared with any other (Table 5-3). However, for specific situations there are specific arguments. **Captopril** seems best for acute severe hypertension because it has the most rapid onset of action. Furthermore, a short duration of action is an advantage when testing the agent in CHF. There are certain borderline indications where the SH-group may possibly be an advantage, such as associated rheumatoid arthritis, the development of nitrate tolerance, and, hypothetically, reperfusion damage. Captopril is chosen for the test dose in all situations because not being a pro-drug it has a rapid onset of action. On the other hand, captopril has certain side-effects specific to the SH-group, including high-dose renal damage, ageusia, and neutropenia. **Enalapril** has a longer duration of action so that it can be given once or twice a day for hypertension with greater confidence, although prolonged hypotension may be a disadvantage in CHF associated with poor renal function. **Lisinopril** is clearly a once-a-day preparation with simple metabolism, with water solubility, with no liver transformation, and with renal excretion, making it an easy drug to use and understand. It should have advantages when SH groups should be avoided or when several other agents are being administered, because there is no risk of hepatic pharmacokinetic interactions.

NITRATE-LIKE VASODILATORS

Nitroprusside (References from Previous Editions)

IV nitroprusside (Nitride) remains the reference vasodilator for severe low output left-sided heart failure provided that the arterial pressure is reasonably maintained, because it acts rapidly and has a balanced effect, dilating both arterioles and veins. Nitroprusside seems particularly useful for increasing LV stroke work in severe refractory heart failure caused by mitral or aortic incompetence. Hemodynamic and clinical improvement also are observed in patients with severe pump failure complicating AMI, in heart failure after cardiac surgery, and in patients with acute exacerbation of chronic heart failure. Because of the increased stroke volume there may be considerable hemodynamic improvement without much hypotension; but, in general, some hypotension accompanies and may limit the therapeutic effect of nitroprusside. Because of the need for careful continuous monitoring and its light sensitivity, nitroprusside is being replaced in severe CHF by nitrates or the inotropic dilators, and in hypertensive crises by sublingual nifedipine or IV labetalol.

Pharmacokinetics. With infusion of nitroprusside, the hemodynamic response (direct vasodilation) starts within minutes and stops equally quickly. Nitroprusside given intravenously is converted to cyanmethemoglobin and free cyanide in the red cells; the free cyanide is then converted to thiocyanate in the liver and is cleared by the kidneys (half-life 7 days).

Dose. An initial infusion of 10 µg/min is increased by 10 µg/min every 10 minutes up to 40 to 75 µg/min with a top dose of 300 µg/min.

Precautions. The infusion rate needs careful titration against the blood pressure, which must be continuously monitored to avoid excess hypotension. Nitroprusside must not be abruptly withdrawn because of the danger of rebound hypertension. Extravasation must be avoided. The solution in normal saline (avoid alkaline solutions) must be freshly made and then shielded from light during infusion; it should be discarded when 4 hours old, or before if discolored. Cyanide may accumulate with prolonged high doses of nitroprusside to produce a lactic acidosis. Toxicity can be avoided by monitoring blood lactate and blood thiocyanate (toxic level 100 µg/ml). But in lactic acidosis due to poor tissue perfusion nitroprusside may be beneficial.

Indications. These include the following situations: (1) for hemodynamic improvement in selected patients with myocardial infarction and LV failure; (2) severe CHF with regurgitant valve disease; (3) in hypertensive crises associated with LV failure; (4) in dissecting aneurysm; and (5) after coronary bypass surgery, when patients frequently have reactive hypertension as they are removed from hypothermia, so that nitroprussides or nitrates are routinely given by most cardiovascular surgical units for 24 hours provided that hypotension is no problem.

Contraindications. Pre-existing hypotension (systolic <90 mm Hg, diastolic <60 mm Hg). All vasodilators are contraindicated in severe obstructive valvular heart disease (aortic, mitral, or pulmonic stenosis). In patients with ventricular septal defect, nitro-prusside by peripheral vasodilation can cause a relative increase in pulmonary vascular resistance with increased left-to-right shunt. AMI is a relative contraindication, for fear of adverse effects of excess hypotension.

Side-effects. Overvigorous treatment may cause an excessive drop in LV end-diastolic pressure, severe hypotension, and myocardial ischemia. Fatigue, nausea, vomiting, and disorientation tend to arise especially when treatment continues for more than 48 hours. In patients with renal failure, thiocyanate accumulates with high dose infusions and may produce hypothyroidism after prolonged therapy. Hypoxia may develop (increased ventilation-perfusion mismatch with pulmonary vasodilation).

Combination with Other Agents. Nitroprusside may be combined with inotropic agents such as dopamine and dobutamine and with digitalis to optimize the hemodynamic benefit. Maintaining an adequate ventricular filling pressure is essential with these combined therapies, and invasive monitoring is required.

Nitroprusside, the prototype IV vasodilator, has balanced venous and arteriolar effects. It is a powerful agent that requires invasive monitoring to avoid excess reduction of preload or hypotension, which can develop very rapidly. When no longer required, nitroprusside must be tapered and not abruptly reduced. The use of sublingual nifedipine for acute afterload reduction and the efficacy of nitrates and furosemide for preload reduction, have tended to decrease the indications for nitroprusside, which must be more carefully monitored than the other agents because of its rapid onset and cessation of activity. Nonetheless, nitroprusside is still the vasodilator of choice in many acute emergency situations.

Nitrates

Nitrates are now used in the therapy of both acute LV failure and chronic heart failure (see References from Previous Editions in Chap. 2). Their major effect is venous rather than arteriolar dilation, thus being most suited to patients with raised pulmonary wedge pressure and clinical features of pulmonary congestion. Sublingual nitrates produce a "pharmacologic phlebotomy." Nitrates are not suitable for the therapy of hypertension uncomplicated by CHF. Although nitrate tolerance is a problem during prolonged therapy, isosorbide dinitrate 40 mg 4x daily combined with hydralazine 300 mg daily gave long-term benefits in patients with severe heart failure in a double-blind, randomized trial.[8] Today, a 12-hour nitrate-free interval would probably be the appropriate dosage schedule.

DIRECT ACTING VASODILATORS

Hydralazine

Hydralazine (Apresoline), a drug that has been in and out of favor over the years and was firmly in favor at the time of the first edition of this book (1980), now once again seems to be on the wane. Other vasodilators, such as the calcium antagonists and α-blockers, are superior to hydralazine in hypertension. **Nonetheless, hydralazine is cheap and is still widely used as a third-line agent in hypertension after diuretics and β-blockade. The observation that tolerance occurs during prolonged hydralazine therapy of CHF**[31] **has limited its use in that condition.** Thus, after 9 months of therapy for CHF, tolerance to hydralazine was a specific tachyphylaxis with a maintained response to nitroprusside. Despite these caveats, combined vasodilator treatment of CHF with two drugs (hydralazine and nitrates), both thought to induce tolerance, did achieve long-term benefit.[8]

Pharmacologic Effects. Hydralazine is predominantly an arteriolar dilator and may also have some indirect positive inotropic effect.[24] It causes a marked increase in cardiac output with little or no decrease in pulmonary wedge or right atrial pressures (Fig. 5–4). In healthy subjects, the arteriolar vasodilation causes a reflex tachycardia, but in CHF hydralazine causes little change in the heart rate, perhaps because the failure dampens reflex arcs.[5] Hydralazine is particularly effective in patients with mitral regurgitation. It increases forward stroke volume and decreases regurgitant volume.[6]

Pharmacokinetics. Hydralazine is rapidly absorbed from the gut (peak concentration 1–2 hours). The plasma half-life is 2 to 8 hours, but the hypotensive effect is long-lasting, possibly because hydralazine is taken up avidly by the arterial wall. It is metabolized via acetylation in the liver with subsequent excretion in the urine. In severe renal failure, the dosage should be reduced. Patients with fast acetylation rates need a dose about 25% higher than those with slow rates. Lupus syndrome is more likely to develop in slow acetylators.

Dose and Indications. In **chronic LV failure**, oral hydralazine (50–75 mg every 6 hours, top dose 800 mg/day) is effective for at least 4 to 6 weeks when added to digoxin and diuretics.[16] Longer term benefit is doubtful[31] unless the drug is combined with nitrates.[8] With high doses the risk of lupus must be weighed against possible benefits. Use of hydralazine is particularly well tested in **severe aortic or mitral regurgitation**.

In **dilated cardiomyopathy**, hydralazine therapy leads to a regression of myocardial cellular hypertrophy,[47] perhaps because of the dominant unloading effect.

In **mild to moderate hypertension**, the usual dose is 50 to 75 mg every 6 to 8 hours, but two divided doses a day are equally effective. In **experimental myocardial hypertrophy of hypertension**, hydralazine can bring down the pressure without causing regression of the hypertrophy, presumably because of the partial inotropic effect or the reflex stimulation of the adrenergic nervous system.

In **pregnancy with pre-eclampsia**, IV hydralazine 40 mg can be infused by itself or with diazepam 40 mg (both in 500 ml) to keep the blood pressure below 160/90 mm Hg. Hydralazine is said to improve uterine blood flow, but data are scant. **Dihydralazine** (Nepresol) frequently is used as 6.25 to 12.5 mg IV slowly or infused at 0.1 mg/min to a total of 25 mg. This use is being supplanted by sublingual nifedipine.

In **sinus bradycardia**, hydralazine is one of the options to increase the heart rate.[63]

In **heart failure following cardiac surgery**, hydralazine (test dose 2.5–5.0 mg IV, up to 7.5 mg every 4 to 6 hours) generally gives improvement within 8 hours.[41]

The intramuscular use of dihydralazine or hydralazine unfortunately still occurs but must be avoided because variable rates of absorption may cause unpredictable hypotension with dangerous end-organ underperfusion.

Side-effects. Side-effects include fluid retention (renin release) that may necessitate diuretic therapy. In hypertension, the direct inotropic effect and the tachycardia limit the usefulness of hydralazine in patients with angina pectoris not on b-blockade. In contrast, in CHF reflex tachycardia is unusual, perhaps because reflex arcs are blunted. The lupus syndrome is rare with doses below 200 mg a day or with total doses below 100 g. Patients on higher doses or prolonged therapy should be checked for antinuclear factors. Headache, nausea, and abdominal pain are not unusual at the start of therapy. Postural hypotension is occasionally seen in patients with CHF. Polyneuropathy (usually responsive to pyridoxin) and drug fever are rare side-effects.

Combination of Hydralazine With Other Agents. In hypertension, hydralazine is best combined with β-blockade (to avoid headache, tachycardia, angina) and diuretics (to avoid fluid retention). In heart failure, long-term combination with isosorbide dinitrate reduces the mortality rate.[8]

Minoxidil

Minoxidil (Loniten) is a powerful arteriolar vasodilator acting by potassium channel opening with potentially serious side-effects, seldom used except in the therapy of **resistant hypertension;** even then, there are now so many other effective agents that the risk of hirsutism or rare pericardial disease seems not worthwhile, unless other vasodilators have failed. Minoxidil can be more effective than hydralazine.[23] Acting differently from the calcium antagonists, it may be combined with them and an α-blocker for maximum vasodilator therapy for severe hypertension. Concomitant β-blockade is required to reduce tachycardia, and diuretics are required to avoid fluid retention. In CHF, controlled studies failed to demonstrate any improvement in maximum oxygen consumption and exercise tolerance, despite increased cardiac output in monoxidil-treated patients.[17] Furthermore, almost all patients developed edema and required increased diuretics. Thus, minoxidil has little value in the management of chronic CHF. The **oral dose** for hypertension is up to 40 mg/day (usually once daily; sometimes twice daily doses are required in severe hypertension). There is renal excretion without hepatic metabolism, and the biologic half-life is 1 to 4 days.

Diazoxide

Diazoxide is now only very occasionally used as IV emergency treatment of hypertensive crises, and its use is being replaced by IV labetalol or sublingual nifedipine. Controlled infusions (5 mg/kg at 15 mg/min) are safest. The hypotensive effect may be excessive. Chronic oral treatment may cause diabetes mellitus, fluid retention, and vascular tolerance.

α-RECEPTOR ANTAGONISTS

Two types of α-receptors have been defined—the presynaptic α_2-receptors and the post-synaptic or vascular α_1-receptors. Sustained α_1-blockade may lead to tolerance, especially with prazosin.[25] This tolerance may in part depend on the complexity of the feedback loops, whereby unimpaired α_2-receptor stimulation inhibits the release of NE from the terminal adrenergic neurons. Presently the major use of these agents is against hypertension and not chronic heart failure. Besides presynaptic α_2-receptors, there are postsynaptic α_2-receptors that may permit vasoconstriction via a process inhibited by calcium antagonists; no specific α_2-receptor blockers are yet available for clinical use.

Prazosin

Prazosin (Minipress) is widely used in the therapy of hypertension, both in combination with diuretics-β-blockers and as monotherapy. A specific attraction is the favorable effect on the lipid profile (see

Table 10-2). During chronic therapy the dose may have to be increased, possibly the result of tachyphylaxis. In CHF, prazosin is one of the agents that can be used acutely, but the long-term effect is similar to that of placebo.

Pharmacology. Prazosin dilates both peripheral arterial and venous systems, thus acting as an "oral nitroprusside" to decrease the blood pressure, to reduce the preload, and to increase the cardiac output. The venous effects may account for first-dose syncope, unless a low dose is used. Arteriolar dilation should cause a reflex tachycardia, yet for some reason the heart rate rises little in hypertension or in CHF, so for a given fall of blood pressure prazosin produces less increase in the cardiac output than does nitroprusside, so that a negative inotropic effect has been suspected.[30] Besides blocking the post-synaptic α_1-receptors, prazosin may also decrease release of epinephrine by peripheral and central mechanisms.[75]

Pharmacokinetics. Prazosin has to be given orally and is well absorbed. The plasma half-life is 3 to 4 hours, yet the antihypertensive effect is prolonged. Although 3x daily doses are conventional, 2x daily doses suffice. Prazosin can be used in renal failure because renal blood flow is not altered, and the drug is chiefly excreted in the feces. Substantial first-pass liver metabolism indicates the need for caution in patients with liver disease.

Dose. The initial dose should be low and taken at night (2 mg for heart failure, 0.5 or 1 mg for hypertension); then 2x daily (previously, 3x daily was recommended). As the dose is worked up to a maximum of 20 mg/day, 1 mg, then 2 mg, then 5 mg tablets 2x daily is convenient. There is no evidence that 30 mg daily gives a better response than 20 mg. Sharp increases in the dose may cause syncope.

Side-effects. First-dose syncope may be due to decreased preload and is especially likely when there is no LV failure or during co-therapy with nitrates or potent diuretics. Chronic postural dizziness is a less frequent side-effect. Several double-blind studies show that prazosin is not effective in the long-term therapy of CHF.[2,8,34] If the clinical response appears inadequate or blunted, there are several practical approaches, such as changing to an ACE inhibitor (because prazosin can activate the angiotensin-renin system[9]) or giving prazosin intermittently or in alternation with other vasodilators. Diuretic doses may need reduction if the LV filling pressure becomes too low. Conversely, weight gain and edema may call for more diuretics.

Tachyphylaxis has now also been described in the therapy of hypertension[25] and may explain why upward adjustment of the dose of prazosin is so frequently needed.

Non-specific side-effects include drowsiness, lack of energy, nasal congestion, depression, and occasional retrograde ejaculation. Tachycardia is usually not common but in some patients can be troublesome. Positive antinuclear factors may develop without clinical lupus.

Combination With Other Agents. In hypertension, prazosin may be combined with β-blockers or with centrally acting agents such as methyldopa and clonidine. Fluid and sodium retention may necessitate the addition of diuretics. Prazosin is sometimes used together with other vasodilators, such as hydralazine, nifedipine, and verapamil. There may be an added interaction between prazosin and calcium antagonists so that excess or added hypotension results.[21,35] In patients with angina and ischemic heart disease, both nitrates and prazosin may cause syncope so that combinations require care; prazosin plus β-blockers or verapamil may be better therapy. In CHF, prazosin in combination with the ACE inhibitors can produce better hemodynamic and clinical effects at the risk of enhanced hypotension.

New α_1-blockers

Terazosin (Hytrin), now available in the USA, is similar in kinetic properties to prazosin (see Tables 7-1 and 7-2).

Doxazosin (Cardura), available in Europe, is a long-acting agent with a half-life of 11 to 13 hours, which can be given once daily. It is claimed to have minimal effect on plasma renin activity.[79]

Labetalol

This β-antagonist agent (Trandate, Normodyne)(see Table 1-2) with added α-antagonist activity is a vasodilatory β-blocker well documented in the use of hypertension. It acts much more rapidly than pure β-blockade in the therapy of acute hypertension (see Table 7-3), even though the α-antagonist activity is much less than the β-antagonist activity. There is not enough α-antagonism for the management of intense α-adrenergic activity, as in some patients with pheochromocytoma or clonidine withdrawal, although labetalol is not contraindicated in pheochromocytoma as are other β-blockers. Labetalol may have a special role in the treatment of black hypertensives who require vasodilation in addition to β-blockade, and for the acute control of severe pregnancy hypertension.

Indoramin

This α_1-blocking agent (Barotec in UK; Wydora in Germany) seems to have a different spectrum of side-effects[42] than prazosin, with more prominent sedation, dizziness, and dry mouth, and less first-dose syncope. These potential differences, however, are not well documented.

Phentolamine

Phentolamine specifically blocks both α_1- and α_2-adrenoceptors, especially the α_2-receptors. Release of NE from the terminal neurons could account for the tachycardia and inotropic effect. In low-output LV failure, large IV doses are required (10 to 20 mg/kg/min) for continuous vasodilation at high expense. Phentolamine is now used only in hypertensive crises when there is excess sympathetic α-stimulation as in pheochromocytoma, clonidine withdrawal, or excess use of sympathomimetic agents, or when breakdown of NE by monoamine oxidase (MAO) is inhibited (hypertensive crisis caused by MAO inhibitors).

Phenoxybenzamine

Phenoxybenzamine is a powerful α-blocking agent with a slow mode of action but with long-lasting effects, used chiefly in the management of pheochromocytoma. The IV dose is 15 to 40 mg given slowly or up to 100 mg. The solution should be freshly diluted and clear.

CALCIUM ANTAGONISTS

Although these agents are strictly vasodilators, they differ from α-blockers and direct vasodilators by being effective in angina, in which hydralazine is contraindicated. They also have a mild diuretic effect, so that co-administration of diuretics is not required so often. They differ from nitrates by being afterload reducers and much more effective for hypertension.

In **CHF**, the calcium antagonists are not generally used because of the potential negative inotropic effect. For example, one-third of patients may deteriorate in response to nifedipine, presumably because the negative inotropic effect is not adequately controlled by peripheral vasodilation.[14] The new calcium antagonist, **felodipine**,[45] appears to be a potent vasodilator and improves cardiac function significantly, even in the presence of severe heart failure; further experience will be required to establish its value. **Presently calcium antagonists should be considered chiefly in patients with mild to moderate heart failure associated with angina or hypertension**.

OTHER VASODILATORS

Adrenergic Blockers

Guanethidine. This agent blocks postganglion sympathetic but not parasympathetic transmission and causes hypotension that is mainly postural. The initial dose is 10 to 20 mg/day; usual dose 50 to 75 mg/day, up to 400 mg/day. Onset of action is 2 to 3 days. Hypertensive crises used to be managed with 10 to 20 mg given intramuscularly or slowly intravenously. **Clonidine** and **methyldopa** stimulate the central α_2-receptors to inhibit the peripheral release of NE and could theoretically be useful in CHF besides their established use in hypertension.

Trimethaphan. Trimethaphan blocks both sympathetic and parasympathetic ganglionic transmission and is largely used for controlling surgical hypertension and in the management of **aortic dissection** (infusion starts at 3 mg/min) because of the rapidity of onset and cessation of action.

Furosemide (≈ Frusemide). Furosemide (Lasix), when injected intravenously in standard doses, can rapidly improve the acute pulmonary edema (in patients with AMI, even before there is an increase in urinary output[6]). The probable mechanism of this early effect is venodilation. In chronic CHF, LV function may transiently deteriorate as plasma renin activity increases following IV furosemide[18] to limit the early benefit (for dose, see Table 4-2).

Phosphodiesterase Inhibitors. The phosphodiesterase inhibitors **amrinone**, **milrinone**, **enoximone**, and **pimobendan** (see Chap. 6) act in CHF largely by peripheral vasodilation, although they also have a direct inotropic effect, being inotropic dilators. Acutely, both these agents work well; during prolonged therapy, efficacy seems to fall and side-effects may arise.

NEW MODES OF VASODILATION

β-Adrenergic Agonists

The β-agonists act on the vascular receptors to cause peripheral vasodilation. Their direct cardiac effect makes them unsuitable for use in hypertension. Dobutamine and dopamine (see Figs. 6-3 and 6-4) may owe part of their beneficial effect in heart failure to β-mediated vasodilation. The following β-agonists are under assessment:

Salbutamol (= albuterol in the USA; Ventolin; Proventil) is a selective β_2-agonist chiefly used as a bronchodilator. (Its use as a vasodilator is investigational in the USA.) It improves indices of contractility when infused (0.5 mg/min/kg) into patients with congestive cardiomyopathy who have already received digitalis and diuretics.[39] Thus it is potentially useful, especially in patients with CHF and obstructive lung disease. In patients with myocardial infarction and severe LV failure, IV salbutamol may improve cardiac output, although the heart rate rises only slightly.

Xamoterol (Corwin, available in Europe) is another combined β-stimulator-blocker with predominant stimulant properties. Xamoterol is, however, β₁-specific, thus being a pure inotropic agent and not a vasodilator. In the UK it is approved for use in mild CHF, but contraindicated in severe heart failure. (See Chap. 1, Ref. 82.)

Other New Vasodilators

Dopamine Receptor Stimulators. These agents are now becoming available in oral form and may have the special advantage of prominent renal vasodilation with little or no effect on the heart rate. **Fenoldopam** is a dopamine₁-agonist, able to reduce blood pressure in severe hypertension with a sodium diuresis, in contrast to sodium nitroprusside, which causes sodium retention.[55]

Serotonin Antagonists. The prototype of these agents is **ketanserin**, known to be an antihypertensive agent. Ketanserin, despite its serotonin-S₂-receptor antagonism and marked antiplatelet activity, was unable to improve claudication distance and ankle systolic pressure in a massive recent trial.[69] Ketanserin, in addition, has α₁-antagonist activity and prolongs the action potential duration so that it should not be given together with diuretic therapy.

Atrial natriuretic peptide (= atrial natriuretic factor: ANP or ANF). This is the peptide that is secreted by the cardiac atria in response to volume distension. It is the natural hypovolemic agent, which acts on the renal vasculature to cause a powerful vasodilation and diuresis. Thus the polyuria frequently associated with paroxysmal supraventricular tachycardia can be explained. ANP acts on vascular cells to produce vasodilatory cyclic GMP. ANP therapy is likely to be of limited benefit in CHF because levels of ANP are already high and downgrading of ANP receptors may also occur.

Flosequinan. This is a direct-acting vasodilator, with both arteriolar and venodilating properties. It decreases pulmonary and systemic venous pressures and increases cardiac output in CHF. With long duration of action, it benefits both acute and chronic heart failure.[73] Long-term efficacy needs to be established.

CHOICE OF VASODILATOR

Until the factors regulating exercise tolerance in CHF are better understood, choosing the most appropriate agent is to some extent a pragmatic procedure. Nonetheless, ACE inhibitors seem likely better to counter the overall metabolic-hormonal abnormalities in severe heart failure, whereas nitrates seem likely better to reduce pulmonary congestion, and afterload reducers such as hydralazine or ACE inhibitors may be best to improve renal blood flow. As ACE inhibitors provide some theoretical advantages over other vasodilators, these agents should be considered as the next step after diuretic therapy. Their superiority to prazosin is particularly well documented.[2,8,34] Patients who develop hypotension may benefit from other vasodilators, such as a combination of an arteriolar dilator (hydralazine) and a venodilator (nitrates) with documented long-term benefit,[8] or may require inotropic support. A reasonable short-term alternate therapy is prazosin, which acutely benefits many patients with heart failure, especially if overdiuresis is avoided. Intermittent nocturnal nitrates may improve nocturnal dyspnea. In contrast, intermittent dobutamine can no longer be considered acceptable. **It needs to be emphasized that there is accumulating evidence that vasodilator therapy improves the prognosis of patients with chronic heart failure**.

End-Stage Heart Failure

Special management may be required in this condition, when the myocardium is largely destroyed and, in addition, the number of β-adrenoceptor sites falls, probably as a result of prolonged excessive and increasing adrenergic stimulation as the CHF intensifies, so that the receptors become "downgraded." To restore the number of binding sites, circulating catecholamines must be diminished, as can theoretically be achieved by vasodilator therapy (especially ACE inhibition), while sympathomimetic stimulation is avoided. Recently, carefully given low-dose β-antagonists have been used to up-regulate the β-receptors in an attempt to improve CHF. Logically, mixed β-agonists-antagonists may be novel and desirable therapy. However, xamoterol therapy was associated with increased deaths in severe CHF, so that it is indicated in the UK only for mild CHF. **In general, vasodilator therapy earlier in the course of CHF could be an advantage in avoiding end-stage heart failure, although there are no firm data to support this proposal**.

SUMMARY

ACE inhibitors, in contrast to other vasodilators, act directly on the renin-angiotensin axis. Initially used only in refractory cases of hypertension and CHF, they are now employed earlier and earlier in those conditions, especially with the emergence of much safer, new low-dose regimes for captopril and the development of structurally different compounds, such as enalapril, lisinopril, and many others. The major side-effect of ACE inhibitors is excess hypotension. The major contraindications are pre-existing hypotension or severe renal impairment or (in the case of captopril) collagen vascular disease. The major danger is renal impairment, especially when hypotension occurs in the presence of pre-existing renal damage, as in severe heart failure or renal artery stenosis (particularly when bilateral). Perhaps unexpectedly, ACE inhibitors ameliorate early renal damage as found, for example, in diabetic subjects. When compared with diuretics, they have a much more favorable metabolic profile, particularly in relation to indices of glucose impairment and lipid abnormalities. A major advantage of ACE inhibitors is that they favorably modify the basic neurohumoral abnormalities in CHF, thus representing a distinct advantage over traditional vasodilators. In mild to moderate hypertension, the major advantage of ACE inhibitors is the absence of side-effects—such as fatigue, mental or sexual impairment, or exercise limitation—so that a feeling of well-being is usual. However, cough can be a troublesome side-effect.

In hypertension, there are many alternative vasodilators, including the calcium antagonists, the α_1-adrenergic blockers, the non-specific agents such as hydralazine, and the potassium channel openers, such as minoxidil, cromakalim, and pinacidil. The choice between these agents is to some extent a matter of physician preference and to some extent a question of patient profiling (see Chap. 7).

In CHF, the only vasodilators thus far well tested, besides the ACE inhibitors, are nitrates combined with hydralazine. Agents such as milrinone should be considered as combined vasodilator-inotropic agents. Among the newer vasodilators, flosequinan appears to be promising.

REFERENCES

References from Previous Editions

1. Bauer JH, Jones LB: Am J Kidney Dis 4:55–62, 1984
2. Bayliss J, Canepa-Anson R, Norell MS, et al: Br Heart J 55:265–273, 1986
3. Bender W, La France N, Walker WG: Hypertension 6(suppl I):I-193–I-197, 1984

4. Captopril Multicenter Research Group: J Am Coll Cardiol 2:755–763, 1983
5. Chatterjee K, Massie B, Rubin S, et al: Am J Med 65:134–145, 1978
6. Chatterjee K, Parmley WW: J Am Coll Cardiol 1:133–153, 1983
7. Cleland JGF, Dargie HJ, Ball SG, et al: Br Heart J 54:305–312, 1985
8. Cohn JN, Archibald DG, Ziesche S, et al: N Engl J Med 314:1547–1552, 1986
9. Colucci WS: Ann Intern Med 97:67–77, 1982
10. Cooper WD, Doyle GD, Donohoe J, et al: J Hypertens 3(suppl 3):S471–S474, 1985
11. Creager MA, Faxon DP, Cutler SS, et al: J Am Coll Cardiol 7:758–765, 1986
12. Croog SH, Levine S, Testa MA, et al: N Engl J Med 314:1657–1664, 1986
13. DiCarlo L, Chatterjee K, Parmley WW, et al: J Am Coll Cardiol 2:865–871, 1983
14. Elkayam U, Weber L, Torkan B, et al: Am J Cardiol 52:1041–1045, 1983
15. Ferguson RK, Turini GA, Brunner HR, et al: Lancet 1:775–778, 1977
16. Fitchett DM, Marin JA, Oakley CM, et al: Am J Cardiol 44:303–309, 1979
17. Franciosa JA, Jordan RA, Wilen MM, et al: Circulation 70:63–68, 1984
18. Francis GS, Siegel RM, Goldsmith SR, et al: Ann Intern Med 10:1–6, 1985
19. Frohlich ED, Cooper RA, Lewis EJ: Arch Intern Med 144:1441–1444, 1984
20. Jaffe IA: Am J Med 80:471–476, 1986
21. Jee LD, Opie LH: Br Med J 287:1514–1516, 1983
22. Jenkins AC, Dreslinski GR, Tadros SS, et al: J Cardiovasc Pharmacol 7:S96–S101, 1985
23. Johnson BF, Black HR, Beckner R, et al: J Hypertens 1:103–107, 1983
24. Khatri I, Uemara N, Notargiacomo A, et al: Am J Cardiol 40:38–42, 1977
25. Khatri IM, Levinson P, Notargiacomo A, et al: Am J Cardiol 55:1015–1018, 1985
26. LeJemtel TH, Maskin CS, Mancini D, et al: Circulation 72:364–369, 1985
27. Mettauer B, Rouleau J-L, Bichet D, et al: Circulation 73:492–502, 1986
28. Myers BD, Moran SM: N Engl J Med 314:97–105, 1986
29. Navis GJ, De Jong PE, Kallenberg CGM, et al: Lancet 1:1017, 1984
30. Packer M, Meller J, Gorlin R, et al: Am J Cardiol 44:310–317, 1979
31. Packer M, Meller J, Medina N, et al: N Engl J Med 306:57–62, 1982
32. Packer M, Medina N, Yushak M: J Am Coll Cardiol 3:1035–1043, 1984
33. Packer M, Medina N, Yushak M, et al: Am Heart J 109:1293–1299, 1985
34. Packer M, Lee WH, Medina N, et al: J Am Coll Cardiol 7:70A, 1986
35. Pasanisi F, Elliott HL, Meredith PA, et al: Clin Pharmacol Ther 36:716–723, 1984
36. Reyes AJ, Leary WP, Acosta-Barrios TN: J Cardiovasc Pharmacol 7:S16–S19, 1985
37. Salvetti A, Pedrinelli R, Magagna A, et al: J Cardiovasc Pharmacol 7:S25–S29, 1985
38. Schwartz JB, Taylor A, Abernethy D, et al: J Cardiovasc Pharmacol 7:767–776, 1985
39. Sharma B, Goodwin JF: Circulation 58:449–460, 1978
40. Sharpe DN, Murphy J, Coxon R, et al: Circulation 70:271–278, 1984
41. Sladen RN, Rosenthal MH: J Thorac Cardiovasc Surg 78:195–202, 1979
42. Stannard M, Cohen M, Marrott PK, et al: J Cardiovasc Pharmacol 8(suppl 2):S48–S52, 1986
43. Sweet CS, Ulm EH: New Drugs Ann: Cardiovasc Drugs 2:1–17, 1984
44. Taguma Y, Kitamoto Y, Futaki G, et al: N Engl J Med 313:1617–1620, 1985
45. Timmis AD, Jewitt DE: Drugs 29(suppl 2):66–75, 1985
46. Tschollar W, Belz GG: Lancet 2:34–35, 1985
47. Unverferth DV, Mehegan JP, Magorien RD, et al: Am J Cardiol 51:1392–1398, 1983
48. Webster J, Newnham DM, Petrie JC: Br Med J 290:1623–1624, 1985
49. Witzgall H, Hirsch F, Scherer B: Clin Sci 62:611–615, 1982

New References

50. Belz GG, Essig J, Erb K, et al: Pharmacokinetic and pharmacodynamic interactions between the ACE inhibitor cilazapril and β-adrenoceptor antagonist propranolol in healthy subjects and in hypertensive patients. Br J Clin Pharmacol 27:317S–322S, 1989
51. Brilla CG, Kramer B, Hoffmeister HM, et al: Low-dose enalapril in severe chronic heart failure. Cardiovasc Drugs Ther 3:211–218, 1989
52. Chalmers JP, West MJ, Cyran J, et al: Placebo-controlled study of lisinopril in congestive heart failure: A multicentre study. J Cardiovasc Pharmacol 9(suppl 3):S89–S97, 1987

53. Consensus Trial Study Group: Effects of enalapril on mortality in severe congestive heart failure: Results of the Cooperative North Scandinavian Enalapril Survival Study (CONSENSUS). N Engl J Med 316:1429–1435, 1987

54. Dzau V, Hollenberg N: Renal response to captopril in severe heart failure: Role of frusemide in natriuresis and reversal of hyponatremia. Ann Intern Med 6:777–782, 1984

55. Elliott WJ, Weber RR, Nelson KS, et al: Renal and hemodynamic effects of intravenous fenoldopam versus nitroprusside in severe hypertension. Circulation 81:970–977, 1990

56. Ferner RE, Simpson JM, Rawlins MD: Effects of intradermal bradykinin after inhibition of angiotensin converting enzyme. Br Med J 294:1119–1120, 1987

57. Flapan AD, Shaw TRD, Stewart S, et al: Duration of endocrine and haemodynamic effects of enalapril and captopril in heart failure. Br Heart J 57:82–83, 1987

58. Fleckenstein A, Fleckenstein–Grun G, Frey M, Zorn J: Calcium antagonism and ACE inhibition: Two outstandingly effective means of interference with cardiovascular calcium overload, high blood pressure, and arteriosclerosis in spontaneously hypertensive rats. Am J Hypertens 2:194–204, 1989

59. Gadsboll N, Hoilund-Carlsen P-F, Badsberg JS, et al: Late ventricular dilatation in survivors of acute myocardial infarction. Am J Cardiol 64:961–966, 1989

60. Gheorghiade M, Hall V, Lakier JB, Goldstein S: Comparative hemodynamic and neurohumoral effects of intravenous captopril and digoxin and their combinations in patients with severe heart failure. J Am Coll Cardiol 13:134–142, 1989

61. Harris P: Congestive cardiac failure: Central role of the arterial blood pressure. Br Heart J 58:190–203, 1987

62. Levy WS, Katz RJ, Buff L, Wasserman AG: Nitroglycerin tolerance is modified by angiotensin converting enzyme inhibitors (abstract). Circulation 80(suppl II):II-214, 1989

63. Lewis BS, Rozenman Y, Merdler A, et al: Chronotropic effect of hydralazine and its mechanism in symptomatic sinus bradycardia. Am J Cardiol 59:93–96, 1987

64. Lichter I, Richardson PJ, Wyke MA: Differential effects of atenolol and enalapril on memory during treatment for essential hypertension. Br J Clin Pharmacol 21:641–645, 1986

65. McEwan JR, Choudry NB, Fuller RW: A role for prostaglandins in angiotensin converting enzyme inhibitor cough (abstract). Circulation 80(suppl II):II-128, 1989

66. Mimran A, Insua A, Ribstein J, et al: Contrasting effects of captopril and nifedipine in normotensive patients with incipient diabetic nephropathy. J Hypertens 6:919–923, 1988

67. Nishimura H, Kubo S, Ueyama M, et al: Peripheral hemodynamic effects of captopril in patients with congestive heart failure. Am Heart J 117:100–105, 1989

68. Odemuyiwa O, Gilmartin J, Kenny D, Hall RJC: Captopril and the diuretic requirements in moderate and severe chronic heart failure. Eur Heart J 10:586–590, 1989

69. PACK Claudication Substudy Investigators: Randomized placebo-controlled, double-blind trial of ketanserin in claudicants: Changes in claudication distance and ankle systolic pressure. Circulation 80:1544–1548, 1989

70. Pfeffer MA, Lamas GA, Vaughan DE, et al: Effect of captopril on progressive ventricular dilatation after anterior myocardial infarction. N Engl J Med 319:80–86, 1988

71. Pollare T, Lithell H, Berne C: A comparison of the effects of hydrochlorothiazide and captopril on glucose and lipid metabolism in patients with hypertension. N Engl J Med 321:868–873, 1989

72. Raya TE, Gay RG, Aguirre M, Goldman S: Importance of venodilatation in prevention of left ventricular dilatation after chronic large myocardial infarction in rats: A comparison of captopril and hydralazine. Circ Res 64:330–337, 1989

73. Remme WJ: Vasodilator therapy without converting-enzyme inhibition in congestive heart failure—usefulness and limitations. Cardiovasc Drugs Ther 3:375–396, 1989

74. Richardson A, Bayliss J, Scriven AJ, et al: Double-blind comparison of captopril alone against frusemide plus amiloride in mild heart failure. Lancet 2:709–711, 1987

75. Riegger GAJ, Haeske W, Kraus C, et al: Contribution of the renin–angiotensin–aldosterone system to development of tolerance and fluid retention in chronic congestive heart failure during prazosin treatment. Am J Cardiol 59:906–910, 1987

76. Salvetti A, Arzilli F: Chronic dose–response curve of enalapril in essential hypertensives. An Italian Multicenter Study. Am J Hypertens 2:352–354, 1989

77. Sassano P, Chatellier G, Billaud E, et al: Comparison of increase in the enalapril dose and addition of hydrochlorothiazide as second-step treatment of hypertensive patients not controlled by enalapril alone. J Cardiovasc Pharmacol 13:314–319, 1989

78. Sharpe N, Murphy J, Smith H, Hannan S: Treatment of patients with symptomless left ventricular dysfunction after myocardial infarction. Lancet 1:255–259, 1988

79. Shionoiri H, Yasuda G, Yoshimura H, et al: Antihypertensive effects and pharmacokinetics of single and consecutive administration of doxazosin in patients with mild to moderate essential hypertension. J Cardiovasc Pharmacol 10:90–95, 1987

Reviews

80. Uretsky BF: Pharmacologic therapy for congestive heart failure: Lessons from the 1980's, issues for the 1990's. American College of Cardiology, Learning Center Highlights 5:11–18, 1990

81. Williams GH: Converting-enzyme inhibitors in the treatment of hypertension. N Engl J Med 319:1517–1525, 1988

F.I. Marcus
L.H. Opie
E.H. Sonnenblick

6

Digitalis and Other Inotropes

"The good news for now is that digoxin can be used with greater confidence in its efficacy."[98]

DIGITALIS

Role of Digitalis in Congestive Heart Failure (CHF)

In CHF, the aim of therapy is to alleviate present and future symptoms and, hopefully, to prevent progression of the primary disease that has caused the symptoms, so that ultimately mortality is decreased—an aim not yet demonstrated for digitalis. Nonetheless, digitalis compounds, together with diuretics, remain the basis of the therapy for CHF, a role increasingly shared with the ACE inhibitors which, in some European countries, have now come to replace digitalis as second-line therapy

Digitalis has three main effects: (1) the heart rate is slowed, especially when there is atrial fibrillation, so that ventricular filling is improved; (2) there is a positive inotropic effect; and (3) there is the recently described sympatholytic effect (Fig. 6–1). The bradycardic effect is universally regarded as beneficial unless there is digitalis toxicity; the inotropic effect has potential for both harm (increasing the work of the heart and the oxygen demand in the face of myocardial disease) and benefit (decreasing the heart size and heart rate, both of which will decrease myocardial oxygen demand). The decrease in heart size may help prevent progressive ventricular dilation. **The combined inotropic-bradycardic action of digitalis is unique when compared to the many sympathomimetic inotropes, which all tend to cause tachycardia.** Furthermore, no sympathomimetics are currently approved for oral use in the USA. Therefore digitalis, whatever its defects, remains the basic inotrope, despite the narrow therapeutic-toxic margin and the "intensifying myriad of interactions."[50]

Digitalis Versus ACE Inhibitors for CHF

The separate and combined effects of digitalis and captopril in patients with CHF already receiving diuretics have been studied.[85] To achieve marked improvements in hemodynamics at rest and during exercise, both digitalis and captopril needed to be added to the diuretic. When compared with enalapril in patients receiving diuretics, digoxin was at least as effective as the ACE inhibitor and had a lower adverse reaction profile.[76]

129

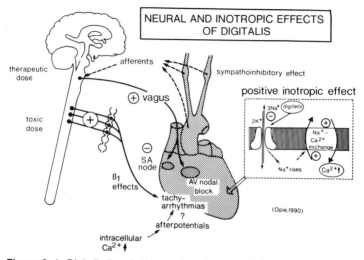

Figure 6–1. Digitalis has both neural and myocardial cellular effects. The inotropic effect of digitalis is due to inhibition of the sodium pump in myocardial cells. Slowing of the heart rate and inhibition of the atrioventricular node is by vagal stimulation (a direct effect on nodal tissue may also play a role). Vagal stimulation also may account for the decreased sympathetic nerve discharge, an important therapeutic benefit. Toxic arrhythmias are less well understood, but may be caused by a combination of sympathomimetic stimulation ($\beta_1 = \beta_1$ adrenoceptor stimulation) and the development of calcium-dependent afterpotentials.

Pharmacologic Properties of Digitalis

Structure. All cardiac glycosides share an aglycone ring wherein the pharmacologic activity resides, usually combined with one to four molecules of sugar, which modify the pharmacokinetic properties. Digoxin is a polar compound with an OH group binding to the steroid nucleus, whereas digitoxin is non-polar, with lesser central nervous penetration.

Mechanism of Action. The myocardial cellular effect of digitalis occurs when it binds to the sarcolemmal receptor, which is the sodium pump (Na/K-ATPase); digitalis inhibits this pump.[1] The result is an enhanced transient increase in intracellular sodium close to the sarcolemma, which in turn enhances calcium influx by the sodium-calcium exchange mechanism, so that an increased cytosolic calcium ion concentration results.[39] The result is enhanced myocardial contractility.

The **autonomic nervous system** is involved in both the therapeutic and toxic effects of digitalis. Parasympathetic activation results in two therapeutic effects—sinus slowing and atrioventricular (AV) nodal inhibition. Thus the inhibitory effect on the AV node depends partly on the degree of vagal tone, which varies from person to person.[37] An ill-understood direct depression of nodal tissue may account for those effects of digitalis still found after vagal blockade.[26]

Sympathetic inhibition may play an important role in the effects of digitalis in CHF. Digitalis inhibits muscle sympathetic nerve activity, an effect that occurs before any observed hemodynamic changes. A similar effect could not be achieved by dobutamine infusion.[82]

In contrast, part of the toxic effects of digoxin are explained by sympathomimetic effects (site of action near the floor of the fourth ventricle), which probably act together with intracellular calcium overload to cause the toxic arrhythmias.

The **hemodynamic effects** of IV digoxin were first described in a classic paper by McMichael and Sharpey-Schafer,[53] who showed that acute digitalization improved cardiac output and heart failure. The

TABLE 6–1 DIGOXIN PHARMACOKINETICS

1. 75% of oral dose rapidly absorbed; rest inactivated in lower gut to digoxin reduction products by bacteria.
2. Circulates in blood, unbound to plasma proteins; "therapeutic level" 1–2 ng/mL; blood half-life about 36 hr.
3. Binds to tissue receptors in heart and skeletal muscle.
4. Lipid-soluble; brain penetration.
5. Most of absorbed digoxin excreted unchanged in urine (tubular excretion and glomerular filtration). About 25% undergoes non-renal clearance.
6. In chronic renal failure, reduced volume of distribution.
7. With small lean body mass, reduced total binding to skeletal muscle.

fall in the venous pressure they found is probably best explained by a decreased sympathetic drive as heart failure improves; the direct effect of digitalis on peripheral veins and arteries is mild vasoconstriction (increase of intracellular calcium). The action of digitalis on AV conduction, which it slows, and on the AV refractory period, which it prolongs, is dependent primarily on vagal tone and only to a minor extent on the direct inhibitory effect of digitalis.[63] The inhibitory effect on the AV node is usually preceded by the inotropic effect; the two effects differ in their mechanisms.

Pharmacokinetics of Digoxin (Table 6-1). The serum half-life is 1.5 days. The major portion is ultimately excreted by the kidneys unchanged. About 18 to 28% is excreted by non-renal routes (stools, hepatic metabolism) in patients with normal renal function.[58] In approximately 10% of patients, intestinal bacteria convert digoxin to an inactive reduction product, dihydrodigoxin; in such patients, the blood level stays low unless the gut flora are inhibited by antibiotics such as erythromycin or tetracycline, which cause the blood digoxin levels to increase.[87] Multiple pharmacokinetic factors influence the blood level obtained with a given dose of digoxin (Tables 6-2 and 6-3). If renal function is subnormal, excretion is impaired and the maintenance dose is lower. The body weight governs the loading dose because a low skeletal mass means less binding to skeletal muscle receptors, so that the blood level for any given loading dose is higher as, for example, in a thin old man.

Dose of Digoxin. Various nomograms have been designed for calculation of the dose, taking into account lean body mass and renal function,[32,72] but none appears to be more effective than the experienced physician's intuitive estimation of the correct digoxin dosage.[34]

A **loading dose** may be required for urgent indications because a certain amount of digoxin is required to saturate the skeletal muscle receptors throughout the body and for tissue penetration until equilibrium is reached. Thus the loading dose is governed by the lean body weight (reduced in old age and severe renal insufficiency). The usual IV loading dose of digoxin is 0.75 to 1 mg which gives transient peak plasma digoxin levels as high as 95 ng/ml without toxic effects (which usually arise only when steady-state levels exceed 2 ng/ml). An oral

TABLE 6–2 CAUSES OF LOW SERUM DIGOXIN LEVEL

Dose too low or not taken.

Poor absorption
    Malabsorption, high bran diet
    Drug interference: cholestyramine, sulfasalazine, neomycin, PAS, kaolin-pectin, rifampin (= rifampicin)
    Hyperthyroidism (additional mechanisms possible)
    Enhanced intestinal conversion to inactive metabolites

Enhanced renal secretion
    Improved GFR* as vasodilator therapy enhances renal blood flow

*GFR = glomerular filtration rate.

TABLE 6–3 DRUG INTERACTIONS AND OTHER CAUSES OF HIGH SERUM DIGOXIN LEVELS

Excess initial dose for body mass (small lean body mass)

Decreased renal excretion
    Severe hypokalemia (<3 mEq/L)
    Concurrent cardiac drugs (**quinidine, verapamil, amiodarone**)
    Depressed renal blood flow (congestive heart failure, β-blockers)
    Depressed GFR (elderly patients, renal disease)

Decreased non-renal clearance
    Antiarrhythmic drugs (**quinidine, verapamil, amiodarone, propafenone**)
    Calcium antagonists (**verapamil** and possibly others)

Decreased conversion in gut to digoxin reduction products
    Destruction by antibiotics of bacteria converting digoxin to inactive
        reduction products (**erythromycin, tetracycline**)

loading dose of 1 mg produces peak blood levels of over 1 ng/ml in about 1 to 5 hours and a maximum inotropic effect at 4 to 6 hours.

Digitalization is now commonly started with multiple doses over a longer period (0.5 mg 2x daily for 2 days or 0.5 mg 3x daily for 1 day followed by 0.25 mg daily) to allow for variable gastrointestinal (GI) absorption, variable cardiac responses, and possible drug interactions. When no loading dose is given, steady-state plasma and tissue concentrations are achieved in 5 to 7 days. **Rapid digitalization** can be achieved with a combination of IV digoxin (0.5 mg IV, followed by oral digoxin 0.25 mg, one or two doses) to a total of 0.75-1.0 mg.

The usual **maintenance dose** remains 0.25 mg daily, even with a wide range of renal and hepatic function.[15] The optimal dose required varies from 0.1 to 0.75 mg daily,[30] and renal function is the most important determinant.[15] We advise a **single evening dose** to allow a steady-state situation for blood digoxin assays in the morning; timing in relation to meals is not important. Each patient's dose must be individually adjusted. Generally, the highest possible dose tolerated is no longer acceptable practice; rather the dose is adjusted according to the blood digoxin level. In **atrial fibrillation**, the aim is for a resting apical rate less than 90 beats/min and a mild post-exercise rise. In the absence of CHF, added verapamil or β-blockade may be needed (see Chap. 11).

Digitalis Indications and Contraindications

Indications. The most solid indication for digitalis is still **the combination of chronic CHF with atrial fibrillation.** It is also used for atrial fibrillation from other causes and sometimes for the treatment of acute supraventricular tachycardias. In such arrhythmias, it may be used alone or in combination with verapamil, diltiazem, or β-blocking drugs. It is preferred to these other drugs if there is heart failure. However, toxicity must be excluded prior to electrical cardioversion.

In the approach to the management of **low-output heart failure** with sinus rhythm, digitalis has gone through three phases.[88] First, it was regarded with the diuretics as essential first-line therapy. Thereafter reports on ineffectiveness or development of tolerance came in, so that its use declined, especially in the UK. More recently, the benefits of digitalis have been re-established as a result of three well-controlled blind studies. In mild to moderate CHF with ejection fractions in the range of 25 to 30%, digitalis improved and maintained exercise performance.[79] In one study, the ejection fraction increased somewhat. In the comparison with xamoterol,[84] digitalis caused minor but definite lessening of the symptoms. Since **some but not all patients with**

chronic CHF benefit from long-term digitalis therapy, the challenge for clinicians is to identify patients who will best benefit from long-term digitalization.

In **recent-onset atrial fibrillation** (less than 1 week) in patients without overt CHF, digoxin was no better than placebo in conversion to sinus rhythm.[81]

Atrial flutter may not respond to digitalis except in high doses, which induce direct atrioventricular blockade with variable degrees of AV block or conversion to atrial fibrillation. In contrast, atrial fibrillation is slowed with moderate dosage due to enhanced vagal tone and partial AV nodal inhibition.

In **mitral stenosis with sinus rhythm**, "prophylactic" digitalis is sometimes used to avoid the harmful effects of sudden atrial fibrillation and to slow the sinus rate to improve ventricular filling. However, (1) the acute onset of atrial fibrillation is usually accompanied by a rapid ventricular response despite prophylactic digitalis; and (2) the inhibitory effect on the sinus node is not very powerful and not as effective as β-blockade.

Acute left ventricular (LV) failure is generally treated by more potent inotropic drugs, such as dopamine, dobutamine, amrinone, or diuretics, before digitalis is considered. In valvular heart disease with failure, digitalization is conventionally the first line of treatment, but patients with regurgitation may do better with vasodilators.

In **children**, digitalis is preferred to diuretics as first-line treatment of heart failure even in high-output states with left or right shunts.[6] Nevertheless, its efficacy is not without dispute.[3]

Contraindications. (1) **Hypertrophic obstructive cardiomyopathy** (hypertrophic subaortic stenosis, asymmetrical septal hypertrophy) is a contraindication (unless there is atrial fibrillation and severe myocardial failure), because the inotropic effect can worsen outflow obstruction. (2) The possibility of **digitalis toxicity** is a frequent contraindication, pending a full history of digitalis dosage, renal function tests, and measurement of serum digoxin. (3) In some cases of **Wolff-Parkinson-White (WPW) syndrome**, digitalization may accelerate antegrade conduction over the bypass tract to precipitate ventricular tachycardia (VT) or ventricular fibrillation (VF);[64] expert evaluation is needed before digitalis is considered in these patients. (4) Significant **AV nodal heart block**. Intermittent complete heart block or second degree AV block may be worsened by digitalis, especially if there is a history of Stokes-Adams attacks or when conduction is likely to be unstable, as in acute myocardial infarction (AMI) or acute myocarditis. (5) **Diastolic dysfunction**, seen most notably with severe ventricular hypertrophy and characterized by a normal or high ejection fraction, nonetheless with elevated filling pressures and reduced filling rates, probably does not respond to digitalis.

Relative Contraindications. (1) If a poor response can be expected, as when low-output states are caused by valvular stenosis, in chronic pericarditis, in chronic cor pulmonale, in high-output states,[52] or when atrial fibrillation is caused by thyrotoxicosis; (2) all conditions increasing digitalis sensitivity to apparently therapeutic levels, such as hypokalemia, chronic pulmonary disease, myxedema, or acute hypoxemia; (3) early AMI and post-infarct (see p 135); (4) renal failure—a lower dose, monitoring of plasma potassium, and a watch for digitalis toxicity are needed; (5) sinus bradycardia or sick sinus syndrome—occasional patients will show a marked fall in sinus rate or sinus pauses;[61] a prolonged PR-interval is usually not a contraindication;[7] (6) combination with other drugs causing sinus bradycardia, such as β-blockers, diltiazem, amiodarone, reserpine, methyldopa, and clonidine; (7) other drugs inhibiting AV conduction (verapamil, diltiazem, β-blockers, amiodarone); here IV digoxin may be hazardous; (8) heart failure accompanying acute glomerulonephritis because renal excretion of digoxin is impaired; (9) severe

TABLE 6–4 FACTORS ALTERING SENSITIVITY TO DIGITALIS AT APPARENTLY THERAPEUTIC LEVELS

Systemic factors or disorders
    Renal failure (reduced volume of distribution and excretion)
    Low lean body mass (reduced binding to skeletal muscle)
    Chronic pulmonary disease (hypoxia, acid-base changes)
    Myxedema (? prolonged half-life)
    Acute hypoxemia (sensitizes to digitalis arrhythmias)

Electrolyte disorders
    Hypokalemia (sensitizes to toxic effects)
    Hyperkalemia (protects from digitalis arrhythmias)
    Hypomagnesemia (sensitizes to toxic effects)
    Hypercalcemia (increases sensitivity to digitalis)
    Hypocalcemia (decreases sensitivity)

Cardiac disorders
    Acute myocardial infarction (may cause increased sensitivity)
    Acute rheumatic or viral carditis (danger of conduction block)
    Thyrotoxic heart disease (decreased sensitivity)

Concomitant drug therapy
    Diuretics with K^+ loss (increased sensitivity via hypokalemia)
    Drugs with added effects on SA or AV nodes (verapamil, diltiazem,
      β-blockers, clonidine, methyldopa, or amiodarone)

myocarditis may predispose to digitalis-induced arrhythmias and decreased digitalis effect; (10) cardioversion—the digoxin level should be in the therapeutic range to avoid post-conversion ventricular arrhythmias. If digitalis toxicity is suspected, elective cardioversion should be delayed. If cardioversion is required, the energy level should be minimal at first and carefully increased.

Clinical States Altering Digitalis Activity

Digitalis in the Elderly. Dall[12] suggested that three-quarters of elderly British patients receiving digoxin did not need it; often the dose was too high, more often it was too low and compliance was poor. There is much to be said for a trial withdrawal of digitalis in the elderly unless it is obviously needed (as in atrial fibrillation with LV failure) while the patient is carefully observed for any clinical deterioration.

The pharmacokinetics of digitalis in the elderly have been well studied.[2] Digoxin absorption is delayed but not decreased. A decreased skeletal muscle and lean body mass causes increased digoxin levels (Table 6-4). The latter are also promoted by a decreasing glomerular filtration rate (GFR), especially after the fifth and sixth decades. Creatinine clearance may be substantially reduced before a rise in serum creatinine alerts the clinician. Digoxin half-life is prolonged to a mean of 73 hours in the elderly, depending on renal function. There is no solid evidence of any alteration in myocardial sensitivity or response to cardiac glycosides in older individuals.

Digoxin and Renal Function. The most important determinant of the daily digoxin dosage in all age groups is renal function (as measured by creatinine clearance or radionuclide GFR). The clinician usually relies upon measurement of the blood urea nitrogen or serum creatinine. These parameters are influenced by factors other than glomerular filtration. For example, serum creatinine may be normal in an elderly patient with a GFR that is half normal if there is a marked decrease in muscle mass, because the amount of creatinine released daily is diminished. Even the GFR provides only a rough estimate of the renal excretion of digoxin, since it is also excreted by tubular secretion. In severe renal insufficiency, there is a decrease in the volume of distribution of digoxin,[22,35] so that it is not exact to use a nomogram to estimate the maintenance dose based on creatinine clearance.[36] One practical policy is to start with a maintenance dose of 0.125 mg/day in patients with severe renal insufficiency and rely on serum digoxin levels for dose adjustment.

In less severe renal insufficiency, a "guestimate" of the digoxin dose can be made as follows: the creatinine clearance can be estimated from age, sex, body weight, and serum creatinine if direct measurement is impractical. In elderly patients with renal impairment, the following approximations hold:[56]

Creatinine clearance	Approximate digoxin dose
10–25 mL/min	0.125 mg/day
26–49 mL/min	0.1875 mg/day
50–79 mL/min	0.25 mg/day

As an example, for a 70-kg male aged 70, the "guestimated" digoxin dose is 0.25 mg for serum creatinine up to about 1.5 mg/dl (140 μmole/L) and 0.125 mg when the creatinine exceeds about 3.0 mg/dl (275 μmole/L). These values are rough approximations, stressing the important role of renal function in determining digoxin dosage. In this situation, nothing can improve on regular monitoring of blood digoxin levels. Digitoxin, which is not eliminated by the kidneys, is an alternative, given in maintenance doses of 0.1 mg 5 days a week.

DIGITALIS AND PULMONARY HEART DISEASE

Not only is digitalis not beneficial in patients with right heart failure due to cor pulmonale, but it may be especially hazardous since such patients may exhibit a sensitivity to digitalis intoxication, even in the absence of hypokalemia, because of hypoxia, electrolyte disturbances, and sympathetic discharge.[55] When right ventricular failure is the result of LV failure, digitalis is indicated.[19]

DIGITALIS AND MYOCARDIAL INFARCTION

When **atrial fibrillation** develops with a rapid ventricular response, digitalis is often the drug of choice for chronic therapy, because these arrhythmias frequently accompany or precipitate CHF. Acutely, verapamil or esmolol more quickly reduces the ventricular rate and may be given while awaiting the effect of digitalis. When CHF is controlled in patients with atrial fibrillation, verapamil or β-blocker is often added to help control the ventricular response in exercise.

When **mild to moderate CHF** that persists for several days complicates AMI, digitalis exerts a modest but detectable inotropic effect. This benefit may be achieved without decreasing myocardial perfusion or an apparent increase in infarct size.[55] However, now a common combination for this situation is the addition of ACE inhibitors to diuretics.

Combination therapy may, however, be used since (1) the inotropic effects of digoxin 0.5 mg IV can be magnified by vasodilator therapy; (2) added β-receptor stimulation may achieve more marked hemodynamic effects.[8]

Chronic Ischemic Heart Disease and β-Blockade. In anginal patients with cardiomegaly, digitalization may avert the precipitation of cardiac failure by β-blockade.[66] In the large dilated hearts of chronic ischemic cardiomyopathy, the response to digitalis is variable.

POST-INFARCTION DIGOXIN

In the absence of substantial ventricular dysfunction characterized by significant reduction of ejection fraction (e.g., <35%), present data suggest that post-infarction digoxin may increase mortality,[99] presumably acting by induction of arrhythmias or by increasing the myocardial oxygen demand. In the absence of a randomized controlled

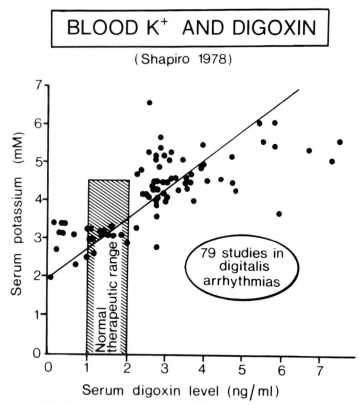

Figure 6–2. As the serum potassium falls, the heart is sensitized to the arrhythmias of digitalis toxicity. Conversely, as the serum potassium rises, a higher serum digoxin level is tolerated. Modified from Shapiro W: Am J Cardiol 41:852–859, 1978, with permission.

trial, finality cannot be reached. It is prudent to use digoxin in post-infarction patients only when strictly required and with frequent checks of serum digoxin levels and potassium. A suitable patient would be one with dilated ventricles, systolic dysfunction, and a third heart sound despite therapy by diuretics and ACE inhibitors.

In general, the reduction of ejection fraction that follows an acute myocardial infarction is directly related to the size of the infarction. Following an extensive infarction, the diastolic size of the heart tends to increase slowly but progressively over months. Prevention of this dilation may help prevent late heart failure. Initial studies suggest that ACE inhibitors may be useful in this regard (Chap. 5); any additional role for digitalis glycosides requires further study.

Ideal Serum Digoxin Levels

Can serum digoxin levels help assessment of the therapeutic effect? The usual therapeutic level ranges between 1 and 2 ng/ml (= 1.3–2.6 nmole/L).[32,68,72] Although values above that range may indicate digitalis toxicity and values below may indicate underdigitalization, there are numerous problems in relating digoxin levels to digoxin therapy (Table 6-4). For example, digitalis-induced arrhythmias can arise in the presence of hypokalemia even when serum levels are well within the therapeutic range, whereas with a normal potassium, serum digoxin levels of 2.0 ng/ml or more are usually required[65,68] (Fig. 6–2). In supraventricular arrhythmias being treated with digoxin, a serum level of 2 to 4 ng/ml (achieved by a higher dose) may be needed to stimulate the vagus enough to control the ventricular rate,

**TABLE 6–5 ANTIARRHYTHMIC DRUGS THAT HAVE NO
PHARMACOKINETIC INTERACTIONS WITH DIGOXIN**

Class IA agents:	procainamide, disopyramide
Class IB agents:	lidocaine, phenytoin, tocainide, mexiletine, ethmozine
Class IC agents:	encainide
Class II agents:	β-blockade, unless renal blood flow critical
Class III agents:	sotalol (not amiodarone)
Class IV agent:	diltiazem (modest elevation compared with verapamil)

which is the best guide to dosage during the therapy of atrial fibrillation. Nonetheless, addition of oral verapamil or diltiazem or β-adrenergic blocking drugs seems preferable to pushing digoxin so high. Conversely, patients with acute hypoxia, as in cor pulmonale, may get digitalis arrhythmias at lower serum levels.

The pharmacokinetics of digoxin also influence interpretation of serum levels. The blood should not be taken less than 4 hours after an IV dose, 6 to 8 hours after an oral dose, or 10 to 12 hours after an intramuscular dose. The multiplicity of factors altering the effects of any given digoxin level (Table 6-4) needs to be taken into account in deciding whether the serum level is inappropriately high or low for that particular patient. With sinus rhythm the digoxin dose cannot be determined from serum levels alone, and suggestions of toxicity, such as early arrhythmias, should lead to dose reduction.

Drug Interactions with Digoxin

The **quinidine-digoxin** interaction is best known. The concomitant administration of quinidine causes the blood digoxin level to approximately double, probably by reducing both renal and extrarenal clearance; such patients should be given about half the previous dose of digoxin, and the clinical course and plasma digoxin should be monitored. **Quinine**, an agent sometimes used in the therapy of muscle cramps, acts likewise. The **verapamil-digoxin** interaction is equally important; similar rules apply. However, verapamil does not alter the volume of distribution of digoxin so that the loading dose of digoxin is unaltered.[57] Other **calcium antagonists** have less effect so that adjustment of the digoxin dose with diltiazem or nifedipine is seldom necessary. However, no simple rules can be made for these agents. For example, nitrendipine may double digoxin levels, whereas isradipine and amlodipine are claimed to have no effect. **Amiodarone** and propafenone (Chap. 8) also elevate serum digoxin levels. With quinidine, verapamil, amiodarone, and possibly propafenone (Chap. 8), digitalis toxicity is more likely to be precipitated. In the case of quinidine, tachyarrhythmias become more likely; in the case of amiodarone and verapamil, the ventricular arrhythmias of digitalis toxicity seem to be suppressed, so that bradycardia and AV block become more likely.[50] Other antiarrhythmics, including procainamide, have no interaction with digoxin (Table 6-5).

Diuretics may induce hypokalemia, which (1) sensitizes the heart to digitalis toxicity and (2) nearly shuts off the tubular secretion of digoxin when the plasma potassium falls to below 2 to 3 mEq/L. **Potassium-depleting corticosteroids** may act likewise. **Potassium-sparing diuretics**, such as amiloride, triamterene, and spironolactone, may all, through diverse mechanisms, decrease digoxin clearance by about 20 to 30%; hence the blood digoxin level ideally needs to be rechecked.[50]

ACE inhibitors, frequently combined with digoxin in the therapy of CHF, decrease the renal excretion of digoxin, thereby increasing blood levels.[77] In addition, by decreasing aldosterone secretion, ACE inhibitors limit potassium loss and help to replenish magnesium stores; both effects may help to reduce digitalis-related arrhythmias and to enhance the safety of digitalis.

Drugs altering GI absorption of digoxin include the following. First, **cholestyramine** decreases digoxin levels, probably by binding of digoxin to the resin with impaired uptake from the GI tract; this interaction can be minimized by giving the digoxin several hours before the resin or by prescribing digoxin solution in a gelatin capsule (Lanoxicaps; 0.2 mg = 0.25 mg of digoxin; same precautions as for digoxin). The latter preparation likewise reduces the risk of (1) kaolin-pectate-induced reduction of GI uptake of digoxin; and (2) **antibiotic-induced increase** in digoxin level (mechanism: erythromycin and tetracycline inhibit the GI flora that convert digoxin to inactive digoxin reduction products). **Cancer chemotherapeutic agents** also depress the GI uptake of digoxin, probably by damaging the intestinal mucosa. **Antacid gels** and a **high bran** diet may also impair the GI uptake of digoxin; here the remedy is to give the digoxin at a different time. Agents altering the **motility of the gut** such as propantheline (Pro-Banthine) do not alter digoxin uptake,[50] contrary to the package insert. The **antimicrobial** agents neomycin, sulfasalazine, and para-aminosalicylic acid (PAS) all delay digoxin uptake by the gut; this effect cannot be avoided by giving digoxin at a different time.

Rifampin (rifampicin) accelerates the hepatic metabolism of many drugs, including digoxin; this may cause a marked reduction in digoxin levels in patients with renal failure, where non-renal clearance becomes important. **Cimetidine** may decrease digoxin levels (controversial). **Vasodilators** (hydralazine, nitroprusside) by enhancing renal blood flow may increase renal excretion of digoxin.

DIGITALIS TOXICITY

The typical patient with digitalis toxicity (Table 6-6) is usually elderly with advanced heart disease and atrial fibrillation, often associated with pulmonary disease and abnormal renal function. Digitalis toxicity should, however, be considered in any patient receiving digitalis who presents with a new GI, ocular, or CNS complaint, or in whom a new arrhythmia or AV conduction disturbance develops. Symptoms do not necessarily precede serious cardiac arrhythmias. The cellular mechanism of digitalis toxicity resides in part in (1) intracellular calcium overload that predisposes to calcium-dependent delayed afterdepolarizations, which, in turn, may develop into ventricular automaticity; (2) excessive vagal stimulation, predisposing to AV block; (3) an added "direct" depressive effect of digitalis on nodal tissue; and (4) sympathetic stimulation.

Typical Digitalis Arrhythmias. A slow pulse, although a traditional indicator of digitalis toxicity, is only a useful alerting signal.[74] Digitalis toxicity may result in second or third degree AV block and increases the automaticity of junctional and His-Purkinje tissue. **Thus accelerated junctional or ventricular arrhythmias may result and, when combined with AV nodal block, are highly suggestive of digitalis toxicity** (Fig. 6–3). The most common cardiac arrhythmias[16] are PVCs, including bigeminy (total, 45%), AV junctional escape beats or tachycardia (40%), second or third degree heart block (25%), atrial tachycardia with block (15%), VT (10%), and SA node or sinus arrest (5%; all figures rounded off).

TABLE 6–6 FEATURES OF DIGITALIS TOXICITY

System	Symptoms and Signs
Gastrointestinal	Anorexia, nausea, vomiting, diarrhea
Neurologic	Malaise, fatigue, confusion, facial pain, insomnia, depression, vertigo, colored vision (green or yellow halos around lights)
Cardiologic	Palpitations, arrhythmias, syncope
Blood	High digoxin level, especially with low potassium; check magnesium, urea, creatinine

DIGITALIS TOXICITY : Ca^{2+} OVERLOAD

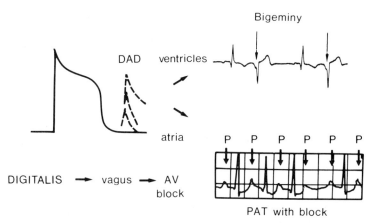

Figure 6–3. The cellular basis of the arrhythmias of digitalis toxicity lies in calcium overload, as a result of excess inhibition of the sodium pump (see Fig. 6–1). The result is the formation of delayed afterdepolarizations (DADs) and risk of ventricular ectopy, typically bigeminy, or atrial arrhythmias, such as paroxysmal atrial tachycardia (PAT). Added excess vagal stimulation (see Fig. 6–1) causes the typical ECG of PAT with block, as shown above. Figure copyright L.H. Opie.

The **diagnosis** of digitalis toxicity is confirmed if the arrhythmias resolve when the drug is discontinued or if the digoxin blood level is inappropriately high for the patient in the presence of suspicious clinical features. Provided that hypokalemia is excluded (see Fig. 6–2), an inappropriately low plasma digoxin level strongly suggests that an arrhythmia or conduction disturbance is not due to digitalis toxicity.

Treatment of Digitalis Toxicity. Much depends on the clinical severity. With only suggestive symptoms, withdrawal of digoxin is sufficient while awaiting confirmation by elevated plasma levels. With dangerous arrhythmias and a low plasma potassium, potassium chloride may be infused intravenously very cautiously as 30 to 40 mEq in 20 to 50 ml of saline at 0.5 to 1 mEq/min into a large vein through a plastic catheter (infiltration of potassium solution can cause tissue necrosis, and infusion into small veins causes local irritation and pain). **Oral potassium** (4 to 6 g of potassium chloride, 50 to 80 mEq) may be given orally in divided doses when arrhythmias are not urgent (e.g., PVCs). Potassium is contraindicated if AV conduction block or hyperkalemia is present, because potassium further increases AV block.[18]

Lidocaine is usually chosen for ventricular ectopy since it does not impair the AV conduction frequently present. Phenytoin, in addition, reverses the high degree AV block, possibly acting by a central mechanism.[21] Class IA agents, such as quinidine, disopyramide, and procainamide, all depress automaticity and may enhance AV block. Quinidine is seldom given intravenously and disopyramide can have a marked negative inotropic effect.

If the patient is already receiving any drugs elevating the blood digoxin, these should be stopped (verapamil, quinidine), as also should β-blockade. On the other hand, because of the long half-life, there is little point in stopping amiodarone.

Temporary transvenous ventricular pacing may be required for marked sinus bradycardia or advanced heart block not responsive to atropine.

Digoxin-specific antibodies, which are now commercially available, are effective therapy for life-threatening digitalis intoxication; the reversal of toxicity is rapid and not accompanied by adverse effects except that anaphylactic shock is theoretically possible. This therapy is usually reserved for the management of toxicity unresponsive to conventional measures, but specialized centers are using it more and more.[73]

Digitoxin

The pharmacokinetics include virtually complete absorption, so that the oral and IV digitalizing doses are the same. Because it is chiefly metabolized or excreted in the gut, **blood levels are not much altered by poor renal function**. However, active metabolites may accumulate in renal failure. Hypokalemia predisposes to toxicity as for digoxin. The great disadvantage is the long half-life (6 to 7 days, compared with 36 hours for digoxin), which complicates the treatment of toxicity.

Digitalization is usually started with a loading dose since otherwise it would take over a month to achieve a steady-state plasma level or serum level. The loading dose ranges from 0.8 to 1.2 mg in 24 hours given in four divided doses 6 hours apart. The maintenance dose is usually 0.1 to 0.15 mg of digitoxin daily. As with digoxin, the dose may need individual adjustment (usual range, 0.05 to 0.20 mg—the smaller dose preferred in the elderly). Therapeutic levels are 15 to 25 ng/ml and toxic levels over 35 ng/ml.

The management of digitalis toxicity changes in patients given digitoxin because of (1) the much longer half-life than that of digoxin and (2) the enterohepatic circulation with 25% recycled, so that cholestyramine or activated charcoal can be given to promote excretion of digitoxin by the gut.[15,59]

Digitalis—Summary

These compounds, by their unique combination of a positive inotropic effect and vagally induced bradycardia with inhibition of AV nodal conduction, remain the oral inotropic agents of choice. A thorough understanding of their pharmacokinetics, numerous interactions with other drugs, and correct use in various clinical situations is mandatory. Chronic digitalis therapy should be undertaken only for clearly defined indications, in the absence of which the benefit will be limited yet involve the risk of digitalis toxicity.

SYMPATHOMIMETIC INOTROPES AND VASODILATORS

Adrenergic Receptors and Inotropic Effects

Norepinephrine (NE) is the endogenous catecholamine that is synthesized and stored in granules in adrenergic nerve endings in the myocardium. When sympathetic nerves to the heart are activated, NE is released from its stores and stimulates specific sites on the myocardial cell surface, termed β_1-**adrenergic receptors** (see Fig. 1–1). Stimulation of these β_1-receptors increases the rate of discharge of the sinoatrial node, thereby augmenting heart rate, enhances AV conduction, and increases the force and speed of contraction of atrial and ventricular myocardium. Most of the released NE is subsequently taken up by the same adrenergic nerve endings and stored for renewed release. Smaller amounts are metabolized. NE also has effects that are exerted largely on the peripheral arterioles, termed α-receptors, and these cause vasoconstriction, raise the blood pressure, and cause reflex bradycardia.

Another type of β-sympathomimetic effect, termed β_2, causes dilation of the smooth muscles of the bronchi, blood vessels, and uterus. A subpopulation of β_2-**receptors** is also found in the heart with effects similar to those of the β_1-receptors; in severe CHF β_2-receptors dominate.[9] Sympathomimetic agents could thus benefit the failing heart: β_1-stimulation by an inotropic effect, β_2-stimulation by afterload reduction (peripheral arterial vasodilation), and α-stimulation by restoring pressure in hypotensive states. Experimental work unfortunately shows that catecholamine stimulation as exemplified by NE infusion should be used with caution in the low output state of AMI, because β_1-effects may precipitate arrhythmias and tachycardia, which can potentially increase ischemia, while excessive α-effects increase the afterload as the blood pressure rises beyond what is required for adequate perfusion. While β_2-stimulation achieves beneficial vasodilation and also mediates some inotropic effect, β-stimulation also causes hypokalemia with enhanced risk of arrhythmias. A further and serious problem is that prolonged or vigorous β-stimulation leads to receptor downgrading with a diminished inotropic response. Consequently, there is an ongoing search for catecholamine-like agents, including phosphodiesterase inhibitors, that lack the undesirable effects.

α-Adrenergic stimulation may also induce a limited calcium-mediated inotropic effect, to contribute to the total effect of adrenergic stimulation.

Inotropic Effect Versus Vasodilation

An intracellular elevation of cyclic AMP, the second messenger of β-adrenergic stimulation, causes the inotropic effect, the chronotropic effect, and peripheral vasodilation (Fig. 6–4). A crucial fact is that

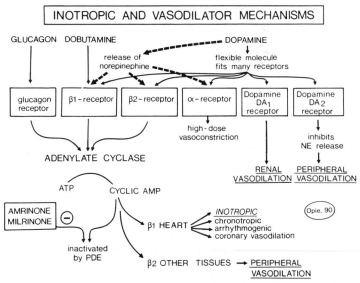

Figure 6–4. The basic mechanisms for combined inotropic and vasodilator effects are (1) stimulation of adenylate cyclase to elevate cyclic AMP, which has a positive inotropic and vasodilatory effect; (2) modulation of release of norepinephrine by dopamine-receptor stimulation; and (3) inhibition of phosphodiesterase (PDE), which increases myocardial and vascular cyclic AMP. (NE = noradrenaline)

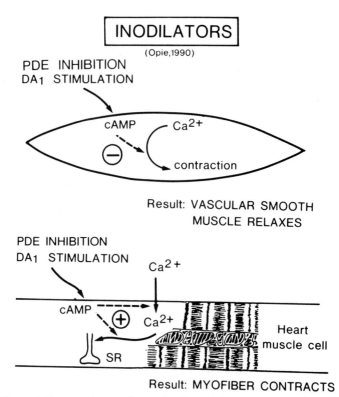

Figure 6–5. Inotropic vasodilators (inodilators) have as their mechanisms of action an increase of cyclic AMP in vascular smooth muscle (top) and in myocardium (bottom). (For cellular mode of action of cyclic AMP in vascular smooth muscle, see Fig. 5–1.) PDE=phosphodiesterase; DA_1=dopaminergic postsynaptic receptor.

cyclic AMP has opposing effects on vascular smooth muscle and on the myocardium (Fig. 6–5). The therapeutic effects that are generally needed are the inotropic and vasodilatory effects. Specific β_1-stimulation will not have a pure inotropic effect without direct vasodilation. β_2-stimulators and phosphodiesterase inhibitors will generally increase cyclic AMP in the heart and in peripheral vessels to cause both vasodilation and a positive inotropic effect. Dopamine, by releasing NE, has mixed β-receptor stimulatory effects and in addition causes specific vasodilation by enhancing the activity of dopaminergic receptors. Compounds such as dopamine and the phosphodi-esterase inhibitors are **mixed inotropic-vasodilators ("inodilators")**. The properties of some of these agents are highlighted in Tables 6-7 and 6-8.

β_1-SELECTIVE STIMULATION

Dobutamine

Dobutamine (Dobutrex), a synthetic analog of dopamine, is a β-adrenergic stimulating agent. It acts directly on β_1-adrenergic receptors to cause a stronger inotropic than chronotropic effect.[33,69] Dobutamine does not directly release NE, as does dopamine, nor does it affect the dopamine receptors. Effects on β_2-receptors are less than those of isoproterenol and effects on α-receptors are less than those of NE. Dobutamine can be used cautiously as an inotropic agent in heart failure to increase cardiac output while reducing ventricular filling pressures. It may also be used in selected cases of evolving myocardial infarction with heart failure and low output, without great risk of increasing infarct size or inducing arrhythmias.[23] Dobutamine directly stimulates the β_1-receptor and does not require the presence of NE stores, which may be depleted in chronic heart failure. Dobutamine also causes modest peripheral vasodilation. The mechanism is unlikely to be via direct stimulation of the vascular β-receptors (β_2) but rather by relief of sympathetic discharge following improvement in heart failure.

Pharmacokinetics. An infusion is rapidly cleared (half-life 2.4 minutes).

Dose. The standard IV dose is 2.5 to 10 μ g/kg/min, occasionally up to 40 μ g/kg/min.[24] The drug can be infused for up to 72 hours with monitoring. There is no oral preparation.

Indications. Refractory heart failure; severe acute forward failure (AMI, after cardiac surgery); cardiogenic shock; excess β-blockade.

Side-effects. In severe CHF, dobutamine causes tachycardia,[24] but there is a dose-related increase in cardiac output.[33] Although there may be less tachycardia and arrhythmias than with dopamine or isoproterenol, all inotropic agents have risk of enhanced arrhythmias.

Precautions. Dilute in sterile water, dextrose, or saline, not in alkaline solutions. Use within 24 hours. Hemodynamic monitoring of patient is required. Check blood potassium.

Clinical Use. The ideal candidate for dobutamine therapy is the patient who has severely depressed LV function with a low cardiac index and elevated LV filling pressure, but in whom extreme hypotension is not present (mean arterial BP not <70 mm Hg).[20,40,46,71] The potential disadvantages of dobutamine are (1) that in severe CHF the β-receptors may be downgraded so that dobutamine may not be as effective as anticipated, (2) prolonged therapy with dobutamine itself could cause receptor downgrading, and (3) dobutamine is not specifically vasodilatory, although relief of CHF may improve peripheral blood flow and enhance renal function indirectly.

An interesting concept for chronic CHF is that infusion of dobutamine for only 4 hr/week may produce a "conditioning effect" with enhanced exercise tolerance and increased functional classification.[41] Possibly intermittent inotropic therapy may improve β-receptor activity as CHF improves, at the same time avoiding drug-induced receptor downgrading. However, a double-blind trial of intermittent IV dobutamine had to be stopped prematurely by the manufacturers because an increased mortality was found in the active treatment group.[80]

Isoproterenol (Isoprenaline)

This relatively pure β-stimulant ($\beta_1 > \beta_2$) is still sometimes used, particularly when cost is a problem. The IV dose is 0.5 to 10 μ g/min, the $T^1/_2$ about 2 minutes, and the major problem lies in the risk of tachycardia and arrhythmias. Other side-effects are headache, tremor, and sweating. Contraindications include myocardial ischemia, which can be worsened, and arrhythmias.

MIXED β_1-β_2-RECEPTOR STIMULATION

Epinephrine

Epinephrine (Adrenaline) gives mixed β-stimulation with some added α-mediated effects. It is used chiefly when combined inotropic/chronotropic stimulation is urgently desired, as in cardiac arrest when the added α-stimulatory effect helps to maintain the blood pressure

TABLE 6–7 EXTENDED CLASSIFICATION OF INODILATORS AND RELATED SUBSTANCES

	Receptor Stimulation Involved in Inodilation	Mechanism
Possible receptors involved	DA_1, DA_2, β_1, β_2	DA_1 = vasodilatory DA_2 = inhibition of presynaptic NE release β_1 = positive inotropic β_2 = vasodilator (and some inotropic effect)
β-Agonists and cyclic AMP		
isoprenaline (isoproterenol)	$\beta_1 + \beta_2$	Increase in myocardial and vascular cyclic AMP (disadvantage: tachycardias and arrhythmias; receptor downgrading)
epinephrine	β_1 greater than β_2	Myocardial greater than vascular cyclic AMP May show disadvantages of isoproterenol
pirbuterol	β_2 greater than β_1	Vascular greater than myocardial cyclic AMP
salbutamol	β_2 greater than β_1	Vascular greater than myocardial cyclic AMP
dibutyryl cyclic AMP	Non-selective[89]	Combined myocardial and vascular effects (disadvantages: tachycardia, arrhythmias; advantage: no receptor downgrading)
PDE inhibitors amrinone milrinone enoximine (MDL 17043) OPC-8490 piroximine 17043 benzimidazole derivatives including sulmazole and pimobendan	No receptors involved	Inhibition of PDE leads to accumulation of cyclic AMP in myocardium and vasculature; risk of arrhythmias

Dopaminergic inodilator agents		
levodopa	$DA_1 + DA_2 + \beta_1$	Vascular cyclic AMP increased, decreased neuronal release of norepinephrine, myocardial cyclic AMP increased
ibopamine	$DA_1 + DA_2 + \beta_1 + \beta_2$	Vascular cyclic AMP increased, decreased neuronal release of norepinephrine, myocardial cyclic AMP increased
dopexamine	$DA_1 + \beta_2 + \beta_1$ (via block of NE uptake)[86]	Vasodilator with some direct inotropic effect (β_2)
Dopaminergic vasodilator agents (non-inotropic)		
fenoldopam	DA_1	Vasodilator without direct inotropic effect
bromocriptine	$DA_1 + DA_2$	Vasodilator without direct inotropic effect
Sympatho-inhibitory inotropes		
digitalis	Na^+/K^+ pump and baroreflex activation	Increased myocardial Ca^{2+} and inhibition of sympathetic outflow in patients with CHF[82]

Adapted from Opie[91] with permission.
Abbreviations:
PDE = phosphodiesterase.
NE = norepinephrine.
CHF = congestive heart failure.
DA_1 = dopaminergic postsynaptic vasodilatory receptor.
DA_2 = dopaminergic presynaptic receptor with inhibition of NE release.
β_1 = β-adrenergic type 1 receptors.
β_2 = β-adrenergic type 2 receptors.

TABLE 6-8 OVERALL PROPERTIES OF β-STIMULANTS AND INOTROPIC VASODILATORS (INODILATORS)

	α>β	β₁-Stimulation	β₁>β₂	Mixed β₁,β₂ Effects	β₂>>β₁	β₁-Agonist Effects	Mixed α,β Effects	PDE inhibitors	Dopaminergic
Drug examples	NE	Dobutamine (also some β₂)	Isoproterenol	Epinephrine (also some α)	Salbutamol (albuterol)	Xamoterol*	Labetalol	Amrinone Milrinone	Dopamine Ibopamine*
Inotropic effect	+	++	+++	++	+	Variable, 0/++	0	+	++
Arteriolar vasodilation	0	+	+	+	++	0	+	++	++
Vasoconstriction	++	0	0	+	0	0	0	0	+
Chronotropic effect	+	0/+	+++	++	0/–	0/+	0	++	0/+
Effect on BP	+	0/+	+SBP	0/+	0/–	0	–	+/–	(high-dose dopamine)
Direct diuretic effect	+	0	0	0	0	0	0	0	++
Arrhythmia risk	+	+/++	+++	+++	+/0	0	0	+/++	0/+ (high-dose dopamine)
Use in CHF	+	++	0	0	+	++	0	++	++
Use in resuscitation	+	++	+/0	+/0	0	0	0	0	++ (dopamine)

+ = increase; 0 = no effect; – = negative effect.

Abbreviations:

NE = norepinephrine.
CHF = congestive heart failure.
PDE = phosphodiesterase.
SBP = systolic blood pressure.
* = not FDA-approved.

despite the peripheral vasodilation achieved by β_2-receptor stimulation. The **dose** is 500 μ g subcutaneously or IM (0.5 ml of 1 in 1000), or 0.5 to 1.0 mg into the central veins, or 100 to 200 μ g intracardiac. The **T½** is 2 minutes. **Side-effects** include tachycardia, arrhythmias, anxiety, headaches, cold extremities, cerebral hemorrhage, and pulmonary edema. **Contraindications** include myocardial ischemia.

Norepinephrine

Norepinephrine (Noradrenaline) is given in an **IV dose** of 8 to 12 μ g/min. It has a **T½** of 3 minutes and produces both α- and β-receptor stimulation. Norepinephrine chiefly stimulates α-receptors in the periphery (with more marked α effects than epinephrine) and β-receptors in the heart. **Side-effects** include headache, tachycardia, bradycardia, and hypertension. Note the risk of necrosis with extravasation. **Contraindications** include late pregnancy because of risk of inducing uterine contractions and myocardial ischemia.

MIXED AGONIST-ANTAGONIST EFFECT
(β-BLOCKERS WITH HIGH ISA)

β-Blockers that also have a high degree of β-receptor stimulation (high intrinsic sympathomimetic activity [ISA] see Fig. 1–5) have significant β-mediated inotropic effect. Oral prenalterol has now been withdrawn because of carcinogenicity in animals. **Xamoterol** (Corwin, available in Europe) compared well with digoxin in the German and Austrian Xamoterol Study Group[84] of mild to moderate CHF; the dose was 200 mg 2x daily. However, xamoterol is contra-indicated in severe CHF because an excess of deaths occurred in xamoterol-treated patients (mechanism uncertain, presumably effects of β-blockade inhibiting the sinus rate and inotropic state). The mechanism of its benefit in mild to moderate (Class II and III) CHF is likely to be a combination of a modest positive inotropic effect (agonist action) and a reduction of the exercise heart rate by its β-blocking effect.[97] These agents have complex and sometimes unpredictable effects dependent on the level of sympathetic tone in CHF. They are orally active and do not increase the heart rate (β-blocking effect). Possible receptor downgrading during prolonged use requires caution.[11] End-points of long-term efficacy have been difficult to establish and evaluate (see also p 19).

MIXED INOTROPIC-VASODILATOR AGENTS
("INODILATORS")

Although "inodilation" is a term recently coined,[91] the rationale goes back at least to 1978 when Stemple and coworkers[95] tried to combine the advantages of the vasodilator effects of nitroprusside with the inotropic effect of dopamine. More recently, recognition of the sympathoinhibitory properties of digitalis[82] leads to inclusion of these compounds in the group of inodilators. Nonetheless, it is the PDE inhibitors that are the prototypical inodilator agents.

Phosphodiesterase-III Inhibitors

These agents, epitomized by amrinone and milrinone, inhibit the breakdown of cyclic AMP and cardiac and peripheral vascular smooth muscle, resulting in augmented myocardial contractility and peripheral arterial and venous vasodilation.[11] These effects occur with relatively little change in heart rate or blood pressure. The added dilator component may explain relative conservation of the myocardial oxygen consumption.[28] Nonetheless, the increase of myocardial cyclic AMP may predispose to ventricular arrhythmias, which could explain the findings in the recent milrinone-digoxin trial in which milrinone was no better than digoxin and led to an increase in ventricular arrhythmias.[79]

Amrinone

Amrinone (Inocor Lactate) is a phosphodiesterase-III inhibitor with both inotropic and vasodilating properties. The IV preparation has recently been approved by the Food and Drug Administration (FDA) for patients with severe CHF not adequately responsive to digitalis, diuretics, or vasodilators. Although the drug is orally active, a multicenter investigation[14] showed no improvement in cardiac function beyond that provided by standard treatment (see acute versus chronic effects of sympathomimetics and vasodilators).

Pharmacology and Pharmacokinetics. By inhibition of phosphodiesterase-III, a combined inotropic and vasodilator effect can be obtained. In patients with severe CHF, the vasodilator effect dominates with a variable direct positive inotropic effect contribution.[17,29,38,75] IV amrinone is rapidly distributed in the circulation with an elimination half-life of 4 hours (prolonged in CHF). About 20 to 40% is plasma bound and the therapeutic plasma level is about $3 \mu g/mL$. Most is excreted unchanged in the urine, some is metabolized, and some is excreted in the feces.

Dose. Intravenously, therapy is initiated with 0.75 mg/kg bolus over 2 to 3 minutes, followed by an infusion of 5 to 10 μ g/kg/min. An added bolus dose may be given 30 minutes later. Higher infusion doses have also been used (10 to 20 μ g/kg/min).[29] Orally (not approved in the USA), amrinone may be given as 100 mg 8-hourly.

Precautions. Amrinone ampules should be protected from the light, and amrinone should not be mixed with glucose (dextrose) for infusion. Predrug and frequently repeated platelet counts are required (decrease drug or discontinue if platelets fall below 150 000/ mm^3). Monitor fluid balance and blood potassium (risk of added hypokalemia). Monitor liver and renal function.

Indications. Severe CHF resistant to conventional therapy; acute LV failure; AMI with cardiogenic shock when dopamine or dobutamine is ineffective (but see contraindications). For the same increase in cardiac output, amrinone is more potent than these other agents in reducing both right and left filling pressures.

Contraindications. AMI (risk of arrhythmias); aortic or pulmonic stenosis (as for all vasodilators); hypertrophic cardiomyopathy (may aggravate obstruction).

Side-effects. Serious side-effects, which are rare during IV use, include thrombocytopenia, ventricular arrhythmias, hepatotoxicity, hypotension, and possibly hypersensitivity reactions. The hypotension may be due to excessive reduction in filling pressure which should generally be maintained at 15 mm Hg or more. However, during acute use adverse effects may be slight.[48]

Drug Interactions. The effects of amrinone and dobutamine are additive in augmenting cardiac output and reducing filling pressure.[28]

Combination Therapy. Amrinone has been combined with digitalis (check blood digoxin and K+ levels for risk of arrhythmias), diuretics (monitor blood K+), and vasodilators such as captopril, hydralazine, and nitrates (watch for additive hypotension). The combined inotropic-vasodilator effects of amrinone are additive with the effects of dobutamine (different mechanisms of stimulating formation of cyclic AMP), dopamine (different mechanisms of vasodilation), and hydralazine.[48]

AMRINONE—SUMMARY

Although amrinone in the oral form is no longer used, the IV preparation with its inotropic and vasodilator effects should be especially useful in patients with β-receptor downgrading, such as those in severe CHF or prior prolonged therapy with dobutamine or other β₁-stimulants. Although in practice, amrinone is usually confined to acutely ill patients requiring IV therapy, further comparisons with other inotropes and dilators are required. Amrinone and similar agents are likely to find a place in the management of the short-term therapy of heart failure.[11]

Milrinone

Milrinone is approved for intravenous use in the USA and UK (Primacor) although it is not yet released in the USA. It is 20x more potent than amrinone, with a similar mechanism of action, and also with a prominent vasodilatory component,[10,47] and is better tolerated during oral administration. When the drug is given acutely, its inotropic and vasodilator effects occur with only a modest change in heart or blood pressure.[5] Milrinone also gives added benefit to patients already receiving captopril.[43] Wirh chronic administration, only some patients benefit,[67] and there is risk of arrhythmias.[31] A recent double-blind study comparing chronic oral milrinone with digoxin treatment[79] showed a marked superiority of digoxin and an adverse effect of milrinone on heart rhythm. In another study, chronic oral milrinone therapy (25–30 mg daily initial dose) given over 2.5 years reduced symptoms in about half without altering the high baseline mortality of 63% after about 1 year.[4] Yet only 11% of patients had drug-related side-effects.

Enoximone

This investigational agent is being widely evaluated and is now available as Perfan for intravenous use in the UK (90 μg/kg/min over 10 to 30 minutes) against acute heart failure or in bridging situations such as for patients awaiting transplantation. Preliminary reports in chronic heart failure suggest that enoximone (50–100 mg t.d.s.) is equipotent with captopril[78,93] and better than placebo[90] over a 12-week period. However, in a double-blind placebo-controlled multicenter study, enoximone only transiently improved the patients, and 48% of enoximone-treated patients dropped out of the study.[96] Furthermore, in this rather small trial, more patients in the enoximone group died. Thus, it is by no means certain that enoximone has overcome the general problem with phosphodiesterase (PDE) inhibitors, namely the risk of serious arrhythmias.

Pimobendan, an investigational calcium sensitizer, also substantially inhibits PDE.

DOPAMINERGIC AGENTS

Dopamine

Dopamine (Intropin) is a catecholamine-like agent used for therapy of severe heart failure and cardiogenic shock. Physiologically it both is the precursor of NE and releases NE from the stores in the nerve-endings in the heart (Fig. 6–3). However, in the periphery this effect is overridden by the activity of the prejunctional dopaminergic DA₂-receptors, inhibiting NE release and thereby helping to vasodilate.[25] Theoretically, dopamine has the valuable property in severe CHF or shock of specifically increasing blood flow to the renal,[51] mesenteric, coronary, and cerebral beds by activating the specific postjunctional dopamine DA_1-receptors. However, at high doses dopamine causes α-receptor stimulation with peripheral vasoconstriction; the peripheral resistance increases and renal blood flow falls.[24] The dose should therefore be kept as low as possible to achieve the desired ends; a combination of dopamine and vasodilator therapy or dopamine and dobutamine would be better than increasing the dose of dopamine.[54]

Pharmacology. The prejunctional DA_2-receptors inhibit NE release and thereby cause vasodilation. The prejunctional DA_1-receptors cause direct vasodilation in renal, mesenteric, coronary, and cerebral vascular beds.[25] Dopamine, a "flexible molecule," also fits into many receptors to cause direct β_1- and β_2-receptor stimulation, as well as α-stimulation. The latter explains why in high doses dopamine may increase pulmonary capillary wedge pressure.

Pharmacokinetics. Dopamine is inactive orally. IV dopamine is metabolized within minutes by dopamine β-hydroxylase and monoamine oxidase.

Dose and Indications. In **refractory cardiac failure**, dopamine can only be given intravenously, which restricts its use to short-term treatment.[24] The dose starts at 0.5 to 1 μ g/kg/min and is raised until an acceptable urinary flow, blood pressure, or heart rate is achieved; vasoconstriction begins at about 10 μ g/kg/min and calls for an α-blocking agent or sodium nitroprusside. In a few patients vasoconstriction can begin at doses as low as 5 μ g/kg/min. In **cardiogenic shock** or **AMI**, 5 μ g/kg/min of dopamine is enough to give a maximum increase in stroke volume, while renal flow reaches a peak at 7.5 μ g/kg/min, and arrhythmias may appear at 10 μ g/kg/min.[44] In **septic shock**, dopamine has an inotropic effect and increases urine volume.[45] Dopamine is widely used for **myocardial failure** after cardiac surgery.[24] It is sometimes given in **acute renal failure** for diuresis.

Precautions. Dopamine must not be diluted in alkaline solutions. Blood pressure, electrocardiogram, and urine flow must be monitored constantly, with intermittent measurements of cardiac output and pulmonary wedge pressure if possible. For oliguria, first correct hypovolemia; add furosemide.

Side-effects and Interactions. Dopamine is contraindicated in ventricular arrhythmias, in pheochromocytoma, and during the use of cyclopropane or halogenated hydrocarbon anesthetics. Extravasation can cause sloughing, prevented by infusing the drug into a large vein through a plastic catheter, and treated by local infiltration with phentolamine. If the patient has recently taken a monoamine oxidase (MAO) inhibitor, the rate of dopamine metabolism by the tissue will fall and the dose should be cut to one-tenth of the usual.

Clinical Use. Comparison of dopamine and dobutamine after cardiac surgery suggests that dobutamine may be best for the patient with depressed cardiac output with only mild to moderate hypotension, particularly when the patient has sinus tachycardia or ventricular arrhythmias. Dopamine, on the other hand, is preferred in the patient who requires both a pressor effect (high-dose α effect) and increase in cardiac output, and who does not have marked tachycardia or ventricular irritability.[27,70] **Dopamine is especially beneficial when renal blood flow is impaired in severe CHF.**[51] Infusion of equal concentrations of dopamine and dobutamine may afford more advantages than either drug singly in cardiogenic shock.[62] Dopamine can further increase the cardiac output in patients treated by nitroprusside.[54]

Levodopa

An oral dopamine-like agent would be useful, and levodopa has been tried after IV dopamine therapy.[24] It can be increased slowly from 250 mg to 2000 mg 4x daily over 7 days with 50 mg pyridoxine (required to decarboxylate levodopa). However, the ideal oral do-pamine-like agent would not cross the blood-brain barrier, thereby avoiding the centrally induced nausea and vomiting that may occur with levodopa.

New Dopaminergic Agents

Bromocriptine, fenoldopam, and **dopexamine** are vasodilators without direct inotropic effect. Agents such as ibopamine stimulate both types of dopamine receptors and are "inodilators" (Table 6-7) with a hemodynamic profile somewhat similar to amrinone and milrinone (Table 6-8). **Ibopamine**[13] is orally active, already available in Europe (Inopamil; Scandine), and under investigation elsewhere. Chemically, it is a butyric acid ester of methyldopamine (the latter is also called epinine). Once absorbed, the ester is hydrolyzed by non-specific esterases in the bloodstream to release epinine, which has effects very similar to those of IV dopamine. There is a desirable hemodynamic profile with a fall in the peripheral vascular resistance, a modest direct inotropic effect, and almost no increase in the heart rate. The added diuretic effect is also a potential benefit. The dose is 50 to 100 mg orally 2 to 3x daily. A recent double-blind comparison of ibopamine with a diuretic in patients with CHF (Classes II and III), ibopamine 200 mg 2x daily was the approximate equivalent over 3 months of Moduretic 1 to 2 tablets daily;[94] hence, ibopamine is a potential first-line agent in CHF provided that it can be shown that the effects are sustained for even longer.

Long-term studies of these new dopaminergic agents are required to show (1) a sustained benefit, (2) the absence of drug tolerance, and (3) the absence of serious side-effects such as arrhythmias.[83] Whether there really is attenuation of the hemodynamic benefit during chronic therapy, as suggested by Rajfer and colleagues,[60] is controversial.[92]

None of the above agents are yet FDA-approved.

ACUTE VERSUS CHRONIC EFFECTS OF SYMPATHOMIMETICS AND VASODILATORS

In **acute LV failure**, these agents may achieve dramatic short-term benefits to remedy the added deterioration that usually accompanies and promotes the condition. Together with loop diuretics and ni-trates, the positive inotropes or inotropic vasodilators frequently save the patient from drowning in his own secretions. In contrast, in **chronic severe heart failure**, the major limitation is the underlying state of the myocardium, which is usually damaged beyond repair, so that all therapy has inherent limitations.[42] Therapy is now aimed at improving the peripheral circulation[49] so that it is vasodilating rather than inotropic properties that become more important. In a third and intermediate situation, **chronic mild to moderate CHF**, the myocar-dium is still theoretically capable of at least some response to inotropic stimulation and may also be better able to withstand possible side-effects of inotropic agents, such as arrhythmias and aggravation of ischemia. In this setting, prevention of further cardiac dilation and resultant functional mitral regurgitation may help to prevent or delay ventricular deterioration. It is in this category that there is most potential for new oral inotropic agents.

ACUTE VERSUS CHRONIC HEART FAILURE

In acute and chronic heart failure, the aims of therapy differ. In acute heart failure, reduction of pulmonary capillary pressure and right atrial filling pressure is sought along with an elevation of cardiac output, if the latter is also reduced. These aims can be achieved by a variety of inotropes, including dopamine, dobutamine, amrinone, and their newer derivatives. Some of these, such as dopamine and amrinone, have a prominent vasodilator component to their action (inodilators). Such inotropic-dilator therapy should be combined with diuretics and sometimes with digitalis.

In **chronic heart failure**, digoxin is no longer compulsory early therapy with diuretics. Rather, ACE inhibitors and diuretics are often combined in mild early heart failure, not because digoxin won't work, but because of its numerous interactions and precautions, so that ACE inhibitors are simpler to use. In more severe heart failure, triple therapy with diuretics, ACE inhibitors, and digoxin has now become standard practice. The aim of therapy is to translate the hemodynamic benefits of inotropic-vasodilator therapy into improved functional capacity, without shortening the duration of life or impairing its quality. Digoxin, a weak inotropic drug, only partially fulfills these criteria. Digoxin does, however, slow the heart rate and decreases the size of the failing heart, thus lessening myocardial oxygen demands. Clearly, the use of digoxin requires thorough knowledge of the multiple factors governing its efficacy and toxicity, including numerous drug interactions. Today, digoxin is no longer the first-line of therapy for acute severe heart failure, but still usually prescribed for chronic LV failure, especially after full therapy by diuretics.

REFERENCES

References from Previous Editions

1. Akera T, Brody TM: Pharmacol Rev 29:187–218, 1978
2. Algeo S, Fenster PE, Marcus FI: Geriatrics 38:93–101, 1983
3. Alpert BS, Barfield JA, Taylor WJ: J Pediatr 106:66–68, 1985
4. Baim DS, Colucci WS, Monrad ES, et al: J Am Coll Cardiol 7:661–670, 1986
5. Benotti JR, Lesko LJ, McCue JE, et al: Am J Cardiol 56:685–689, 1985
6. Berman WR Jr, Yebak SM, Dillon T, et al: N Engl J Med 308:363–366, 1983
7. Blumgart HL, Altschule MD: Am J Med Sci 198:455–463, 1939
8. Bostrom PA, Andersson J, Johansson BW, et al: Eur J Clin Invest 14:175–180, 1984
9. Bristow MR, Ginsburg R, Umans V, et al: Circ Res 59:297–309, 1986
10. Cody RJ, Muller FB, Kubo SH, et al: Circulation 73:124–129, 1986
11. Colucci WS, Wright RF, Braunwald E: N Engl J Med 314:290–299; 349–358, 1986
12. Dall JLC: Br Med J 2:705–706, 1970
13. Dei Cas L, Bolognesi R, Cucchini F, et al: J Cardiovasc Pharmacol 5:249–253, 1983
14. DiBianco R, Shabetai R, Silverman BD: J Am Coll Cardiol 4:855–866, 1984
15. Dobbs SM, Mawer GE, Rodgers EM, et al: Br J Clin Pharmacol 3:231–237, 1976
16. Ewy GA, Marcus FI, Fillmore SJ, et al: In Melmon KL (ed): Cardiovascular Drug Therapy. FA Davis, Philadelphia, 1974, 153–174
17. Feldman M, Gwathmey J, Copelas L, et al: Circulation 72:(suppl III):III-404, 1985
18. Fisch C, Martz BL, Priebe FH: J Clin Invest 39:1885–1893, 1960
19. Fleg JL, Gottlieb SH, Lakatta EG: Am J Med 73:244–250, 1982
20. Francis GS, Sharma B, Hodges M: Am Heart J 103:995–1000, 1982
21. Garan H, Ruskin JN, Powell WJ Jr: Am J Physiol 241:H67–H72, 1981
22. Gault MH, Churchill DN, Kalras J: Br J Clin Pharmacol 9:593–597, 1980
23. Gillespie TA, Ambos HT, Sobel BE, et al:. Am J Cardiol 39:588–594, 1977
24. Goldberg LI, Hsieh Y-Y, Resnekov L: Prog Cardiovasc Dis 19:327–340, 1977
25. Goldberg LI, Rajfer SI: Circulation 72:245–248, 1985
26. Gomes JAC, Kang PS, El–Sherif N: Am J Cardiol 48:783–788, 1981
27. Gray R, Shah PK, Singh B, et al: Chest 80:16–22, 1981
28. Grose R, Strain J, Greenberg M, et al: J Am Coll Cardiol 7:1107–1113, 1986

29. Hermiller JB, Leithe ME, Magorien RD, et al: J Pharmacol Exp Ther 228:319–326, 1984
30. Hoechsen RJ, Cuddy TE: Am J Cardiol 35:469–472, 1975
31. Holmes JR, Kubo SH, Cody RJ, et al: Am Heart J 110:800–806, 1985
32. Jelliffe RW, Brooker G: Am J Med 57:63–68, 1974
33. Jewitt DE, Birkhead J, Mitchell A, et al: Lancet 2:363–367, 1974
34. Johnston GD: Drugs 20:494–499, 1980
35. Jusko WG, Weintraub M: Clin Pharmacol Ther 18:449–454, 1974
36. Keller F, Molzahn M, Ingerowski R: Eur J Clin Pharmacol 18:433–441, 1980
37. Kim YI, Noble RJ, Zipes DP: Am J Cardiol 36:459–467, 1975
38. Konstam MA, Cohen SR, Weiland DS, et al: Am J Cardiol 57:242–248, 1986
39. Lee CO, Abete P, Pecker M, et al: J Mol Cell Cardiol 17:1043–1053, 1985
40. Leier CV, Heban PT, Huss P, et al: Circulation 58:466–475, 1978
41. Leier CV, Huss P, Lewis RP, et al: Circulation 65:1382–1387, 1982
42. LeJemtel TH, Sonnenblick EH: N Engl J Med 310:1384–1385, 1984
43. LeJemtel TH, Maskin CS, Mancini D, et al: Circulation 72:364–369, 1985
44. Levine PA, McGillivray M, Klein MD: Circulation 51/52 (abstr):208, 1975
45. Loeb HS, Winslow EBJ, Rahimtoola SH, et al: Circulation 44:163–173, 1971
46. Loeb HS, Bredakis J, Gunnar RM: Circulation 55:375–381, 1977
47. Ludmer PL, Wright RF, Arnold MO, et al: Circulation 73:130–137, 1986
48. Mancini D, LeJemtel T, Sonnenblick E: Am J Cardiol 56:8B–15B, 1985
49. Mancini DM, LeJemtel TH, Factor S, et al: Am J Med 80:2–13, 1986
50. Marcus FI: J Am Coll Cardiol 5:82A–90A, 1985
51. Maskin C, Ocken S, Chadwick B, et al: Circulation 72:846–852, 1985
52. Mathur PM, Powles P, Pugsley SO, et al: Ann Intern Med 95:283–288, 1981
53. McMichael J, Sharpey-Schafer EP: Qrtly J Med 53:123–135, 1944
54. Miller RR, Awan NA, Joye JA, et al: Circulation 55:881–884, 1977
55. Morrison J, Caromilas J, Robins M, et al: Circulation 62:8–16, 1980
56. Opie LH: Lancet 1:912–918, 1980
57. Pedersen KE: Acta Med Scand (suppl 697):12–40, 1985
58. Peters U: Eur Heart J 3(suppl D):65–78, 1982
59. Pond S, Jacobs M, Marks J, et al: Lancet 2:1177–1178, 1981
60. Rajfer SI, Rossen JD, Douglas F, et al: Circulation 73:740–748, 1986
61. Reiffel JH, Bigger JT Jr, Cramer M: Am J Cardiol 43:983–994, 1979
62. Richard C, Ricome JL, Rimailho A, et al: Circulation 67:620–626, 1983
63. Schaal SF, Sugimoto T, Wallace AG, et al: Cardiovasc Res 2:356–359, 1968
64. Sellers TD Jr, Bayshore TM, Gallagher JJ: Circulation 1977; 56:260–267.
65. Shapiro W: Am J Cardiol 41:852–859, 1978
66. Sharma B, Majid PA, Meeran MK, et al: Br Heart J 34:631–637, 1972
67. Sinoway LS, Maskin CS, Chadwick B, et al: J Am Coll Cardiol 2:327–331, 1983
68. Smith TW, Haber E: N Engl J Med 289:945–952; 1010–1015; 1063–1072; 1125–1129, 1973
69. Sonnenblick EH, Frishman WH, LeJemtel TH: N Engl J Med 300:17–22, 1979
70. Steen PA, Tinker JH, Pluth JR, et al: Circulation 57:378–384, 1978
71. Stoner JD, Bolen JL, Harrison DC: Br Heart J 39:536–539, 1977
72. Sumner DJ, Russell AJ, Whiting B: Br J Clin Pharmacol 3:221–229, 1976
73. Wenger TL, Butler VP Jr, Haber E, et al: J Am Coll Cardiol 5:118A–123A, 1985
74. Williams P, Aronson J, Sleight P: Lancet 2:1340–1342, 1978
75. Wilmshurst PT, Walker JM, Fry CH, et al: Cardiovasc Res 18:302–309, 1984

New References

76. Beaune J, for the Enalapril vs Digoxin French Multicenter Study Group: Comparison of enalapril vs digoxin for congestive heart failure. Am J Cardiol 63:22D–25D, 1989
77. Cleland JGF, Dargie HJ, Pettigrew A, et al: The effects of captopril on serum digoxin and urinary urea and digoxin clearances in patients with congestive heart failure. Am Heart J 112:130–135, 1986
78. Crawford MH, Deedwania P, Massie B, et al: Comparative efficacy of enoximone versus captopril in moderate heart failure (abstr). Circulation 80(suppl II):II–175, 1989

79.   DiBianco R, Shabetai R, Kostuk W, et al: A comparison of oral milrinone, digoxin and their combination in the treatment of patients with chronic heart failure. N Engl J Med 320:677–683, 1989

80.   Dies F, Krell MJ, Whitlow P, et al: Intermittent dobutamine in ambulatory out-patients with chronic cardiac failure. Circulation 74(suppl II):II-39, 1986

81.   Falk RH, Knowlton AA, Bernard SA: Digoxin for converting recent-onset atrial fibrillation to sinus rhythm. Ann Intern Med 106:503–506, 1987

82.   Ferguson DW, Berg WJ, Sanders JS, et al: Sympatho-inhibitory responses to digitalis glycosides in heart failure patients: Direct evidence from sympathetic neural recordings. Circulation 80:65–77, 1989

83.   Furlanello F, Aguglia C, Brusoni B, et al: Influence of ibopamine on heart rate and arrhythmic pattern in patients with congestive heart failure. A double-blind multicentre study. G Ital Cardiol 19:71–80, 1989

84.   German and Austrian Xamoterol Study Group: Double-blind placebo-controlled comparison of digoxin and xamoterol in chronic heart failure. Lancet 1:489–493, 1988

85.   Gheorghiade M, Hall V, Lakier JB, et al: Comparative hemodynamic and neurohumoral effects of intravenous captopril and digoxin and their combinations in patients with severe heart failure. J Am Coll Cardiol 13:134–142, 1989

86.   Goldberg LI, Bass AS: Relative significance of dopamine receptors, beta adrenoceptors and norepinephrine uptake inhibition in the cardiovascular actions of dopexamine hydrochloride. Am J Cardiol 62:37C–40C, 1988

87.   Lindenbaum J, Rund DG, Butler VP, et al: Inactivation of digoxin by the gut flora: Reversal by antibiotic therapy. N Engl J Med 305:789–794, 1981

88.   Marcus FI: The use of digitalis for the treatment of congestive heart failure: A tale of its decline and resurrection. Cardiovasc Drugs Ther 3:473–476, 1989

89.   Miyagi Y, Sasayama S, Nakajima H, et al: Comparative hemodynamic effects of intravenous dobutamine and dibutyryl cyclic AMP, a new inotropic agent, in severe congestive heart failure. J Cardiovasc Pharmacol 15:138–143, 1990

90.   Narahara KA and the Western Enoximone Study Group: Enoximone versus placebo: A double-blind trial in chronic congestive heart failure (abstr). Circulation 80(suppl II):II–175, 1989

91.   Opie LH: Inodilators. Lancet 1:1336, 1989

92.   Opie LH: Pharmacologic profile of ibopamine and related dopamine-like inodilators. Cardiovasc Drugs Ther 3:1041–1054, 1989

93.   Orie JE, Rakho PS, Brookfield L, et al: A double blind comparison of enoximone (Enox) and captopril (Cap) in CHF (abstr). Circulation 80(suppl II):II-175, 1989

94.   SK+F Ibopamine Working Group: Ibopamine versus hydrochloro-thiazide/amiloride in patients with mild congestive heart failure. Cardiovasc Drugs Ther 3:897–902, 1989

95.   Stemple DR, Kleiman JH, Harrison DC: Combined nitroprusside-dopamine therapy in severe chronic congestive heart failure. Dose-related hemodynamic advantages over single drug infusions. Am J Cardiol 42:267–275, 1978

96.   Uretsky BF, Jessup M, Konstam MA, et al: Multicenter trial of oral enoximone in patients with moderately severe congestive heart failure: Lack of benefit compared to placebo (abstr). Circulation 80(suppl II):II-175, 1989

97.   Vigholt-Sorenson E, Faergeman O, Snow HM: Effects of xamoterol, a β_1–adrenoceptor partial agonist, in patients with ischaemic dysfunction of the left ventricle. Br Heart J 62:335–341, 1989

Reviews

98.   Cohn J: Inotropic therapy for heart failure: Paradise postponed. N Engl J Med 320:729–731, 1989

99.   Poole-Wilson PA, Robinson K: Digoxin—A redundant drug in congestive cardiac failure. Cardiovasc Drugs Ther 2:733–741, 1989

N.M. Kaplan
L.H. Opie

Antihypertensive Drugs

Because the blood pressure (BP) is the product of the cardiac output and the peripheral vascular resistance (BP = CO x PVR), all antihypertensive drugs must act by reducing either the CO (as do the β-blockers) or the peripheral vascular resistance (as do all the others, and perhaps a late effect of β-blockade). Diuretics act chiefly as volume depletors, thereby reducing the CO, and also as indirect vasodilators. All antihypertensive drugs, except the centrally active agents and ganglion blockers, have other uses and therefore have already been discussed in earlier chapters of this book. Despite the host of potential agents, the therapy of hypertension is usually simple, since many patients have minimally or moderately elevated pressures that usually respond adequately to one or two drugs (Table 7-1). More effective, less bothersome, and longer-acting agents have become available, so that for most hypertensives one or two pills every morning work quite well. Asymptomatic patients, however, often will not stay on therapy, particularly if it makes them feel weak, sleepy, forgetful, or impotent. A small proportion have resistant hypertension, which may only respond to multiple therapies. It must be considered that hypertension is usually multifactorial in etiology, that different drugs act by different mechanisms (Fig. 7–1), and that the aim is to match the drug to the patient.

THE DECISION TO TREAT: NON-DRUG THERAPY

Before any drug is started, persistence of the patient's hypertension should be ascertained by multiple measurements over at least a few weeks, preferably at home and at work, unless the pressure is so high (e.g., >180/110 mm Hg) as to mandate immediate therapy. Non-drug therapies should be standard in all hypertensives, particularly weight reduction for the obese and moderate dietary **sodium restriction** such as 80 to 100 mmole/day or about 5 to 6 g sodium chloride or 2 g sodium;[65] sodium restriction should be used before drugs in those with marginal elevations. **Weight reduction** can be crucial in offsetting the increased cardiovascular risk from the cholesterol increase associated with diuretic use.[77] Furthermore, **obesity** is an independent risk factor for coronary heart disease in women.[66] **Fish oil supplements** have a modest antihypertensive effect.[46] **Other measures** include increased aerobic exercise,[43] cessation of smoking, and decreased alcohol. Drugs should be reserved for those with higher BP levels, especially in the presence of additional risk factors.

In the USA, an aggressive approach to the active drug therapy of even **minimally elevated pressures**, such as diastolics in the 90 to

TABLE 7–1 SPECIFICS ABOUT ORALLY EFFECTIVE ANTIHYPERTENSIVE DRUGS

Drug	Registered Trade Name (in USA)	Dose Range (mg/day)	Doses/Day
Diuretics (see Table 6–3)			
Hydrochlorothiazide	HydroDIURIL, Esidrix	12.5–50	1
Combination agents	Dyazide, Maxzide, Moduretic	$^1/_2$–1 tablet	1
β-Blockers			
Acebutolol	Sectral	400–800	1
Atenolol	Tenormin	50–100	2
Labetalol	Normodyne, Trandate	200–800	2
Metoprolol	Lopressor	100–400	2
Nadolol	Corgard	40–320	1
Pindolol	Visken	10–60	2
Propranolol	Inderal	80–480	2
Timolol	Blocadren	20–60	2
ACE inhibitors			
Captopril	Capoten	25–150	2–3
Enalapril	Vasotec	5–40	1–2
Lisinopril	Zestril, Prinivil	10–60	1
Calcium antagonists			
Diltiazem SR	Cardizem SR	180–360	2
Nicardipine	Cardene	60–120	3
Nifedipine XL	Procardia XL	30–90	1
Nifedipine	Procardia, Adalat	20–120	2–3
Verapamil SR	Isoptin SR, Calan SR	240–480	1–2
α-Blockers			
Prazosin	Minipress	2–20	2
Terazosin	Hytrin	1–20	1
Doxazosin	Cardura	1–16	1
Direct vasodilators			
Hydralazine	Apresoline	50–200	2–3
Minoxidil	Loniten	5–40	1
Non-receptor adrenergic inhibitors			
Reserpine	Serpasil	0.05–0.25	1
Rauwolfia whole root	Raudixin	50–100	1
Centrally active:			
Methyldopa	Aldomet	500–1500	2
Clonidine	Catapres	0.5–1.5	1–2
Clonidine transdermal	Catapres-TTS	1 patch	(Once weekly)
Guanabenz	Wytensin	8–64	2
Guanfacine	Tenex	1–3	1
Peripheral:			
Guanethidine	Ismelin	10–150 or more	1
Guanadrel	Hylorel	10–75	2

100 mm Hg range, has become "accepted medical practice." In most of the rest of the world, drug therapy is usually reserved for those with diastolics over 100 mm Hg.[94] When in doubt about a marginal BP level, multiple out-of-the-office readings should be obtained, either by inexpensive home blood pressure devices or by **ambulatory BP monitoring**. As hypertension is merely one of several risk factors for coronary artery disease or stroke, it makes sense to treat at lower BP values in the presence of higher blood cholesterols or in smokers or diabetics. Conversely, in very low risk groups (non-smoking middle-aged females) there may not be much advantage in treatment of mild to moderate hypertension. Consequently, voices for a less aggressive approach are being heard in the USA and elsewhere, and the current therapeutic over-enthusiasm may cool.

The efficacy of antihypertensive treatment depends not only on the control of the BP, but on the co-existence of other risk factors. Whereas in low risk groups, many hundreds of patients must be treated to prevent one stroke, in very high risk groups, such as the

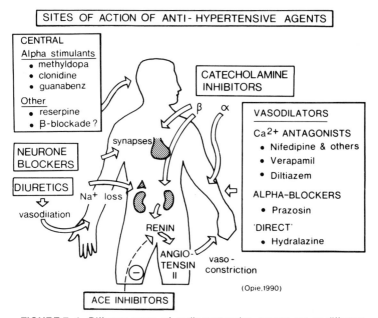

FIGURE 7–1. Different types of antihypertensive agents act at different sites. Because hypertension is frequently multifactorial in origin, it may be difficult to find the ideal drug for a given patient. Drug combinations often are used.

elderly, only 20 to 40 patients need to be treated for 1 year to prevent one cardiovascular event, including stroke. Because the majority of patients with mild to moderate hypertension are entirely asymptomatic, it is essential to match the drug to the patient and to realize that many existing therapies, including especially diuretics and β-blockade, in some way impair the quality of life or bring about undesirable changes in blood chemistry, including blood lipids. Although **virtually all recommendations for treatment, including those of the World Health Organization, are based on a cut-off diastolic blood pressure level, it clearly makes sense to alter that level according to the degree of concomitant estimated risk for coronary artery disease, stroke, or renal failure. Moreover, systolic levels should be considered, particularly in the elderly. At all ages, they are even more predictive of risk than are diastolic levels.** The cost, both financial and in terms of expected side-effects, needs to be balanced against the expected benefits. Even with agents such as the angiotension converting enzyme (ACE) inhibitors and calcium antagonists, which have no central effects and relatively preserve the quality of life, evaluation of the cost-benefit ratio is not easy and requires specific attention to the needs of each patient.

OVERALL AIMS OF TREATMENT

Lowering the BP should never be the sole aim of therapy. All abnormalities associated with hypertension, including shortened life expectancy, should be reverted to normal. Overall cardiovascular mortality has been reduced by therapy, primarily through a decrease in stroke mortality.[49] Yet thus far in no convincing single trial has mortality from coronary disease been improved. Why are excess risks for coronary disease associated with elevated BP not fully removed by prolonged reduction of the pressure to levels seen in untreated people? There are several possibilities, including (1) the multifactorial nature of coronary heart disease, (2) the short duration of treatment, (3) the

TABLE 7–2 PERSPECTIVES ON ORALLY EFFECTIVE ANTIHYPERTENSIVE AGENTS

Advantages	Disadvantages
Thiazides and other diuretics	
Once a day (usually)	Effectiveness reduced by heavy sodium
Potentiate effects of other agents,	intake or renal insufficiency
especially ACE inhibitors	(furosemide and metolazone still
Prevent reactive fluid retention	effective)
	Hypokalemia–arrhythmias
	Hypercholesterolemia — atherosclerosis
	Abnormal glucose tolerance — diabetes
	Hyperuricemia — gout
Potassium-sparing agents	
Given in combination with diuretic	Potential for hyperkalemia, particularly
Few overt side-effects	in renal insufficiency or with ACE
	inhibitors
β–Blockers	
Many once a day: e.g., atenolol,	Serious side effects: bronchospasm,
nadolol	prolongation of insulin-induced
	hypoglycemia, heart failure, impotence
Relief from anxiety-related symptoms	Others: cold extremities, reduced
Little volume retention	exercise tolerance, fatigue, insomnia,
Antianginal and antiarrhythmic	memory deficit
Post-infarct protection	Unknown consequences: increased
(Side-effects may be diminished	triglycerides, decreased HDL —
by choice of agent, e.g., cardio-	cholesterol
selective, vasodilatory)	Less effective in blacks (unless
	vasodilatory in type or with diuretic)
ACE inhibitors	
Captopril	Side-effects: cough, hypotension, rash,
No sedation, lipid neutral, good	loss of taste, renal
quality of life vs propranolol	
Renal protective effect	Rare: proteinuria, leukopenia
Enalapril, lisinopril	Side-effects: cough, hypotension, renal
Similar effects, longer acting	
Calcium antagonists	
Nifedipine, nicardipine, amlodipine	Headaches, flushing, pedal edema
Anti-anginal	
Easy combination with β-blockers	
Lipid neutral	
Verapamil	Headache, constipation, AV block,
Anti-anginal	negatively inotropic (care with
Lipid neutral	β-blockade)
Diltiazem	Headache, bradycardia (care with
Anti-anginal; lipid	β-blockade), AV block
neutral	

lack of adequate control of blood pressure, (4) the metabolic side-effects or other hazards of the drugs used, and (5) overtreatment in susceptible patients. Several trials have suggested a J-shaped curve indicating an increase of coronary complications in patients whose diastolic BP was reduced below 90 mm Hg (or about 95 mm Hg in the elderly). Reduction of diastolics below 95 mm Hg during treatment has been associated with only a marginally lower incidence of stroke or coronary events than reduction of higher values.[20] Therefore, the effort involved, the discomfort to the patient, and the cost in achieving lower diastolics might not be worth it, especially because a fall of only 5 mm Hg of the usual DBP removes at least one-third the risk of stroke and one-fifth that of coronary heart disease.[49]

CHOICE OF INITIAL DRUG (Table 7–2)

Until recently a **diuretic** has been the first drug advocated by authorities and chosen by most practitioners.[4,24,33,39] β-Blockers have, since

**TABLE 7–2 PERSPECTIVES ON ORALLY EFFECTIVE
ANTIHYPERTENSIVE AGENTS** (Continued)

Advantages	Disadvantages
α–Blockers: prazosin, terazosin, doxazosin	

Lack of sedation or dry mouth
  Decrease in peripheral resistance
  No fall in cardiac output
  May benefit plasma lipids
	First-dose hypotension (minimized by
	  small doses and deletion of diuretics)
	Lassitude
	Tolerance may require titration

Direct vasodilators	

Hydralazine
  Increase in cardiac output and
  renal blood flow
	Reflex sympathetic tachycardia and
	  increased cardiac output — prevent
	  by adrenergic inhibitor
	Lupus-like (rare below 200 mg/day)

Minoxidil
  Once a day
  Greater potency
  Effective in renal failure
	Reactive fluid retention
	Reflex sympathetic stimulation
	Hirsutism in 80%

Non-receptor adrenergic inhibitors	

Reserpine (central and peripheral)
  Ultralong NE depletion
  Inexpensive
  Minimal titration needed
	Slow onset. Sedation, nasal stuffiness
	Rare: depression, increased gastric
	  acidity

Clonidine (central)
  Available in patch for once-a-week
  use
  No immune side-effects
	Common side-effects: sedation, dry
	  mouth
	Rare: rebound of blood pressure

Guanabenz (central)
  Twice a day
  May cause less reactive fluid
  retention
	Side effects: sedation, dry mouth

Guanfacine (central) Once daily	Side-effects: sedation, dry mouth

Methyldopa (central)
  Hemodynamics unchanged
  Proven long-term effects
	Common side-effects: sedation, dry
	  mouth
	Rare: autoimmune reactions

Guanadrel (peripheral)
  No central nervous effects
	Side-effects: Similar but less severe
	  than guanethidine. Not with MAO
	  inhibitors

Guanethidine (peripheral)
  Steep dose-response curve
  Once a day
  No central effects
	Frequent orthostatic hypotension
	Occasional diarrhea, retrograde
	  ejaculation
	Not with MAO inhibitors

MAO inhibitors = monoamine oxidase inhibitors, such as isocarboxazid (Marplan), phenelzine (Nardil), and tranylcypromine (Parnate). NE = norepinephrine.

then, gained in popularity. Although an overall meta-analysis of 14 major trials involving over 37,000 patients has demonstrated a modest protection against coronary disease by both diuretics and beta-blockers, these agents were only about half as effective as they should have been, taking into account the BP reduction found.[49] Since diuretics and β-blockers induce complex metabolic changes, and β-blockers have many contraindications besides frequent subjective symptoms, such as fatigue, attention is now focusing on those drugs that have no central effect, that are metabolically neutral, and that act on the peripheral vascular resistance—namely the ACE inhibitors and the calcium antagonists. Although these categories of agents are logical choices, there are unfortunately no long-term outcome trials to prove their efficacy on morbidity or mortality.

The choice of drugs should not be automatic, based upon habit (e.g., the continued widespread use of methyldopa), or based upon the intensity of promotional advertisement (e.g., the minimal use of low-dose reserpine, which has no commercial advocates, or the excess use of ACE inhibitors, currently heavily promoted). Increasingly,

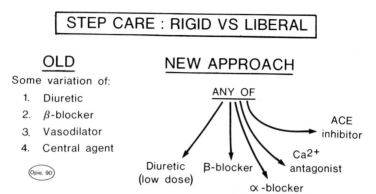

STEP CARE : RIGID VS LIBERAL

OLD
Some variation of:
1. Diuretic
2. β-blocker
3. Vasodilator
4. Central agent

(Opie, 90)

NEW APPROACH

ANY OF

Diuretic (low dose) β-blocker α-blocker Ca2+ antagonist ACE inhibitor

FIGURE 7–2. The previous rigid step-care, almost always starting with a diuretic and going on to a β-blocker before a vasodilator, is now being replaced by a more liberal approach. Any of five agents can be chosen as first-line therapy, thereafter proceeding to combinations of those agents, progressively increasing the number of agents used, as required.

instead of automatically going through a rigid "step-care" procedure, **the drug should be tailored to the patient** (Fig. 7–2). For example, in the presence of a family history of diabetes or gout, thiazide diuretics are contraindicated, whereas ACE inhibitors and calcium antagonists are metabolically "neutral." In patients with a very stressful early morning, additional acute therapy by a short-acting anti-adrenergic drug such as labetalol might be useful. In patients with anxiety and a resting tachycardia, β-blockade remains first choice.

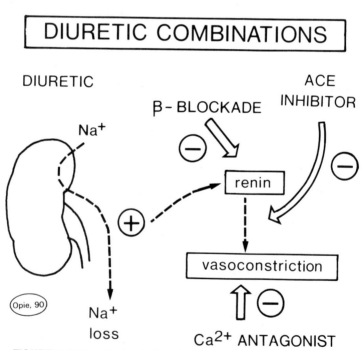

DIURETIC COMBINATIONS

DIURETIC

β - BLOCKADE

ACE INHIBITOR

Na+

renin

vasoconstriction

(Opie, 90)

Na+ loss

Ca2+ ANTAGONIST

FIGURE 7–3. Diuretics, basically acting by sodium loss, cause an increased circulating renin, which results in angiotensin-mediated vasoconstriction. Diuretics therefore combine well with β-blockers, which inhibit the release of renin; with ACE inhibitors, which inhibit the formation of angiotensin-II; and with calcium antagonists, which directly oppose diuretic-induced vasoconstriction. Because, however, calcium antagonists are mildly diuretic in themselves, the combination with diuretics is only logical in the presence of high salt intake.

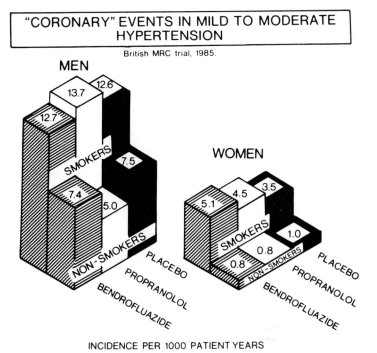

FIGURE 7–4. Note that in the large, placebo-controlled Medical Research Council (MRC) trial, the major factors governing occurrences of coronary events are smoking and male gender. A high dose of the diuretic bendrofluazide used in this trial left coronary events unaltered. Propranolol decreased coronary events only in non-smoking males. These data emphasize the inability of high-dose diuretics to decrease coronary events. Medical Research Council Working Party: Br Med J 291:97–104, 1985.

In addition to the specific individual factors, certain generalizations can be made. A moderate dose of any of these drugs will lower the blood pressure to about the same degree in most patients.[4] Blacks may be more responsive to diuretics or to vasodilators and less responsive to β-blockers. Older or low renin patients may respond slightly better to calcium antagonists. Patients with very high renin levels may do better with renin inhibition by an ACE inhibitor. Patients with abnormal blood lipid profiles may require an α-blocker. The **response rate** to each of these five major groups of agents—calcium antagonists, diuretics, β-blockers, ACE inhibitors, and α-blockers—may be no more than about 50 to 60%, depending on the criteria used and the dose given.

DIURETICS FOR HYPERTENSION

The diuretic first "step-care" approach has been used in most large therapeutic trials in the USA, and diuretics are still the drugs most often used either as monotherapy or in combination (Fig. 7–3). The vascular complications more directly related to the height of the blood pressure per se (strokes and CHF) have been reduced, but the frequency of the most common cause of disease and death among hypertensives, namely coronary artery disease, has not been significantly altered (Fig. 7–4). Increasingly the metabolic side-effects of diuretics are regarded as undesirable or harmful. Although a single morning dose of 25 mg of **hydrochlorothiazide** or its equivalent will provide a 10 mm Hg fall in the blood pressure of most uncomplicated hypertensives within several weeks, even that dose is probably too high. Lower doses (12.5 mg hydrochlorothiazide) have been shown to be equally effective especially when combined with β-blockade.[28] Nevertheless, only 12.5 mg hydrochlorothiazide may still induce blood lipid abnormalities,[69] even though the blood sugar does not rise.[48] Even lower doses may be effectively antihypertensive. The equivalent of 9 mg of hydrochlorothiazide provided all of the antihypertensive effect of a dose 4x larger with less hypokalemia, no hyperuricemia, and surprisingly no rise in plasma renin activity;[71] apparently, there were also no changes in blood lipid levels (data not yet reported). Higher doses of diuretics lead to only slightly greater falls in BP and may enhance side-effects. High doses may actually cause excess Na^+ depletion, especially when combined with excessively strict low sodium diets, with risk of reflex adrenergic activation.[87] High doses of thiazide are contained in many combination agents. In the case of longer-acting diuretics, such as **chlorthalidone**, a lower dose of 15 mg daily is almost as good as 25 mg and less hypokalemic.[95] Chlorthalidone 25 mg daily raises serum cholesterol by 8 to 10%.[77] The shorter-acting loop diuretics, furosemide or bumetanide, usually reserved for those with edema or renal insufficiency, are also effective antihypertensives in other patients, but require multiple daily doses. Metolazone may provide as much diuretic potency on a once-a-day basis.

Although the modified thiazide **indapamide** (Lozol, Natrilix) is claimed to have no metabolic side-effects, one study showed that it may be no better than hydrochlorothiazide-amiloride (Moduretic) as a third-line agent after β-blockade and diuretics.[82] In another study, indapamide 2.5 mg daily avoided blood lipid changes, yet the K^+ fell and uric acid rose.[58]

Despite these reservations, **diuretics remain among the preferred initial treatment in elderly, obese, or black patients**. Furthermore, when compared with placebo, they have been shown to reduce stroke in mild to moderate hypertension, although high doses were used in that study.[29] Strictly speaking, we do not know that the low doses of diuretics currently used really result in patient benefit unless certain assumptions are made.[49]

Potassium-sparing agents may add a few cents to the cost but save a good deal more by the prevention of diuretic-induced hypokalemia. All should be combined with another diuretic. The combinations of triamterene (Dyazide, Maxzide) or amiloride (Moduretic) with hydrochlorothiazide are usually chosen rather than spironolactone (Aldactazide) because the latter decreases testosterone synthesis. The dose of hydrochlorothiazide in one tablet of Dyazide is 25 mg, but only about half is absorbed. Standard Moduretic contains 50 mg, but in Europe, a "mini-Moduretic" (Moduret) with half the standard thiazide dose is now marketed to overcome this objection. However, even these doses may be too high.

β-BLOCKERS FOR HYPERTENSION

For initial therapy of hypertension, β-blockade is particularly suitable for patients with "increased adrenergic drive," those with associated angina pectoris, or in post-infarct patients. In young hypertensives, the cardiac output is high and the systemic vascular resistance is not increased,[63] so that β-blockade should theoretically be ideal treatment, although no formal studies can prove this point. In patients with mild to moderate hypertension, 50 to 70% respond to "average" doses of β-blockers,[36,37,40] but the optimal dose is hard to predict in the individual patient. A pragmatic rule is that if a standard dose of a standard β-blocker does not work within a week, it is useless to try another β-blocker.

β-Blockers are particularly well tested for "quality of life" (better kept with atenolol than with propranolol or pindolol).

In **black patients**, vasodilation or sodium loss seems to be the key to successful treatment; hence, logical first choices are diuretics[36] or the vasodilatory β-blocker, labetalol,[14] or other vasodilators.

Outcome trials comparing a β-blocker with placebo are few in number. In the case of propranolol, long-term outcome trials are available showing that a reduction of coronary events and strokes occurs chiefly in non-smokers; in non-smoking women, event rates were very low indeed, even during placebo treatment (see Fig. 7–4).

Dose. It is best to start with a low dose to lessen the chances of initial fatigue, which is probably due in part to the fall in cardiac output. For propranolol there is little, if any, additional antihypertensive effect with doses above 80 mg/day, given either once or twice per day.[13,15,31] The current trend is to use relatively low doses of all β-blockers. If the response to ordinary doses of β-blocker is inadequate, the preferred action is to change to another type of agent, such as a diuretic, calcium antagonist, or an ACE inhibitor, before going on to combination therapy.

Pharmacokinetics. Dose adjustment is more likely to be required with more lipid-soluble (lipophilic) agents, which have a high "first-pass" liver metabolism that may result in active metabolites (4-hydroxypropranolol, diacetolol metabolite of acebutolol); the rate of formation will depend on liver blood flow and function.

The **ideal β-blocker for hypertension** would be long-acting, cardioselective (see Fig. 1–4), and usually effective in a standard dose; there would also be simple pharmacokinetics (no liver metabolism, little protein binding, no lipid-solubility, and no active metabolites). Sometimes added vasodilation should be an advantage although, when a vasodilatory β-blocker was compared with atenolol over 1 year, there was no difference in the overall effects on the patients.[42] The ideal drug would be "lipid neutral." Of the existing agents, atenolol probably comes closest to providing this profile. If a truly long-acting β-blocker is required, nadolol is the agent of choice. In practice, once-a-day therapy is satisfactory with atenolol, sotalol, nadolol, penbutolol, dilevalol, and adequate doses of acebutolol, metoprolol, pindolol, propranolol, and oxprenolol, especially when the dose is high or when slow-release preparations (available for propranolol worldwide and for oxprenolol in Europe) are used.

Combination Therapy with Blockade for Hypertension. Combinations of β-blockers with one or another agent from all other classes have been successful in the therapy of hypertension.

In the case of **diuretics plus β-blockers**, the total daily dose of β-blocker-thiazide combination should ideally contain no more than 12.5 mg hydrochlorothiazide, 2.5 mg bendrofluazide, or a similar low dose of another diuretic.[28] Such low doses are not available as combination tablets with standard β-blocking doses. Double the ideal diuretic doses are provided in the USA by **Timolide** (10 mg timolol, 25 mg hydrochlorothiazide) or **Corzide** (80 mg nadolol, 5 mg bendrofluazide). Neither combination agent has a potassium-retaining component, provided in Europe by **Kalten** with 50 mg atenolol, 25 mg hydrochlorothiazide, and 2.5 mg amiloride.

β-Blocker-nifedipine is a hemodynamically sound combination, with powerful afterload reduction achieved by nifedipine offsetting the bradycardia and negative inotropic effects of β-blockade. There is an added hypotensive effect. Such combination therapy may be used both in mild to moderate hypertension not responding to monotherapy[11] and in severe or refractory hypertension, when further combination with a diuretic is usual.[23] In Europe, combination acebutolol with nifedipine is available, as well as atenolol-nifedipine (**Tenif** or **Beta-Adalat**, consisting of atenolol 50 mg and slow-release nifedipine 20 mg; the dose is 1–2 capsules daily for hypertension). In a large, randomized controlled study, nifedipine was more effective than atenolol in lowering systolic blood pressure, both drugs were

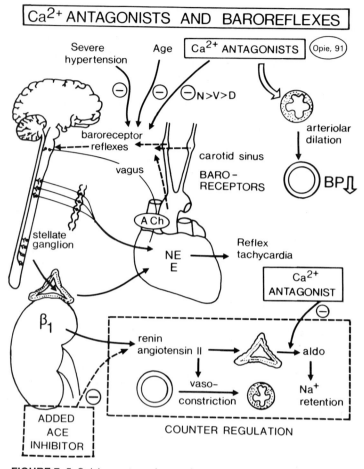

FIGURE 7–5. Calcium antagonists evoke counter-regulatory mechanisms, dependent on stimulation of renin and formation of angiotensin, as well as on reflex release of norepinephrine. The baroreceptor reflexes are inhibited by severe hypertension, by increasing age, and by continued use of the calcium-antagonist drugs (nifedipine more so than verapamil, in turn, more so than diltiazem). The concomitant use of ACE inhibitors is logical because ACE inhibitors decrease peripheral vasoconstriction and indirectly act as sympatholytic agents (see Fig. 5-5).

equally effective in lowering diastolic blood pressure, and, when patients failed to respond to atenolol or nifedipine alone, the combination showed further reduction in blood pressure.[59]

CALCIUM ANTAGONISTS FOR HYPERTENSION

Calcium antagonists compare well in their hypotensive effect with the established first-line agents, diuretics or β-blockers. Calcium antagonists act primarily to reduce peripheral vascular resistance, aided by an initial diuretic effect that persists, at least in the case of isradipine. No negative inotropic effect can be detected in patients with initially normal myocardial function. All three prototypical calcium antagonists, especially nifedipine, tend modestly to increase plasma catecholamines with a borderline elevation of plasma renin activity caused by the counter-regulatory effect (Fig. 7–5). There are no long-term outcome studies available on calcium antagonists in hypertension. As a group, calcium antagonists, and especially nifedipine and verapamil, are well tested in patients with severe hypertension. These agents are particularly effective in elderly patients and are equally effective in blacks and non-blacks. Calcium antagonists may be selected as initial monotherapy, especially if there are other indications for these agents, such as angina pectoris, Raynaud's phenomenon, or supraventricular tachycardia (Table 3-6).

Choice of Agent. Nifedipine is among the most effective antihypertensives in severe hypertension, and its use for mild to moderate hypertension will doubtless increase with the introduction of extended once-daily tablets (**Procardia XL**). Headache and ankle swelling are likely to remain the limiting side-effects. Other dihydropyridines effective on a once-a-day basis, such as **amlodipine**, are now also becoming available. The mild diuretic effect of the dihydropyridines contributes to the long-term benefit. Verapamil and diltiazem are also increasingly chosen as first-line antihypertensive agents, especially if angina is associated. Frequent constipation with verapamil is a disadvantage, especially in the elderly, although in patients on high fiber diets, verapamil can obviate diarrhea. Diltiazem monotherapy reduces BP in a dose-responsive way, with a mean fall of 12 mm Hg at a dose of 360 mg daily (given as 180 mg slow-release formulation twice daily[48]).

Compared with diuretics (also advocated for elderly or black patients), calcium antagonists are more expensive; however, calcium antagonists cause little or no metabolic disturbances in potassium, glucose, uric acid, or lipid metabolism, nor does aldosterone increase, whereas renin rises only slightly or not at all. Patients on calcium antagonists do not require intermittent blood chemistry checks. There is no evidence that calcium antagonists cause impairment of renal function, as is found with thiazide diuretics; rather, they may improve renal function. However, when hypertension is caused by chronic renal disease it is frequently volume-dependent, and diuretics are more logical therapy than calcium antagonists.

Compared with β-blockers, calcium antagonists cause less fatigue and little or no interference with normal cardiovascular dynamics, especially during exercise. Calcium antagonists have fewer contraindications and can, for example, be used safely in asthmatics, cause little or no interference with diabetic control, and are not contraindicated in peripheral vascular disease or in borderline heart failure (especially not nifedipine). However, β-blockers have established post-infarction protection and are usually preferred in post-infarct hypertension. Nonetheless, diltiazem benefits post-infarct hypertension in those without pulmonary congestion during the actual infarct.[76]

Of the **combinations**, calcium antagonist–β-blocker therapy has been well studied and is especially safe in the case of nifedipine. Although the addition of a diuretic has been claimed to add no benefit in the case of nifedipine,[64] a well-controlled study demonstrates an additive effect in the case of diltiazem.[48] A sustained natriuretic effect is probably best documented in the case of nifedipine-like agents. Calcium antagonists are thought to be most effective in the same groups in which diuretics are effective (elderly, blacks) and may have inherent diuretic properties. Therefore the combination of calcium antagonists with β-blockers seems more logical than that of calcium antagonists with diuretics, unless there is a persisting high sodium intake.[57] There are no comparative outcome studies in which calcium antagonists have been put against β-blockers or diuretics, so that the advantages of choosing a calcium antagonist must be predicted by an equal antihypertensive efficacy and lack of metabolic and central adverse effects.

Calcium antagonists and ACE inhibitors should combine well,[92] without the hemodynamic disadvantages of β-blockade or the metabolic problems caused by diuretics. ACE inhibitors oppose the negative counterregulation induced by the powerful vasodilatory calcium antagonists (see Fig. 7–5). Yet much more information is needed on this combination, particularly outcome studies.

ACE INHIBITORS FOR HYPERTENSION

ACE inhibitors, once reserved for refractory hypertension, especially when renal in origin, have edged their way into a prime position, where they are recognized as one of several agents of first choice. Minimal side-effects (often limited to cough), simplicity of use, a flat dose-response curve, virtual absence of contraindications except for bilateral renal artery stenosis and some related types of renal impairment, and ready combination with other modalities of treatment, as well as acceptability by the elderly, have promoted the increasing use of these agents. Furthermore, a specific case can be made for their preferential use in diabetic hypertensives or patients with hyperuricemia.

Captopril was the first ACE inhibitor, but enalapril and lisinopril are now available, and the list will soon expand to a multiplicity of agents, one from almost every drug company. All are antihypertensive, with a few practical differences (see Table 5-3). Heavy promotion has encouraged heavy use; nonetheless, as with other agents, a minority of hypertensive patients (possibly about 40%) do not respond fully for reasons not well understood.

In **mild to moderate hypertension**, captopril, enalapril, lisinopril, or any other ACE inhibitor can be used as monotherapy, even in low-renin patients,[41] or in combination with thiazide diuretics,[38] β-blockers, or calcium antagonists. High-dose captopril and enalapril are equipotent.[38] About 50 to 75% of mild to moderate hypertensives respond to monotherapy with ACE inhibition,[16] which is as effective as β-blockade or hydrochlorothiazide with fewer adverse subjective, metabolic, hypovolemic effects.[2,8,17] Combination captopril or enalapril with a thiazide diuretic achieves an additive antihypertensive effect while decreasing the thiazide-induced hypokalemia (Chap. 4).

In **renovascular hypertension,** where circulating renin is high and is a critical part of the hypotensive mechanism, ACE inhibition is logical first-line therapy. Because the hypotensive response may be dramatic, a low test dose is essential; because captopril acts quickest and is shortest in its duration of action, the **test dose** for ACE inhibitors should be 6.25 mg captopril. With standard doses of captopril or enalapril, the GFR falls acutely[3] to largely recover in cases of unilateral, but not bilateral, disease. However, blood flow to the stenotic kidney may remain depressed after removal of the angiotensin-II support, and progressive ischemic atrophy is possible.[81] This mechanism is quite different from the immune-based renal toxicity caused by captopril in the early high-dose studies. Logically, ACE inhibitors should be given only with greatest care (if at all) when there is pre-existing bilateral renal artery disease or unilateral disease in a solitary kidney, or when renal failure complicates renal artery stenosis. It may prove safe in those with unilateral renovascular disease, but careful follow-up of renal blood flow or function is required. Angioplasty or surgery is preferable to chronic medical therapy.

In **acute severe hypertension**, sublingual (chewed) captopril rapidly brings down the blood pressure,[35] but it is not clear how bilateral renal artery stenosis can be excluded quickly enough to make the speed of action of captopril an important benefit. Furthermore, the safety of such sudden falls of blood pressure in the presence of possible renal impairment (always a risk in severe hypertension) has not been evaluated.

In **hypertension unresponsive to conventional therapy**, renal artery stenosis must be considered, and ACE inhibition may be especially effective in the typical case with unilateral disease (precautions: bilateral disease or low total GFR).

In **diabetic hypertensives**, ACE inhibitors may be better than β-blockade or diuretics because of the potential benefit against progressive glomerulosclerosis[75] and because blood sugar regulation is unaltered. Diabetic hypertension may be a clear indication for preferential use of the ACE inhibitors.[78] In a comparative study, captopril decreased filtration fraction, whereas nifedipine increased it; correspondingly, captopril reduced albuminuria, whereas nifedipine increased it,[74] suggesting that the site of vasodilation might be important. Pre-glomerular vasodilation by calcium antagonists may increase intraglomerular pressure and albuminuria, whereas post-glomerular dilation by the ACE inhibitors may be beneficial. Proper clinical study of this potential difference is needed.

In **early renal failure** of hypertension, ACE inhibitors are being tested for a possible beneficial reduction of intrarenal hypertension.

In **elderly hypertensives**, ACE inhibitors were originally thought not to work so well because of the trend to a low renin status in that group. Several studies have now documented the benefit of ACE inhibition therapy in the elderly, although in many studies a diuretic was added.[78]

In **black hypertensives**, ACE inhibitors seem less effective than thiazides[78] and, again, an added diuretic may be required.

ACE Inhibitors: Antihypertensive Drug Combinations and Interactions

ACE Inhibitors Plus Diuretics. ACE inhibitors may be combined with thiazide diuretics to enhance hypotensive effects (see Fig. 7–3) and to lessen metabolic side-effects,[2] yet with some diuretic-induced loss of "quality of life."[8] This combination is logical because diuretics increase renin, the effects of which are antagonized by ACE inhibitors (see Fig. 7–3). Combination captopril-hydrochlorothiazide (Capozide) and enalapril-thiazide (Vaseretic) are now available (see Table 4-7). Enalapril 20 mg once daily, combined with only 12.5 mg hydrochlorothiazide, gives as good an antihypertensive effect as is achieved with more hydrochlorothiazide.[9] Such addition of a thiazide is better than increasing the dose of enalapril.[89] When combined with potassium-retaining thiazide diuretics (Dyazide, Moduretic, Maxzide), and especially spironolactone,[32] there is a **risk of hyperkalemia** because ACE inhibitors decrease aldosterone secretion and potassium excretion (see Fig. 7–5).

ACE Inhibitors Plus β-Blockade. This combination has been widely used in hypertension, although it is theoretically not the combination of choice because both agents have an ultimate antirenin effect. Nonetheless, current studies show additive antihypertensive effects.

ACE Inhibitors Plus Calcium Antagonists. This combination, now increasingly used in the therapy of hypertension (see Fig. 7–5), attacks both the renin-angiotensin system and the increased peripheral vascular resistance. Both types of agents are free of central nervous side-effects. However, large-scale studies on the combination are lacking.

α-ADRENERGIC BLOCKERS

Of the α_1-receptor blockers, only **prazosin** (Minipress) and **terazosin** (Hytrin) are available in the USA, but others, such as **indoramin** (Baratol, Wydora) and **doxazosin** (Cardura), are in use elsewhere. Their advantages usually include freedom from the central nervous depression of centrally acting drugs and the lipid perturbations of β-blockers, and a more appropriate physiologic action to lower peripheral resistance. Some patients develop troublesome side-effects:

drowsiness, postural hypotension, and occasional retrograde ejaculation. Tolerance, likely related to fluid retention, may develop during
chronic therapy with α_1-blockers, requiring increased doses[26] or
added diuretics, which explains why the Joint National Council in the
USA has not recommended α-blockers as first-line therapy. Nonetheless, they clearly have a place in initial monotherapy, particularly
in those with some disturbance of the blood lipid profile or in prostatic
men (α-blockade is used in the therapy of prostatism). α-Blockers also
combine well with β-blockers or diuretics. In the case of calcium
antagonists there may be an excess hypotensive response, as the
combination eliminates two of the three major vasoconstrictive
mechanisms, the remaining one being angiotensin-mediated. Thus,
when used with care, α-blockers are often excellent catalysts to calcium antagonists. Little is known of α-blockers plus ACE inhibitors.
Phenoxybenzamine and phentolamine are combined α_1 and α_2-blockers
used only for pheochromocytoma.

DIRECT VASODILATORS

Hydralazine used to be a standard third drug, its effectiveness
enhanced and side-effects removed by concomitant use of a diuretic
and an adrenergic inhibitor. Being inexpensive, hydralazine is still
widely used in the Third World. Elsewhere, fear of lupus and lack of
evidence for regression of left ventricular hypertrophy (LVH) has led
to its replacement by the calcium antagonist vasodilators. **Minoxidil**
is a potent long-acting vasodilator acting on the potassium channel. It
often causes profuse hirsutism so its use is usually limited to men with
severe refractory hypertension or renal insufficiency (it dilates renal
arterioles).

CENTRAL ADRENERGIC INHIBITORS

Of the centrally acting agents, **reserpine** is easiest to use in a low
dose of 0.05 mg/day, which provides almost all of its antihypertensive
action with fewer side-effects than higher doses.[37] Onset and offset of
action are slow and measured in weeks. When cost is crucial, reserpine
and diuretics are the cheapest combination. **Methyldopa**, still widely
used despite adverse central symptoms and potentially serious hepatic and blood side-effects, acts like clonidine on central α_2-receptors
usually without slowing the heart rate.[34] **Clonidine** and **guanabenz**
provide all of the benefits of methyldopa with none of the rare but
serious autoimmune reactions (as with methyldopa, sedation is frequent). A **transdermal form of clonidine** (Catapres-TTS) provides
once-a-week therapy likely minimizing the risks of clonidine withdrawal. **Guanabenz** resembles clonidine but may cause less fluid
retention and reduces serum cholesterol by 5 to 10%. **Guanfacine** is a
similar agent that can be given once daily.

MATCHING THE DRUG TO THE PATIENT

Diuretics and β-blockers are now used less and less for initial
therapy, except diuretic therapy for black, obese, or elderly patients,
with β-blockers kept for those with a prominent anxiety component or
ischemic heart disease. ACE inhibitors or calcium antagonists have
now become first-line agents of choice, particularly since once-a-day
formulations are now available, because they basically leave the
central and autonomic nervous systems' responses unaltered, act

specifically on peripheral resistance, and have few or no significant metabolic side-effects. In patients with blood lipid abnormalities, only an α_1-blocker, guanabenz or guanfacine, improves the lipid profile. The large number of agents now available, their very different side-effects, and the varying response of individual patients means that, increasingly, the old step-care approach is being used less and less; rather, an attempt is made to link the agent chosen to the specific needs of the individual patient.

PATIENT PROFILING

Patients Prone to Coronary Artery Disease. Awareness of the biochemical derangements often induced by chronic diuretic therapy, including an average 0.6 mmol/L fall of serum potassium, a 10 to 20 mg/dl rise in serum cholesterol, and a worsening of glucose tolerance, all of which could add risks for coronary disease, has raised concern over the appropriateness of a diuretic as the routine choice as initial therapy.[25] In an elegant demonstration of the metabolic disadvantages of diuretic therapy, Pollare and colleagues[79] studied carbohydrate and lipid metabolism during therapy with captopril in comparison with an equally antihypertensive dose of hydrochlorothiazide (mean dose 40 mg/day). The ACE inhibitor increased insulin sensitivity by 11%, whereas hydrochlorothiazide decreased it by a similar amount. Whereas the blood lipid profile changed little with captopril, in the hydrochlorothiazide group total serum cholesterol rose, as did low-density lipoprotein, total triglycerides, and very low-density triglycerides. However, there is as yet no proof that antihypertensive treatment by ACE inhibitors will achieve the desired reduction in coronary mortality. Regarding β-blockade, many clinicians assume (without evidence) that the partial protection β-blockers provide against recurrent heart attacks may serve to prevent initial coronary events, but the evidence is not clear-cut, with only one of four trials showing that a β-blocker was better than a diuretic.[83,96] Pooled data suggest a small benefit in men, especially in non-smokers. Perhaps more active weight reduction[77] or control of blood lipids[88] could be crucial in obtaining better reduction in cardiac mortality.

In addition to concern about the overt side-effects of β-blockers (in particular, their reduction of exercise capacity), their covert action to raise serum triglycerides and to lower HDL levels, as well as to impair insulin sensitivity,[79] has prompted advocacy of other agents as initial therapy. As a result, ACE inhibitors, calcium antagonists, and α-blockers are being used earlier and earlier whenever the lipid profile or the glucose tolerance is in question. **Whatever the drug chosen, evaluation of blood cholesterol is essential in all hypertensives and the effects of the agents chosen on the blood lipid profile need consideration**. Hopefully, more vigorous treatment of lipid abnormalities as well as of blood pressure will in time lead to decreased coronary artery disease.[88]

Hypertension in the elderly. What constitutes hypertension in the elderly and indeed what constitutes an elderly population are moot questions. One recent European trial[1] treated patients over 60 with pressures above 160/95 mm Hg initially by a diuretic plus potassium-sparer (Dyazide) and then added **methyldopa** (Aldomet). Results were impressive, with a reduction in stroke and cardiac mortality (from heart failure, not coronary disease); nonetheless, overall mortality was not affected. That trial showed that elderly patients may well require therapy and perhaps should be regarded as a "high risk group." However, treatment of patients with low mean initial blood pressure values (about 160-175/85-95 mm Hg) was actually associated with an increased mortality and a clear benefit of treatment was achieved only in those with initial mean blood pressure of about 180 / 105 mm Hg or more.[93] Hence, unless there are other risk factors present or unless there is end-organ damage, the case for treating mild elevations of blood pressure in the elderly is weak. Diuretics remain first-line treatment because they were successfully used in the European study and, perhaps even more important, they help to prevent osteoporosis, often disabling in the elderly (Chap. 4).

Regarding **β-blockade in the elderly**, most authorities, with the exception of Bühler's group,[47] have come to accept that β-blockade is as effective as in younger patients, with, however, the added risks of greater degrees of sinus or AV node inhibition and the disadvantages of a lower cardiac output resulting from bradycardia. In elderly patients, the vasodilatory β-blockers may be better because of the higher heart rate and maintenance of cardiac output. Thus dilevalol was more effective than atenolol in reducing the blood pressure, the heart rate fell less, and the ejection fraction rose slightly.[56] In a crucial well-designed study, three different regimens had similar BP lowering effects in the "young elderly" (mean age 66): a β-blocker, an ACE inhibitor, and a diuretic. However, exercise time was best on the ACE inhibitor.[61]

In **systolic hypertension in the elderly**, the present trend is to reduce values to below 160 mm Hg if possible. Nonetheless, reduction of systolic blood pressure (SBP) may drop the diastolic blood pressure (DBP) and, if that is already low, dangers of inadequate tissue perfusion become a reality. Hence therapy of systolic hypertension may not be easy, nor is the benefit yet proven. Older patients are likely to have a decreased vessel wall compliance, so for them one might choose a drug acting on the arteriolar wall, such as a calcium antagonist.[10] Diuretics such as chlorthalidone are also effective in systolic hypertension in the elderly[78] and, presumably, are also effective added to other agents such as β-blockers.

Tissue underperfusion in the elderly is a real risk. Indiscriminate reduction of diastolic blood pressure below a certain optimal value may actually increase mortality.[93] This so-called J-shaped curve seems to come into play below DBP values of about 90 mm Hg, or even higher in the elderly. Although the existence of this curve is still highly controversial, it makes sense that tissue underperfusion can lead to adverse effects. In systolic hypertension, any decrease in the systolic value may be accompanied by a fall in the diastolic value, already low in many elderly hypertensives with pure systolic hypertension.

Black Patients. "Within the criteria of the individualized patient profile, the race of the patient should be considered."[91] For reasons not quite evident, black patients seem to respond better to a diuretic,[36] to the vasodilatory β-blocker labetalol,[14] or to a calcium antagonist[68] than to a conventional β-blocker. Smoking, while generally an adverse factor in patients with hypertension, seems specifically to interfere with the effects of propranolol in black hypertensives.[67] When cost is crucial, it is important to know that reserpine plus diuretic is as effective as β-blocker plus diuretic in black patients.[91]

Smokers. The puzzled cardiologist is bound to get lost in the intricacies of the published studies, and the only sure conclusion is that smoking is a very adverse factor in hypertension (see Fig. 7–4).

For example, in two trials, the non-selective β-blockers, propranolol and oxprenolol, were more cardioprotective than a diuretic in non-smokers but not in smokers.[20,72] In the HAPPHY trial[97] there were no such differences; this time a cardioselective agent was the baseline β-blocker. In the MAPHY study,[96] which evolved from the HAPPHY study, the cardioselective β-blocker metoprolol was compared over a mean of 4 years with a high-dose thiazide diuretic (50 mg hydrochlorothiazide)—giving identical control of blood pressure—yet total mortality was lower in the β-blocker group, as a result of fewer deaths from coronary heart disease and stroke. In contrast to other studies, the benefit of the β-blockade was largely found in smokers. The major problem with this study is that the apparent reduction of coronary mortality when comparing metoprolol with a diuretic seems to be an adverse effect of diuretics and smoking in the group treated without metoprolol. Hypothetically, cardioselectivity could allow more favorable hemodynamics (less peripheral vasoconstriction) during β-blockade in smokers than a non-selective β-blocker such as propranolol.[55] Yet in that case why did atenolol not provide benefit in the HAPPHY study?

It is imperative that the patient stop smoking. Smoking, besides being an independent risk factor for coronary artery disease and for stroke (the latter often forgotten), also interacts directly with hypertension. First, smoking helps to promote renovascular and malignant hypertension. Second, smoking results in a short-lived rise in SBP and DBP, extending for 2 hours after smoking 2 cigarettes when combined with 500 ml coffee.[54] Third, smoking interferes with the benefits of propranolol,[67,72] at least in part by decreasing circulating blood levels of propranolol.[12]

Does this negative interaction between smoking and β-blockade extend beyond propranolol? At present, it makes little sense to use propranolol in refractory smokers. Rather, a cardioselective β-blocker should be used, or perhaps an α-blocker or vasodilatory β-blocker.

Obese Hypertensives. Obese hypertensives tend to have an increased extracellular and interstitial fluid volume[85] with an increased plasma volume in borderline obese hypertensives.[73] Thus, failing weight reduction, diuretics are more logical therapy than β-blockade.[70] A complex diet aimed at weight reduction, decreased salt intake, reduction of dietary fat, and increased polyunsaturated fats was less antihypertensive than the β-blocker atenolol, whereas blood lipid profiles responded better to the diet.[45]

Advanced Renal Failure. There is preliminary evidence that in advanced renal failure calcium, antagonists can prevent progression.[52]

Insulin Sensitivity and Diabetic Hypertensives. In **non-diabetic hypertensives**, both thiazides and β-blockers can impair insulin sensitivity.[80] Hypertension is associated with insulin resistance.[53] Therefore, it makes sense to avoid diuretics and β-blockers in the therapy of those prone to diabetes by a personal or family history or in non-insulin-dependent diabetics.

In **hypertensive diabetics** (type II non-insulin-dependent), similar principles apply. The combination of propranolol and hydrochlorothiazide increases the blood sugar by 56%.[50] Calcium antagonists generally leave diabetic control unaltered, although rarely, control may deteriorate. In the specific case of verapamil, glucose tolerance actually improves in non-diabetics.[84] ACE inhibitors have been shown to improve indices of glucose metabolism, especially in comparison with thiazide therapy but, again, the data were on non-diabetics.[79] ACE inhibitors may also bring about specific benefit in diabetic microangiopathy with albuminuria.[75] Furthermore, captopril is better than nifedipine in lessening exercise-induced microalbuminuria.[86]

The most important aim should be to reduce the BP to less than 140/90 mm Hg, and for this a combination of a low-dose diuretic and/or a cardioselective β-blocker and/or an ACE inhibitor as single, dual, or triple therapy is used as required.[75] As the GFR falls, a thiazide must be replaced by a loop diuretic.

SPECIFIC AIMS OF ANTIHYPERTENSIVE THERAPY

Regression of LVH. LVH, preferably diagnosed by echocardiography, is increasingly seen as an important adverse complication of hypertension, particularly in the light of the Framingham study.[60] Apart from increasing the cardiac risk, LVH is associated with abnormalities of diastolic function, which can result in dyspnea or even overt LV failure. An important point is that regression of the BP does not automatically result in decreased LVH, and the evidence that diuretics or hydralazine can lessen LVH is not impressive. On the other hand, in the case of many of the other drugs the studies, although abundant, have often been retrospective or uncontrolled.[90] Among the drugs best documented for their effects on regression of LVH are the β-blockers, with some good studies also favoring calcium antagonists, ACE inhibitors, and clonidine or methyldopa. In an excellent prospective study over 12 months,[90] propranolol was better than labetalol (α-β-blocker). Both propranolol and labetalol reduced LV wall thickness, yet labetalol increased LV cavity size, possibly because of the higher cardiac output with this drug. In other studies, atenolol, acebutolol, and metoprolol have all regressed LV mass,[90] which seems to be a general property of β-blockers.

Prevention of Sexual Dysfunction. Sexual dysfunction has been reported with almost every antihypertensive drug, probably a consequence of reduction of blood flow through genital vessels already sclerotic from the ravages of smoking, hypercholesterolemia, and diabetes.[44] However, there **are** differences between drugs. For example, ACE inhibitors[8] and calcium antagonists appear not to cause impotence. As impotence often has a psychogenic component, it can do no harm to tell the patient that nifedipine will bring blood to the penis on the basis of a few case reports of nifedipine-induced priapism.

Optimal Intellectual Activity . In general, antihypertensives with the exception of centrally active agents should be free of central side-effects. Nevertheless, it is now becoming clear that β-blockers have subtle effects on the intellect (see Table 1-4). Although propranolol is the major culprit, even the lipid-insoluble agent atenolol is not blameless. α-Blockers may invoke drowsiness in some. To be sure of unimpaired intellectual activity, calcium antagonists or ACE inhibitors seem to be the agents of choice. For example, patients on enalapril (20–40 mg daily) showed no change in memory, whereas atenolol (50–100 mg daily) caused mild but consistent impairment.[62]

Maintenance of Physical Activity. β-Blockers may induce fatigue and limit exercise capacity. Diuretics, calcium antagonists, ACE inhibitors, and α-blockers are all preferable. Vasodilatory β-blockers still need evaluation, but are logical choices.

Diurnal Variations. For specific patients, a 24-hour ambulatory BP highlights the hours of high BP, for example in the morning. BP control can be tapered to such patterns by "pulsed therapy," for example, by added short-acting nifedipine or labetalol. In others, a vigorous early morning jog may induce sufficient reactive vasodilation to be effectively antihypertensive through the morning.

Cost Effectiveness. In the Third World and often elsewhere, expensive drugs are a luxury, and the principles of choice are governed by economic necessity. Much can be said for low-dose thiazide diuretics as initial therapy, followed by reserpine. Low-dose generic thiazide diuretic is relatively free of metabolic side-effects (possibly except for effects on lipids). The cost of reserpine is extremely low, it is effectively antihypertensive, and it is relatively free from significant hemodynamic or subjective side-effects. A diuretic-based therapy is also logical in black patients. When compliance is relatively limited by educational handicaps, the very long biologic half-life of reserpine, with catecholamine depletion lasting for many weeks, is a major advantage. Furthermore, a cheap vasodilator (hydralazine) can readily be combined with diuretic-reserpine as the next step to give a poor man's equivalent of the very effective β-blocker–diuretic–calcium antagonist combination.

In the USA, complex and possibly misleading computer calculations[51] suggest that the cost of treatment for 1 year for each life saved with the various agents is $10,900 for propranolol, $16,400 for hydrochlorothiazide (where the greatest cost is in the laboratory blood tests), $20,800 for atenolol, $31,600 for nifedipine, $61,900 for prazosin, and $72,100 for captopril. If, however, the impaired quality of life with propranolol is allowed for, the cost with propranolol becomes $33,300 per quality-adjusted life year. As no allowance has been made for diabetes or gout or loss of quality of life induced by the high diuretic dose (hydrochlorothiazide 75–100 mg), atenolol followed by nifedipine may in the end be most cost-effective.

ACUTE SEVERE HYPERTENSION

For urgent therapy of acute severe hypertension (Table 7-3) the choice used to fall on an IV agent, but sublingual nifedipine is now almost standard therapy. It consistently reduces SBP and DBP by about 20% within 20 to 30 minutes.[6] Such a rapid reduction of hypertension may be safe even in the presence of cerebral symptoms;[5,19] **nevertheless it is prudent to consider whether rapid pressure reduction is really desirable in the presence of cerebral symptoms or symptoms of myocardial ischemia.** Case reports indicating the precipitation of cerebral infarction by acute hypotensive therapy have consistently included therapies that cause excess hypotension,[7,27] whereas nifedipine has very rarely caused "overshoot" in the treatment of acute severe hypertension.[21] Nifedipine is especially useful in the therapy of hypertensive heart failure with pulmonary edema.

Parenteral agents such as nitroprusside are still used extensively. These all require careful monitoring to avoid overshoot. Nitroprusside reduces preload and afterload and has the risk of rebound hypertension. An infusion of nitroprusside is less effective and costs more than sublingual nifedipine (see Chap. 3). Labetalol does not cause tachycardia and gives a smooth dose-related fall in blood pressure; the side-effects of β-blockade, such as heart failure and bronchospasm, may be countered by the added α-blockade and ISA (p 4) of labetalol. Diazoxide is best avoided. Hydralazine and dihydralazine may cause tachycardia and are also best avoided especially in angina, unless there is concomitant therapy with a β-blocker. There is no IV preparation of prazosin, which does, however, have a rapid onset of action when given orally. Starting with an oral β-blocker seems to work well in some patients with acute severe hypertension even in the presence of papilledema.[21] At present, when **the ideal rate of reduction of hypertension requiring urgent therapy is not known**, the simplicity of sublingual nifedipine (10 mg) is increasingly seen as seemingly safe therapy, provided there is no clinical evidence of cerebral or myocardial ischemia or clinically evident renal failure. When such complications are present, careful slow-monitored reduction of blood pressure still seems best.

In **severe hypertension in the elderly**, sublingual nifedipine seems as safe as in younger subjects.[10] Decreased cerebral perfusion in elderly patients is a potentially serious hazard so that, if nifedipine is chosen, an initial dose of 5 mg nifedipine may be better than 10 mg.[22] Where 5-mg capsules are not available (as in the USA), the contents of a 10-mg capsule may be extracted by a syringe and half may be given intraorally. With nifedipine, as with any other effective hypotensive therapy, the risk of precipitating cerebral ischemia must be carefully considered despite the reported cerebral vasodilating effect of nifedipine.

TABLE 7–3 AGENTS FOR USE IN HYPERTENSIVE EMERGENCIES (CAUTION: SEE TEXT FOR IMPORTANT RESERVATIONS)

Agent	Usual Dose	Side-Effects	Comments	Cross Reference
Nifedipine	5–20 mg bite-and-swallow, sublingual or orally, repeat every 4–6 hours; then introduce β-blocker, ACE inhibitor, or diuretic. When stabilized, replace capsules by long-acting nifedipine	Few; "overshoot" seldom ischemia	Simple therapy, usually effective; needs further evaluation and caution in presence of papilledema and hypertensive encephalopathy	Chap. 3, p 61
Captopril	25 mg chewed*	Risk of renal failure, especially in bilateral renal stenosis. Risk of excess hypotension in high renin states	Exclude renal artery stenosis, especially bilateral Test dose 6.25 mg	Chap. 5, p 113
Labetalol	Infuse at 2 mg/min to total of 1–2 mg/kg Oral dose 400 mg start, then 200 mg 6-hourly**	May worsen cardiac failure Usually safe	Avoids tachycardia. IV use gives smooth and rapid dose-related fall in blood pressure. Oral therapy under-used	Chap. 1, p 4
Nitroprusside	Infusion of 40–75 μg/min	Hypotension, must monitor constantly	Especially useful if pulmonary edema or encephalopathy, otherwise avoid	Chap. 5, p 117
Hydralazine	5–10 mg IV every 4–6 hr	Tachycardia, contraindicated in angina, ischemic strokes	Avoid if possible. Tachycardia can be countered by propranolol 1–2 mg IV	Chap. 5, p 118
Dihydralazine	6.25–12.5 mg IV slowly or infuse IV as 0.1 mg/min to total of 25 mg	As above, prefer infusion	As above	Chap. 5, p 119
Furosemide	IV 40–180 mg; oral 40–240 mg	Hypokalemia, hyponatremia	Best for fluid retention, renal failure	Chap. 4, p 75

Modified from Opie LH: Drugs and the Heart. London, Lancet, 1980, p 109.
*Tschollar and Belz: Lancet 2:34–35, 1985.
**Ghose and Sampson: Curr Med Res 5:147, 1977.

MAXIMAL THERAPY

When confronted with the occasional patient who appears to be refractory to all known forms of therapy, the following points are worth considering: (1) Is the patient really compliant with the therapy? (2) Are the blood pressure values taken in the doctor's office really representative of those that the patient lives with (there can be striking differences)? (3) Has the patient developed some complications such as atherosclerotic renal artery stenosis or renal failure? (4) Has the patient upped the salt or alcohol intake or taken NSAIDs or sympathomimetic agents? (5) Are there temporary psychological stresses? (6) Is the therapy really maximal, particularly regarding the diuretic dose, because overfilling of dilated vasculature by reactive sodium retention may also preclude a fall in the peripheral resistance? (Note that low dose diuretic therapy is reluctantly abandoned at this stage.)

Logically, refractory hypertension means that the peripheral vascular resistance has failed to fall. Therefore the emphasis should be on vasodilator therapy, acting on every conceivable mechanism: calcium antagonism, α-blockade, ACE inhibition, K^+ channel-induced vasodilation by minoxidil, and high-dose diuretics. Combination of α-blockade and ACE inhibition together with calcium antagonism blunts the adverse baroreflex response to the calcium antagonism. Potassium channel dilation complements other vasodilatory mechanisms. In addition, a centrally active agent indirectly lessens the release of norepinephrine from the nerve terminals. β-Blockade, by reducing the cardiac output, acts through an entirely different mechanism. Severe hypertension often has a volume-dependent component and reactive sodium retention often accompanies the fall in BP induced by vasodilatory drugs; therefore, the addition of more diuretics, particularly the loop agents, is an important component of maximal therapy. Occasionally, in a patient in whom blood pressure remains elevated despite the above measures, hospital admission with acute intravenous BP lowering, for example by IV verapamil or labetalol, helps to reset the baroreflexes whereupon previously refractory hypertension yields to more standard therapy.

The **ganglion blockers** (**guanethidine** and **guanadrel**), now decidedly out of fashion because of frequent orthostatic hypotension and interference with sexual activity, should therefore be reserved for the last resort.

REFERENCES

References from Previous Edition (Previously Chapter 11)

1. Amery A, Birkenhager W, Brixko P, et al: Lancet 2:1349–1354, 1985
2. Bauer JH, Jones LB: Am J Kidney Dis 4:55–62, 1984
3. Bender W, La France N, Walker WG: Hypertension 6 (suppl I):I-193–I-197, 1984
4. Berglund G, Andersson O: Lancet 1:744–747, 1981
5. Bertel O, Conen D, Radu EW: Br Med J 1:19–21, 1983
6. Conen D, Bertel O, Dubach UC: J Cardiovasc Pharmacol 4:S378–S382, 1982
7. Cove DH, Seddon M, Fletcher RF: Br Med J 2:245–246, 1979
8. Croog SH, Levine S, Testa MA, et al: N Engl J Med 314:1657–1664, 1986
9. Dahlof B, Andren L, Eggertsen R, et al: J Hypertens 3 (suppl 3):S483–S486, 1985
10. Dais K, Jones J, Gooray D, et al: Circulation 72(suppl III):III–50, 1985
11. Daniels AR, Opie LH: Am J Cardiol 57:965–970, 1986
12. Deanfield J, Wright C, Krikler S, et al: N Engl J Med 310:951–954, 1984
13. Douglas-Jones AP, Baber NS, Lee A: Eur J Clin Pharmacol 14:163–166, 1978

14. Flamenbaum W, Weber MA, McMahon FG, et al: J Clin Hypertens 1:56–69, 1985

15. Galloway DB, Glover SC, Hendry WG, et al: Br Med J 2:140–142, 1976

16. Gavras H, Biollaz J, Waeber B, et al: Lancet 2:543–549, 1981

17. Helgeland A, Strommen R, Hagelund CH, et al: Lancet 1:872–875, 1986

18. Hodsman GP, Brown JJ, Cumming AMM, et al: J Hypertens 1(suppl 1):109–117, 1983

19. Huysmans FTM, Sluiter HE, Thien TA, et al: Br J Clin Pharmacol 16:725–727, 1983

20. International Prospective Primary Prevention Study in Hypertension (IPPPSH): J Hypertens 3:379–392, 1985

21. Isles CG, Johnson AOC, Milne FJ: Br J Clin Pharmacol 21:377–383, 1986

22. Ito H, Arakawa M, Shibasaki T, et al: Drug Res 34:630–636, 1984

23. Jennings AA, Jee LD, Smith JA, et al: Am Heart J 111:557-563, 1986

24. Joint National Committee on Detection, Evaluation and Treatment of High Blood Pressure: Arch Intern Med 140:1280-1286, 1980

25. Kaplan NM: In Clinical Hypertension, ed 4: Baltimore, Williams & Wilkins, 1986, pp 180–272

26. Khatri IM, Levinson P, Notargiacomo A, et al: Am J Cardiol 55:1015–1018, 1985

27. Ledingham JCG: Hypertension 5 (suppl 3):114–119, 1983

28. MacGregor GA, Banks RA, Markandu ND, et al: Br Med J 286:1535–1538, 1983

29. Medical Research Council Working Party: Br Med J 291:97–104, 1985

30. Perry HM, Hulley SB, Furberg CD, et al: Circulation 72(suppl III):III-50, 1985

31. Serlin MJ, Orme MLE, Baber NS, et al: Clin Pharmacol Ther 27:586–592, 1980

32. Sharpe DN, Murphy J, Coxon R, et al: Circulation 70:271–278, 1984

33. Stumpe KO, Overlack A: Br J Clin Pharmacol 7(suppl 2):189–197, 1979

34. Struthers AD, Brown MJ, Adams EF, et al: Br J Clin Pharmacol 19:311–317, 1985

35. Tschollar W, Belz GG: Lancet 2:34–35, 1985

36. Veterans Administration Cooperative Study Group on Antihypertensive Agents: JAMA 237:2303–2310, 1977

37. Veterans Administration Participating Medical Centers: JAMA 248:2471–2477, 1982

38. Vlasses PH, Conner DP, Rotmensch HH, et al: J Am Coll Cardiol 7:651–660, 1986

39. Whitworth JA, Kincaid-Smith P: Drugs 23:394–402, 1982

40. Wilcox RG, Hampton JR: Br Heart J 46:498–502, 1981

41. Wilkins LH, Dustan HP, Walker JF, et al: Clin Pharmacol Ther 34:297–302, 1983

New References

42. Ambrosioni E, Birkenhager W, De Leeuw PW, et al: Comparison of a vasodilating β-blocker and a cardioselective β-blocker in long-term treatment of hypertension: A European multicentre study. J Hypertens 7(suppl 6): S266–S267, 1989

43. Baglivo HP, Fabregues G, Burrieza H, et al: Effect of moderate physical training on left ventricular mass in mild hypertensive persons. Hypertension 15(suppl I):I-153–I-156, 1990

44. Bansal S: Sexual dysfunction in hypertensive men: A critical review of the literature. Hypertension 12:1–10, 1988

45. Berglund A, Andersson OK, Berglund G, Fagerberg B: Antihypertensive effect of diet compared with drug treatment in obese men with mild hypertension. Br Med J 299:480–485, 1989

46. Bonaa KH, Bjerve KS, Straume B, et al: Effect of eicosapentaenoic and docosahexaenoic acids on blood pressure in hypertension. A population-based intervention trial from the Tromso Study. N Engl J Med 322:795–801, 1990

47. Bühler F: Antihypertensive treatment according to age, plasma renin, and race. Drugs 35:495-503, 1988

48. Burris JF, Weir MR, Oparil S, et al: An assessment of diltiazem and hydrochlorothiazide in hypertension: Application of factorial trial design to a multicenter clinical trial of combination therapy. JAMA 263:1507–1512, 1990

49. Collins R, Peto R, MacMahon S, et al: Blood pressure, stroke, and coronary heart disease. Part 2: Short-term reductions in blood pressure:

Overview of randomised drug trials in their epidemiological context. Lancet 335:827–838, 1990

50. Dornhorst A, Powell SH, Pensky J: Aggravation by propranolol of hyperglycaemic effect of hydrochlorothiazide in Type II diabetics without alteration of insulin secretion. Lancet 1:123–126, 1985

51. Edelson JT, Weinstein MC, Tosteson ANA, et al: Long-term cost-effectiveness of various initial monotherapies for mild to moderate hypertension. JAMA 263:408–413, 1990

52. Eliahou HE, Cohen D, Ben-David A, et al: The calcium channel blocker nisoldipine delays progression of chronic renal failure in humans (preliminary communication). Cardiovasc Drugs Ther 1:523–528, 1988

53. Ferrannini E, Buzzigoli G, Bonadonna R, et al: Insulin resistance in essential hypertension. N Engl J Med 317: 350–357, 1987

54. Freestone S, Ramsay LE: Effect of coffee and cigarette smoking on the blood pressure of untreated and diuretic-treated hypertensive patients. Am J Med 73:348–353, 1982

55. Freestone S, Ramsay LE: Effect of β-blockade on the pressor response to coffee plus smoking in patients with mild hypertension. Drugs 25(suppl 2):141-145, 1983

56. Frishman WH, Glasser SP, Strom JA, et al: Effects of dilevalol, metoprolol and atenolol on left ventricular mass and function in non-elderly and elderly hypertensive patients. Am J Cardiol 63:69–74, 1989

57. Galletti F, Strazzullo P, Cappuccio FP, et al: Calcium channel blockers and sodium intake: A controlled study in patients with essential hypertension. Cardiovasc Drugs Ther 3:135–140, 1989

58. Gerber A, Weidmann P, Bianchetti MG, et al: Serum lipoproteins during treatment with the antihypertensive agent indapamide. Hypertension 7(suppl II):II-164–II-169, 1985

59. Heagerty AM, Swales J, Baksi A, et al: Nifedipine-Atenolol Study Review Committee: Nifedipine and atenolol singly and combined for treatment of essential hypertension: Comparative multicentre study in general practice in the United Kingdom. Br Med J 296:468–472, 1988

60. Kannel WB, Cupples LA, D'Agostino RB, Stokes J, III: Hypertension, antihypertensive treatment, and sudden coronary death: The Framingham Study. Hypertension 11(suppl II): II-45–II-50, 1988

61. Leonetti G, Mazzola C, Pasotti C, et al: Antihypertensive efficacy and influence on physical activity of three different treatments in elderly hypertensive patients. J Hypertens 7(suppl 6):S304–S305, 1989

62. Lichter I, Richardson PJ, Wyke MA: Differential effects of atenolol and enalapril on memory during treatment for essential hypertension. Br J Clin Pharmacol 21:641–645, 1986

63. Lund-Johansen P: Central haemodynamic in essential hypertension at rest and during exercise: A 20-year follow-up study. J Hypertens 7(suppl 6):S52–S55, 1989

64. MacGregor GA: Nifedipine and hypertension: Roles of vasodilation and sodium balance. Cardiovasc Drugs Ther 3:295–301, 1990

65. MacGregor GA, Markandu ND, Sagnella GA, et al: Double-blind study of three sodium intakes and long-term effects of sodium restriction in essential hypertension. Lancet 2:1244–1247, 1989

66. Manson JE, Colditz GA, Stampfer MJ, et al: A prospective study of obesity and risk of coronary heart disease in women. N Engl J Med 322:882–889, 1990

67. Materson BJ, Reda D, Freis ED, Henderson WG: Cigarette smoking interferes with treatment of hypertension. Arch Intern Med 148:2116–2119, 1988

68. M'Buyamba-Kabangu J-R, Lepira B, Lijnen P, et al: Intracellular sodium and the response to nitrendipine or atenolol in African blacks. Hypertension 11:100–105, 1988

69. McKenney JM, Goodman RP, Wright JT, et al: The effect of low-dose hydrochlorothiazide on blood pressure, serum potassium, and lipoproteins. Pharmacotherapy 6:179–184, 1986

70. McMahon SW, Wilcken DEL, MacDonald GJ: The effect of weight reduction on left ventricular mass: A randomized controlled trial in young, overweight hypertensive patients. N Engl J Med 314:334–339, 1986

71. McVeigh G, Galloway D, Johnston D: The case for low dose diuretics in hypertension: Comparison of low and conventional doses of cyclopenthiazide. Br Med J 297:95–98, 1988

72. Medical Research Council Working Party: Stroke and coronary heart disease in mild hypertension: risk factors and the value of treatment. Br Med J 296:1565–1570, 1988

73. Messerli FH, Ventura HO, Reisin E, et al: Borderline hypertension and obesity: Two prehypertensive states with elevated cardiac output. Circulation 66:55–60, 1982

74. Mimran A, Insua A, Ribstein J, et al: Contrasting effects of captopril and nifedipine in normotensive patients with incipient diabetic nephropathy. J Hypertens 6:919–923, 1988

75. Mogensen CE: Management of diabetic renal involvement and disease. Lancet 1:867–870, 1988

76. Moss AJ, Rubison M, Oakes D, et al: Effect of diltiazem on long-term outcome in post-infarction patients with a history of hypertension (abstract). Circulation 80(suppl II):II-268, 1989

77. Oberman A, Wassertheil-Smoller S, Langford HG, et al: Pharmacologic and nutritional treatment of mild hypertension: Changes in cardiovascular risk status. Ann Intern Med 112:89–95, 1990

78. Perry IJ, Beevers DG: ACE inhibitors compared with thiazide diuretics as first-step antihypertensive therapy. Cardiovasc Drugs Ther 3:815–819, 1989

79. Pollare T, Lithell H, Berne C: A comparison of the effects of hydrochlorothiazide and captopril on glucose and lipid metabolism in patients with hypertension. N Engl J Med 321:868–873, 1989

80. Pollare T, Lithell H, Selinus I, Berne C: Sensitivity to insulin during treatment with atenolol and metoprolol: A randomized, double-blind study of effects on carbohydrate and lipoprotein metabolism in hypertensive patients. Br Med J 298:1152–1157, 1989

81. Postma CT, Hoefnagels WHL, Barentsz JO, et al: Occlusion of unilateral stenosed renal arteries: Relation to medical treatment. J Human Hypertens 3:185–190, 1989

82. Poulsen L, Friberg M, Noer I, et al: Comparison of indapamide and hydrochlorothiazide plus amiloride as a third drug in the treatment of arterial hypertension. Cardiovasc Drugs Ther 3:141–144, 1989

83. Psaty BM, Koepsell TD, LoGergo JP, et al: β-Blockers and primary prevention of coronary heart disease in patients with high blood pressure. JAMA 261:2087–2094, 1989

84. Rojdmark S, Andersson DEH: Influence of verapamil on human glucose tolerance. Am J Cardiol 57:39D–43D, 1986

85. Raison J, Achimastos A, Asmar R, et al: Extracellular and interstitial fluid volume in obesity with and without associated systemic hypertension. Am J Cardiol 57:223–226, 1986

86. Romanelli G, Giustina A, Ababiti-Rosei E, et al: Short-term effect of captopril and nifedipine on micro-albuminuria induced by exercise in hypertensive diabetic patients. J Hypertens 6(suppl 6):S312–S313, 1989

87. Rosenman RH: Results of the multicenter antihypertensive treatment trials: Therapeutic implications and the role of the sympathetic nervous system. Am J Hypertens 2:313S–338S, 1989

88. Samuelsson O, Wilhelmsen L, Andersson OK, et al: Cardiovascular morbidity in relation to change in blood pressure and serum cholesterol levels in treated hypertension: Results from the primary prevention trial in Goteborg, Sweden. JAMA 285:1768–1776, 1987

89. Sassano P, Chatellier G, Billaud E, et al: Comparison of increase in the enalapril dose and addition of hydrochlorothiazide as second-step treatment of hypertensive patients not controlled by enalapril alone. J Cardiovasc Pharmacol 13:314–319, 1989

90. Szlachcic J, Hall WD, Tubau JF, et al: Left ventricular hypertrophy reversal with labetalol and propranolol: A prospective, randomized, double-blind study. Cardiovasc Drugs Ther 4:115–121, 1990

91. Seedat YK: Editorial review. Varying responses to hypotensive agents in different racial groups: Black versus white differences. J Hypertens 7:515–518, 1989

92. Singer DRJ, Markandu ND, Shore AC, MacGregor GA: Captopril and nifedipine in combination for moderate to severe essential hypertension. Hypertension 9:629–633, 1987

93. Staessen J, Bulpitt C, Clement D, et al: Relation between mortality and treated blood pressure in elderly patients with hypertension: Report of the European Working Party on High Blood Pressure in the Elderly. Br Med J 298:1552–1556, 1989

94. Swales JD, Ramsay LE, Coope JR, et al: Regular review: Treating mild hypertension. Br Med J 298:694–698, 1989

95. Vardan S, Mehrotra KG, Mookherjee S, et al: Efficacy and reduced metabolic side-effects of a 15 mg chlorthalidone formulation in the treatment of mild hypertension. JAMA 258:484–488, 1987

96. Wikstrand J, Warnold I, Olsson G, et al: Primary prevention with metoprolol in patients with hypertension: Mortality results from the MAPHY study. JAMA 259:1976–1982, 1988

97. Wilhelmsen L, Berglund G, Elmfeldt D, et al: β-Blockers versus diuretics in hypertensive men: Main results from the HAPPHY trial. J Hypertens 5:561–572, 1987

Book

98. Kaplan, Nm: Clinical hypertension. 5th edition. Baltimore, Williams & Wilkins, 1990

B.N. Singh
L.H. Opie
F.I. Marcus

8

Antiarrhythmic Agents

Arrhythmias require treatment either for alleviating symptoms or for prolonging survival. The wisdom of treating arrhythmias "prophylactically" has been severely questioned by the results of the CAST Study.[168] Although undertaken with Class IC agents, the principle raised is important in that arrhythmias need treatment only when they are symptomatically significant, or when the benefit of treatment clearly outweighs the risks involved.

CLASS IA: QUINIDINE AND SIMILAR COMPOUNDS

There are four established classes of antiarrhythmic agents (Table 8-1). Class IA agents (quinidine, disopyramide, procainamide) lengthen the effective refractory period by two mechanisms in the usual therapeutic concentrations. First, they inhibit the fast sodium current and the upstroke of the action potential; second, they prolong the action potential duration and thereby have a mild Class III effect (Figs. 8–1 and 8–2). Such compounds can cause pro-arrhythmic complications by prolonging the QT-interval in certain predisposed individuals (see QT-Prolongation and Torsades de Pointes), or by depressing conduction and promoting re-entry. Despite newly reported side-effects, quinidine still has a place.

Quinidine

Electrophysiology. Quinidine (Fig. 8–3) is the prototype of Class I agents. It has a wide spectrum of activity against re-entrant as well as ectopic, atrial, and ventricular tachyarrhythmias. It slows conduction and increases refractoriness in the retrograde limb of AV nodal tachycardias and over the anterograde or retrograde limbs of Wolff-Parkinson-White (WPW) syndrome re-entrant tachycardias (Fig. 8–4). Quinidine also prolongs anterograde refractoriness of the accessory pathway, thereby slowing the ventricular response to atrial fibrillation in WPW.

Receptor Effects. Quinidine inhibits peripheral and myocardial α-adrenergic receptors,[78] so that there is risk of hypotension with IV administration. By also inhibiting muscarinic receptors, quinidine has an anticholinergic effect (vagolytic), which may cause sinus tachycardia[71] and facilitate AV conduction to increase the ventricular rate in atrial flutter or fibrillation.

Pharmacokinetics and Therapeutic Levels (Table 8-2). Quinidine is metabolized primarily by hydroxylation in the liver, and a

TABLE 8–1 ANTIARRHYTHMIC DRUG CLASS

Class	Channel Effects	Repolarization Time	Drug Examples
IA	Sodium block Effect ++	Prolongs	Quinidine Disopyramide Procainamide
IB	Sodium block Effect +	Shortens	Lidocaine Phenytoin Mexiletine Tocainide Ethmozine*
IC	Sodium block Effect +++	Unchanged	Flecainide Encainide Propafenone Indecainide Ethmozine*
II	Phase IV (depolarizing current); calcium channel	Unchanged	β-Blockers
III	Repolarizing K$^+$ currents	Markedly prolongs	Amiodarone Sotalol Bretylium
IV	Calcium block Effect ++	Unchanged	Verapamil Diltiazem
	K$^+$ channel openers (hyperpolarization)	Unchanged	Adenosine ATP

*Ethmozine has "mixed" properties and is not easy to classify.
+   = inhibitory effect.
++   = markedly inhibitory effect.
+++ = very major inhibitory effect.

small amount is excreted by the kidneys; mean bioavailability is about 90%, but varies greatly. Quinidine elimination is grossly normal in heart or renal failure, but not in hepatic failure, which results in higher blood levels. The plasma half-life increases with age so that the dose should be reduced. Therapeutic blood levels are 2.3 to 5.0 μ g/ml (= 3–5.5 μ M/L) with specific assays.

Indications. Quinidine is frequently used in attempted pharmacologic conversion of atrial flutter or fibrillation, sometimes combined with verapamil or digoxin to prevent acceleration of ventricular response prior to cardioversion. Post-cardioversion quinidine is often used in the hope of maintaining sinus rhythm with, however, the risk of increased mortality.[126a] It is reasonably effective in reducing recurrences of supraventricular tachycardias, including those of the bypass tract, and recurrent ventricular tachycardia (VT). Quinidine has not been shown to reduce sudden death or to prolong survival.

Dose. A test of 0.2 g of quinidine sulfate is traditionally given while the patient is monitored to check for drug idiosyncrasy, including cardiovascular collapse, although such serious side-effects are seldom seen and the whole procedure is of unproven value. Then sustained oral therapy is started. Conventional dosing is 300 mg or 400 mg **quinidine sulfate** 4x daily or every 6 hours, with a usual total dose of 1.2 to 1.6 g/day with a maximum of 2 g.[103] Long-acting quinidine preparations (similar dose limits) are **quinidine gluconate** (multiples of 330 mg or 325 mg) and **quinidine polygalacturonate** (multiples of 275 mg as Cardioquin 8–12 hourly). The systemic availability is nearly equivalent for the above doses of these three preparations. Marked individual variations in half-life may require monitoring by plasma levels. When a long-acting preparation is started, a loading dose of quinidine sulfate 0.6 to 0.8 g, given 1 hour before the first long-acting dose, will produce an adequate blood level in 3 hours. **IV quinidine** is now rarely used because of hypotension (vasodilator effect).

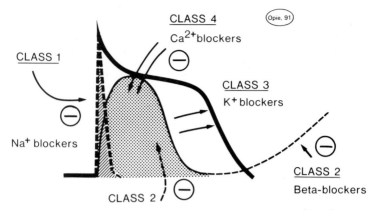

FIGURE 8–1. The classic four types of antiarrhythmic agents. Class I agents decrease phase zero of the rapid depolarization of the action potential (rapid sodium channel). Class II agents, β-blocking drugs, have complex actions including inhibition of spontaneous depolarization (phase 4) and indirect closure of calcium channels, which are less likely to be in the "open" state when not phosphorylated by cyclic AMP. Class III agents block the outward potassium channels to prolong the action potential duration and hence refractoriness. Class IV agents, verapamil and diltiazem, and the indirect calcium antagonist adenosine, inhibit the inward calcium channel, which is most prominent in nodal tissue, particularly the AV node. Most antiarrhythmic drugs have more than one action.

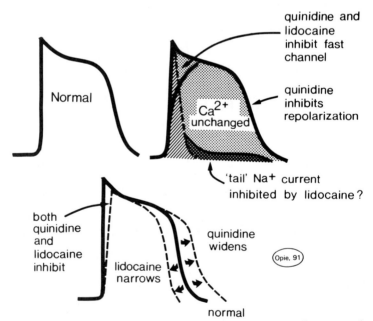

FIGURE 8–2. Both quinidine and lidocaine inhibit the fast sodium channel. The effect on upstroke velocity is exaggerated for diagrammatic purposes. Lidocaine maximally inhibits the fast channel when it is in the inactivated state, as found in ischemic tissue. Lidocaine promotes repolarization to narrow the action potential duration, possibly through inhibition of a "background" sodium current. In contrast, quinidine readily inhibits the sodium channel in its open state, explaining the more marked inhibition of the upstroke velocity of the action potential. Quinidine also prolongs the action potential duration, by inhibition of the repolarizing K+ currents.

QUINIDINE

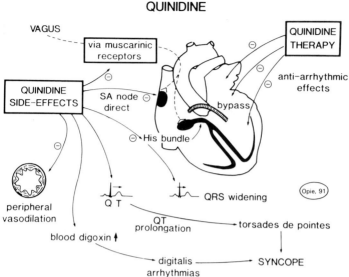

FIGURE 8–3. Schematic proposal for therapeutic and side-effects of quinidine. Note multiple mechanisms, including antiarrhythmic effects, by inhibition of the sodium channel (see Fig. 8–1), direct inhibition of the SA node and the His bundle, a vagolytic effect through the muscarinic receptors, peripheral vasodilation by α-receptor blockade, and an increased blood digoxin level.

Precautions. Quinidine excess is best prevented by serial measurements of QRS-duration and QT-interval on the ECG. **Conduction delay and pro-arrhythmic effects**[74] are potentially serious. Reduce dose or reassess therapy if QRS-duration widens by 50% or 25% in the presence of intraventricular conduction defects, if the total QRS-duration exceeds 140 msec, or if QT- or QTu-prolongation occurs beyond 500 msec. These guidelines, although reasonable, are not well documented. Besides monitoring QRS- and QT-intervals throughout, hypokalemia should be avoided, as it predisposes to torsades de pointes, which is the probable explanation of quinidine syncope. In patients with the **sick sinus syndrome**, a direct depressant effect of quinidine may be seen (Table 8-3); in others, nodal depression is overridden by the vagolytic effect.

Side-effects. Serious side-effects may develop soon after the first dose if there is idiosyncrasy, or gradually from cumulative overdosage. Check QRS and QT. Subjective side-effects were studied in a double-blind trial[72] when 139 patients took quinidine 300 to 400 mg every 6 hours. Most common were diarrhea (33%), nausea (18%), headache (13%), and dizziness (8%). Twenty-one patients discontinued the drug because of these side-effects. Long-term tolerance in those without early side-effects is excellent. Hypersensitivity reactions to quinidine include fever, skin rash, angioedema, thrombocytopenia, agranulocytosis, hepatitis, and lupus erythematosus.

Contraindications. Quinidine is contraindicated when ventricular tachyarrhythmias are associated with or caused by QT-prolongation. Caution is required with a pre-existing prolonged QT-interval or pre-existing QRS-duration or clinical congestive heart failure (CHF), with low initial doses and close monitoring. Other relative contraindications: sick sinus syndrome, bundle branch block, myasthenia gravis, and severe liver failure (altered pharmacokinetics). Watch for drug interactions. Periodic blood counts are advisable during long-term therapy.

Drug Interactions **(Table 8–4). Quinidine increases blood digoxin levels (decrease dose of digoxin, reassess blood levels). Quinidine may enhance the effects of other hypotensive agents or**

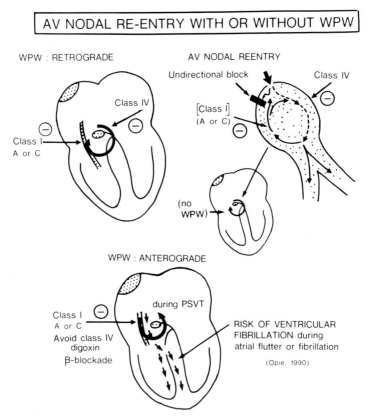

AV NODAL RE-ENTRY WITH OR WITHOUT WPW

WPW : RETROGRADE

AV NODAL REENTRY

Undirectional block

Class IV

Class IV

[Class I]
(A or C)

Class I
A or C

(no WPW)

WPW : ANTEROGRADE

during PSVT

Class I
A or C

Avoid class IV
digoxin
β-blockade

RISK OF VENTRICULAR
FIBRILLATION during
atrial flutter or fibrillation

(Opie, 1990)

FIGURE 8–4. Effects of slow calcium channel blockers (verapamil and diltiazem) and of fast channel blockers in AV nodal re-entry tachycardia (top) or bypass re-entry (bottom). In top right, AV conduction is anterograde (dashed line) followed by retrograde (solid line). In general, slow channel blockers are used in most cases of paroxysmal supraventricular nodal tachycardia, with or without overt bypass conduction, unless anterograde conduction down the bypass tract is expected (bottom).

agents inhibiting the sinus node (β-blockers and some calcium antagonists). The effect of warfarin may be enhanced by a hepatic interaction. Drugs such as phenytoin, barbiturates, and rifampin (rifampicin), which induce hepatic enzymes, may markedly increase the hepatic metabolism of quinidine with decreased steady-state blood levels. Conversely, cimetidine can decrease the metabolism of quinidine with opposite effects.[27] Hypokalemia decreases quinidine efficacy and increases QT- or QTu-prolongation. Concomitant therapy with amiodarone or sotalol or other drugs prolonging the QT-interval requires great care and is best avoided.[66] Quinidine reduces the effects of procedures that enhance vagal activity, such as carotid sinus massage, by its vagolytic effect (this opposes some digitalis effects, such as slowing of the heart). Quinidine also reduces the effects of anticholinesterases in myasthenia gravis (inhibition of muscarinic receptors) and enhances antibiotic-induced muscle weakness.

Treatment of Acute Toxicity. Stop quinidine, reduce plasma potassium if elevated, and acidify urine to encourage excretion. Torsades de pointes or severely disorganized conduction may require temporary ventricular pacing and/or magnesium sulfate.

Procainamide

Procainamide (Pronestyl) is generally effective against a wide variety of supraventricular and ventricular arrhythmias, including VT.

As in the case of quinidine, no effect on mortality or survival has been shown. Although usually given orally, intravenous (IV) procainamide may be tried if lidocaine fails. The oral use is limited by a short half-life and the long-term danger of the lupus syndrome. In contrast, other side-effects are less than with quinidine (GI, QRS or torsades, hypotension), and there is no interaction with digoxin.

Electrophysiology. Procainamide is a Class IA agent, like quinidine, but does not prolong the QT-interval to the same extent and has less interaction with the muscarinic receptors.[71]

Pharmacokinetics. Oral procainamide has to be given frequently in high doses because of the rapid renal elimination (half-life, 3.5 hours with normal renal function). In the elderly with decreased renal function, the dose of procainamide should be reduced by about 50%.[94] In mild heart failure the dose should be reduced by a quarter. IV procainamide should not be given at a dose exceeding 25 mg/min (see Side-effects). Plasma metabolism by acetylation yields the active N-acetylated procainamide (NAPA) with a half-life of 6 to 8 hours and Class III antiarrhythmic activity.

Dose. An **oral** loading dose of procainamide 1 g is followed by up to 500 mg 3-hourly. A slow-release preparation of procainamide (Procan SR) appears to allow 6-hourly dosing intervals. The **IV dose** is 100 mg over 2 minutes, then up to 25 mg/min to a maximum of 1 g in the first hour, then 2 to 6 mg/min.

Indications. In acute myocardial infarction (AMI), even when complicated by cardiac failure or low cardiac output,[9] procainamide can be given slowly intravenously. Continuous blood pressure and ECG monitoring is essential. Koch-Weser and associates[55] reported oral procainamide (oral loading dose 1 g) highly effective in prevention of ventricular arrhythmias early after infarction, but in the long term, 500 mg every 6 hours was not beneficial.[56] Like other Class IA agents, procainamide is also effective against many supraventricular tachyarrhythmias, including those complicating the bypass tract.

Contraindications. Contraindications include shock, myasthenia gravis (see quinidine), heart block, and severe renal failure. Severe heart failure is a relative contraindication.[135]

Side-effects. Hypotension is a common side-effect with IV administration (vasodilator effect), especially with doses exceeding 25 mg/min.[47] Heart block may develop or increase. In atrial fibrillation or flutter, the ventricular rate may increase as the atrial rate slows, so that concomitant digitalization is advisable. The vagolytic effect of procainamide is much weaker than that of quinidine.[71] Pro-arrhythmic effects, including torsades de pointes, may be dose-related.[115] During oral therapy,[56] 9 of 39 patients had early side-effects (rash, fever) and 14 of 16 had late side-effects (arthralgia, rash); fear of the lupus syndrome (likeliest in slow acetylators) limited therapy to 6 months at the most. Despite the efficacy of procainamide, the risk of lupus is about one-third of patients treated for over 6 months, and hence seriously limits the drug's long-term usage. Agranulocytosis may be a late side-effect of procainamide, especially with the slow-release preparation.[25]

Drug Interactions. Cimetidine inhibits the renal clearance of procainamide to prolong the elimination half-life, so that the procainamide dose should be reduced.[17]

Treatment of Acute Toxicity. Treatment is the same as for quinidine.

Disopyramide

Disopyramide is a Class IA antiarrhythmic agent, electrophysiologically like quinidine, with a similar antiarrhythmic profile. Like quinidine, it prolongs the QT-interval with risk of torsades. The crucial differences lie in the side-effects: GI problems are fewer with disopyramide, but there is a much stronger anticholinergic effect

TABLE 8–2 ANTIARRHYTHMIC DRUGS USED IN THERAPY OF VENTRICULAR ARRHYTHMIAS

Agent	Dose (IV = intravenous; IM = intramuscular)	Pharmacokinetics and Metabolism ($T^1/_2$ = plasma half-life; level = therapeutic blood level)	Side-effects and Contraindications	Interactions and Precautions
Quinidine (Class IA)	Orally 1.2–1.6 g/day in divided doses, 4–12 hourly, depending on preparation Not IV (risk of hypotension)	$T^1/_2$ 7–9 hr. Level 2.3–5 µg/ml Hepatic hydroxylation Reduce dose in liver disease	Many side-effects including diarrhea, nausea; torsades de pointes and hypotension. Vagolytic. Monitor QRS, QT, plasma K	Increases digoxin level Enzyme inducers; cimetidine; Class III agents (torsades); diuretics Warfarin (risk of bleeding)
Procainamide (Class IA)	IV 100 mg bolus over 2 min up to 25 mg/min to 1 g in first hr; then 2–6 mg/min Oral 1 g, then up to 500 mg 3-hourly	$T^1/_2$ 3.5 hr. Level 4–10 µg/ml Plasma metabolism to NAPA Rapid renal elimination	Hypotension with IV dose. Limit oral use to 6 months (lupus) Torsades de pointes rare	No digoxin interaction Class III agents (torsades)
Disopyramide (Class IA)	Oral dose 100–200 mg 6-hourly Loading dose 300 mg (less if CHF)	$T^1/_2$ 8 hr. Level 3–6 µg/ml toxic > 7 µg/ml Hepatic metabolism (50%), unchanged urinary excretion (50%)	Hypotension, QRS- or QT- prolongation, torsades, congestive heart failure Prominent vagolytic and negative inotropic effects	No digoxin interaction Class III agents (torsades)
Lidocaine (Class IB)	IV 100–200 mg; then 2–4 mg/min for 24–30 hr (No oral use)	Effect of single bolus lasts only few min, then $T^1/_2$ about 2 hr. Rapid hepatic metabolism Level 1.4–5.0 µg/mL; toxic > 9 µg/ml	Reduce dose by half if liver blood flow low (shock, β-blockade, cirrhosis, cimetidine, severe heart failure). High-dose CNS effects	β-Blockers decrease hepatic blood flow and increase blood levels Cimetidine (decreased hepatic metabolism of lidocaine)
Tocainide (Class IB)	* IV 0.5–0.75 mg/kg/min for 15 min Oral loading 400–800 mg, then 2–3 times daily	$T^1/_2$ 13.5 hr. Level 4–10 µg/ml Unchanged renal excretion (50%)	CNS, GI side-effects. Sometimes immune-based problems (lung fibrosis, blood dyscrasias)	None known
Mexiletine (Class IB)	* IV 100–250 mg at 12.5 mg/min, then 2.0 mg/kg/hr for 3.5 hr, then 0.5 mg/kg/hr Oral 100–400 mg 8 hourly; loading dose 400 mg	$T^1/_2$ 10–17 hr. Level 1–2 µg/ml Hepatic metabolism, inactive metabolites	CNS, GI side-effects. Bradycardia, hypotension especially during co-therapy	Enzyme inducers; disopyramide and β-blockade; increases the theophylline levels

Drug (Class)	Dose	Pharmacokinetics	Side-effects	Interactions
Phenytoin (Class IB)	IV 10–15 mg/kg over 1 hr; Oral 1 g; 500 mg for 2 days; then 400–600 mg daily	$T^{1}/_{2}$ 24 hr. Level 10–18 µg/ml. Hepatic metabolism. Hepatic or renal disease requires reduced doses	Hypotension, vertigo, dysarthria, lethargy, gingivitis, macrocytic anemia, lupus, pulmonary infiltrates	Hepatic enzyme inducers
Flecainide (Class IC)	*IV 1–2 mg/kg over 10 min, then 0.15–0.25 mg/kg/hr; Oral 100–400 mg 2 times daily; Hospitalize	$T^{1}/_{2}$ 13–19 hr. Hepatic (2/3); 1/3 renal excretion unchanged. Keep trough level below 1.0 µg/ml	QRS-prolongation. Pro-arrhythmia Depressed LV function. CNS side-effects. Increased incidence of death post-infarct	Many, especially added inhibition of conduction and nodal tissue
Encainide (Class IC)	25–75 mg 3 times daily; Hospitalize	$T^{1}/_{2}$ 1–2 hr. No levels. Hepatic. Normal phenotype produces long-acting metabolites (3–12 hr)	QRS-prolongation. CNS side-effects. Pro-arrhythmia. Increased incidence of death post-infarct	Probably similar to flecainide. Reduce dose in renal failure
Propafenone (Class IC)	*IV 2 mg/kg then 2 mg/min; Oral 150–300 mg 3 times daily	$T^{1}/_{2}$ variable 2–10 hr, up to 32 hr in non-metabolizers. Level 0.2–3.0 µg/ml. Variable hepatic metabolism (P-450 deficiency slows)	QRS-prolongation. Modest negative inotropic effect. GI side-effects. Pro-arrhythmia	Digoxin level increased. Hepatic inducers.
Sotalol (Class III)	*160–640 mg daily, occasionally higher, may divide doses	Not metabolized. Renal loss	Myocardial depression, sinus bradycardia, AV block. Torsades especially if hypokalemic or if dose too high	Added risk of torsades with IA agents or diuretics
Amiodarone (Class III)	Oral loading dose 1200–1600 mg daily; maintenance 200–400 mg daily, sometimes less; *Occasional IV use (see text)	$T^{1}/_{2}$ 25–110 days. Level 1.0–2.5 µg/ml. Hepatic metabolism. Lipid soluble with extensive distribution in body. Excretion by skin, biliary tract, lacrimal glands	Complex side-effects including pulmonary fibrosis. QT-prolongation. Torsades. Uncommon, but seen especially with hypocalcemia (not systematically dose-related)(keep dose low)	Class IA agents predispose to torsades. β-Blockers predispose to SA and AV nodal depression
Bretylium tosylate (Class III)	IV 5–10 mg/kg, lifting arm, repeat to max 30 mg/kg, then IV 1–2 mg/min or IM 5–10 mg/kg 8-hourly at varying sites (local necrosis)	$T^{1}/_{2}$ 7–9 hr. Level 0.5–1.0 µg/ml	IV: hypotension. Initial sympathomimetic effects	Decrease dose in renal failure

Compiled by LH Opie and modified from previous edition.

*Not in the USA.

V = intravenous; IM = intramuscular; $T^{1}/_{2}$ = plasma half-life; level = therapeutic blood level.

Enzyme hepatic inducers = barbiturates, phenytoin, rifampin, which induce hepatic enzymes, thereby decreasing blood levels of the drug.

TABLE 8–3 EFFECTS AND SIDE-EFFECTS OF SOME ANTIARRHYTHMIC AGENTS ON ELECTROPHYSIOLOGY AND HEMODYNAMICS

Agent	Sinus Node	Sinus Rate	A-His	PR	AV Block	H-P	WPW	QRS	QT	Serious Hemodynamic Effects	Risk of Torsades	Risk of Mono-morphic VT
Quinidine	→	↑	0	0/→	0	→	↓A/R	↑↑	↑↑	IV may cause	++	0,+
Procainamide	0	0/↑	0/↓	0/→	Avoid	→	↓A/R	0/→	↑	Rare	+	0,+
Disopyramide	→	↑	0	0/→	0	0/↓	↓A/R	↑	↑↑	LV marked depression	+	0,+
Lidocaine	0	0	0/↓	0	0	0	↓/0	0	0	Only with toxic doses	0?	0?
Phenytoin	0	0	↑/0	0	Lessens	0	↓/0	0	↓	IV hypotension	0,+	0,+
Mexiletine	0	0	↑/0	0	↓/0	↓/0	↓/0	0/→	0	Only with toxic doses	0,+	0,+
Tocainide	0	0	↓/0	0	↓/0	↓/0	↓/0	0	0	In CHF	0,+	0,+
Flecainide	0/↓	0	↓↓↓	↑	Avoid	↓↓	↓A/R	↑↑	→ (Via QRS)	LV depression	0	+++
Encainide	0/↓	0	↓↓↓	↑	Avoid	↓↓	↓A/R	↑↑	→ (Via QRS)	In CHF	0	+++
Sotalol	↓↓	↓↓	→	↑	Avoid	0	↓A/R	0	↑↑	IV may cause occasionally	++	0,+
Amiodarone	→	→	→	0/→	Avoid	0/↓	↓A/R	0	↑↑↑	Occasional with IV use	+	0,+

Table compiled by LH Opie and modified from previous edition. For hemodynamic effects of procainamide, encainide, and tocainide, see Gottlieb et al (1990).
A-His = Atria-His conduction; H-P = His-Purkinje conduction; WPW = Wolff-Parkinson-White syndrome accessory pathways; LV = left ventricle; R = retrograde; A = antegrade; BBB = bundle branch block; IV = intravenous; ↓ = depresses; → = prolongs; ↑ = increases; ↓↓ = shortens.

TABLE 8–4 INTERACTION OF ANTIARRHYTHMIC DRUGS

Drug	Interaction With	Result
Quinidine	Digoxin	Increased digoxin level
	Other class I antiarrhythmics	Added negative inotropic effect and/or depressed conduction
	β-Blockers, verapamil	Enhanced hypotension, negative inotropic effect
	Amiodarone, sotalol	Increased risk of torsades
	Diuretics	If hypokalemia, risk of torsades
	Verapamil	Increased quinidine level
	Nifedipine	Decreased quinidine level
	Warfarin	Enhanced anticoagulation
	Cimetidine	Increased blood levels
	Enzyme inducers	Decreased blood levels
Procainamide	Cimetidine	Decreased renal clearance
	Class III agents, diuretics	Torsades
Disopyramide	Other class I antiarrhythmics	Depressed conduction
	Amiodarone, sotalol	Torsades
	β-Blockers, verapamil	Enhanced hypotension
	Anticholinergics	Increased anticholinergic effect
	Pyridostigmine	Decreased anticholinergic effect
Lidocaine	β-Blockers, cimetidine, halothane	Reduced liver blood flow (increased blood levels)
	Enzyme inducers	Decreased blood levels
Tocainide	None known	–
Mexiletine	Enzyme inducers	Decreased mexiletine levels
	Disopyramide, β-blockers, theophylline	Negative inotropic potential Theophylline levels increased[165]
Flecainide	Added SA or AV node inhibition (β-blockers, verapamil, diltiazem, digoxin)	SA and AV nodal depression; depressed myocardium; conduction delay
	Added negative inotropic effects (β-blockers, quinidine, disopyramide)	
	Added HV conduction depression (quinidine, procainamide)	
Encainide	See flecainide	See flecainide
Propafenone	As for flecainide (but amiodarone interaction not reported), digoxin, warfarin	Enhanced SA, AV, and myocardial depression Digoxin level increased Anticoagulant effect enhanced[144]
Sotalol	Diuretics, Class IA agents, amiodarone, tricyclics, phenothiazines	Risk of torsades; avoid hypokalemia
Amiodarone	As for sotalol, digoxin, flecainide, warfarin	Risk of torsade Digoxin and flecainide levels increase Increased warfarin effect
Verapamil	β-Blockers, excess digoxin, myocardial depressants, quinidine	Increased myocardial or nodal depression

Enzyme inducers = hepatic enzyme inducers, i.e., barbiturates, phenytoin, rifampin.
For references, see Table 3 in Opie.[153]

because disopyramide is forty times more effective an inhibitor of the muscarinic receptors than is quinidine,[71] so that **(1) anticholinergic side-effects can become a major problem (urinary retention, worsening of glaucoma or myasthenia gravis, or constipation); and (2) there is a relative increase of sympathetic activity so that the direct depressant effects of disopyramide on nodal and conduction tissue may be masked.** A prominent and largely unexplained side-effect of disopyramide is the negative inotropic effect, so marked that disopyramide is now also used in the therapy of hypertrophic obstructive cardiomyopathy;[117] presumably it interferes with excitation contraction coupling.

Pharmacokinetics and Therapeutic Levels. The phosphate salt (Norpace; Dirythmin) and the free base (Rythmodan) have similar bioavailability and pharmacokinetics. Most of the oral dose is bioavailable. About half is metabolized (not in the liver) by *N-dealkylation* and about half excreted unchanged in the urine. The usual half-life is about 8 hours. One metabolite is powerfully anticholinergic. Disopyramide reduces PVCs at a serum concentration of 3 to 8 μ g/ml.[110]   The higher the blood level, the lower the percentage bound to plasma proteins, so that potential toxicity is enhanced.

Dose. The usual **oral dose** is 100 to 200 mg 6-hourly, with an initial loading dose of 300 mg (less if CHF). Several long-acting preparations, including Norpace CR, Rythmodan Retard, and Dirythmin SA, need only 12-hourly dosing. The dose should be reduced in severe renal failure and in the elderly (renal excretion of disopyramide) and in CHF (prolonged half-life). With the IV preparation (not in the USA), optimal blood levels can be rapidly achieved and maintained by giving 0.5 mg/kg over 5 minutes, repeating after 5 minutes (repeat twice more if needed), then 1 mg/kg/hr from 0 to 3 hours and 0.4 mg/kg/hr for 3 to 18 hours.

Indications. Oral disopyramide is approved only for the treatment of **ventricular arrhythmias** in the USA. It prevents induction of VT/VF (ventricular fibrillation) in up to one-third of patients.[61] In paroxysmal VT and other ventricular arrhythmias, disopyramide may be effective when other Class IA agents, such as quinidine or procainamide, fail;[112] the logic for this observation is not clear but may include minor electrophysiologic differences and a different side-effect profile so that relatively higher doses of disopyramide could be given to certain patients. Conversely, quinidine is sometimes effective when disopyramide fails.

In **supraventricular tachycardia**, oral or IV disopyramide may cause reversion to sinus rhythm, especially if the arrhythmia is of recent onset. In the atrial arrhythmias of the WPW syndrome, disopyramide acts by inhibition of both retrograde and antegrade conduction (Fig. 8–5),[106] so that the ventricular response rate is decreased. Disopyramide is better than placebo in reducing recurrent atrial fibrillation after direct current (DC) cardioversion.[38] Disopyramide is probably most effective in the prevention of recurrent atrial arrhythmias, including fibrillation in patients without a history of CHF.

In **hypertrophic cardiomyopathy**, disopyramide acts hemodynamically by its negative inotropic effect[117] and may be better than propranolol.[90,155]

In **AMI**, IV disopyramide (not in the USA) is one of several agents used for lidocaine failures,[102] but the risk of myocardial depression with hypotension is much greater than with lidocaine.

Side-effects. Side-effects include (1) negative inotropic effects; (2) possibly serious anticholinergic activity especially in elderly men (prostatic obstruction), in threatened glaucoma, with myasthenia gravis, or when constipation is a pre-existing problem (verapamil co-therapy); (3) excessive QT-prolongation and torsades de pointes;[70] and (4) occasional hypoglycemia[107] and cholestatic jaundice. Oral cholinesterase inhibitors may decrease side-effects (see Beneficial Drug Interaction).

Contraindications. Uncompensated CHF is an absolute contraindication, as are glaucoma, hypotension, untreated urinary retention, and significant pre-treatment QT-prolongation. Relative contraindications are (1) compensated CHF; (2) prostatism; (3) treated glaucoma or a family history of glaucoma; (4) severe constipation; and (5) sinus node dysfunction[58] and, by analogy, AV nodal block.[4,6] Bundle branch block is not normally a contraindication.[20]

Precautions. Electrocardiographically, disopyramide can increase QT- or QRS-prolongation (as for quinidine); the exact criteria are not known. Development of second or third degree AV block or uni-, bi-, or trifascicular block requires discontinuation of the drug unless an artificial pacemaker is used. Digitalization is indicated for borderline or suspected heart failure or for atrial flutter or fibrillation to avoid sudden acceleration of AV conduction. In pregnancy, disopyramide may stimulate uterine contractions; also it is excreted in human milk.

Drug Interactions. IV disopyramide can substantially **reduce cardiac output** in patients receiving negatively inotropic drugs such as β-blockers or verapamil, or in patients with pre-existing myocardial depression. Combinations with other **drugs likely to depress nodal tissue or conduction,** such as quinidine, digoxin, β-blockade, and methyldopa, are potentially dangerous. Disopyramide is ineffective in digitalis toxicity and should be avoided because of the possibility of added depressant effects on the AV and sinus nodes. There is no interaction between disopyramide and lidocaine. The concomitant use of **other Type 1 antiarrhythmic agents or β-blockers** with disopyramide should be reserved for life-threatening arrhythmias, which are demonstrably unresponsive to single agent antiarrhythmic agents (risk of negative inotropic effects, prolonged conduction). Co-therapy with Class III agents or diuretics increases the risk of torsades de pointes, as does co-therapy with erythromycin.[158] Phenytoin or other inducers of hepatic enzymes may lower disopyramide plasma levels.

Beneficial Drug Interaction. Pyridostigmine bromide (Mestinon Timespan, 90–180 mg 3x daily) or bethanechol[131] may reduce anticholinergic side-effects of disopyramide by inhibition of cholinesterase activity.

CLASS IB: LIDOCAINE (LIGNOCAINE) AND SIMILAR COMPOUNDS

As a group, Class IB agents inhibit the fast sodium current (typical Class I effect) while shortening the action potential duration (see Fig. 8–2). The former has the more powerful effect, whereas the latter might actually predispose to arrhythmias, but ensures that QT-prolongation does not occur. Class IB agents act selectively on diseased or ischemic tissue, where they are thought to promote conduction block, thereby interrupting re-entry circuits. They have a particular affinity for binding with inactivated sodium channels with rapid onset-offset kinetics, which may be why such drugs are ineffective in atrial arrhythmias, since the action potential duration is so short.[146]

Lidocaine (Lignocaine)

Lidocaine (Xylocaine; Xylocard) has become the standard IV agent for suppression of arrhythmias associated with AMI and with cardiac surgery. It has no role in the control of chronic recurrent ventricular arrhythmias. Lidocaine acts preferentially on the ischemic myocardium[32] and is more effective in the presence of a high external potassium;[163] therefore hypokalemia must be corrected for maximum efficacy (also for other Class I agents).

Pharmacokinetics. The bulk of an IV dose of lidocaine is rapidly de-ethylated by liver microsomes. The two critical factors governing lidocaine metabolism and hence its efficacy are liver blood flow (decreased in old age and by heart failure, β-blockade, and cimetidine) and liver microsomal activity (enzyme inducers). Since lidocaine is so rapidly distributed within minutes after an initial IV loading dose, there must be a subsequent infusion or repetitive doses to maintain therapeutic blood levels (1.4–5.0 μ g/ml). Lidocaine metabolites circulate in high concentrations and may contribute to toxic and therapeutic actions.

Dose. A constant infusion would take 5 to 9 hours to achieve therapeutic levels (1.4–5.0 μ g/ml), so standard therapy includes a

LIDOCAINE KINETICS

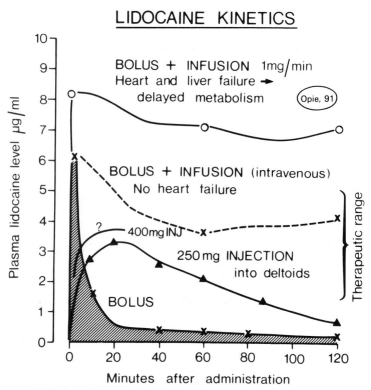

FIGURE 8–5. Lidocaine kinetics. To achieve and maintain an adequate blood level of lidocaine requires an initial bolus, or intramuscular injection, followed by an infusion. For an intramuscular injection to give sustained high blood levels may require a dose of 400 mg. In the presence of cardiac or liver failure, delayed metabolism increases the blood level, with danger of toxic effects.

loading dose of 100 to 200 mg intravenously[36,62] (Fig. 8–5) or 400 mg intramuscularly.[57] Thereafter, lidocaine is infused at 2 to 4 mg/min for 24 to 30 hours, aiming at 3 mg/min, which prevents VF but may cause serious side-effects in about 15% of patients, in half of whom the lidocaine dose may have to be reduced.[62] Poor liver blood flow (low cardiac output or β-blockade), liver disease, or cimetidine or halothane therapy calls for halved dosage. The dose should also be decreased for elderly patients in whom toxicity develops more frequently.

Side-effects. Lidocaine is generally free of hemodynamic depressive side-effects, even in patients with CHF, and it seldom impairs nodal function or conduction. The higher infusion rate of 3 to 4 mg/min may result in drowsiness, numbness, speech disturbances, and dizziness, especially in patients over 60 years of age. Minor adverse neural reactions can occur in about half the patients, even with 2 to 3 mg/min of lidocaine.[2] Occasionally there is SA arrest, especially during co-administration of other drugs, potentially depressing nodal function.

Drug Interactions. In patients receiving cimetidine, propranolol, or halothane, the hepatic clearance of lidocaine is reduced and toxicity may occur more readily, so that the dose should be reduced. With hepatic enzyme inducers (barbiturates, phenytoin, and rifampin) the dose needs to be increased.

Lidocaine Failure. If lidocaine apparently fails, is there hypokalemia? Are there technical errors? If none of these factors is present, a blood level is taken (if available), and the infusion rate can be increased cautiously until development of the central nervous system effects (confusion, slurred speech). Alternatively or concomi-

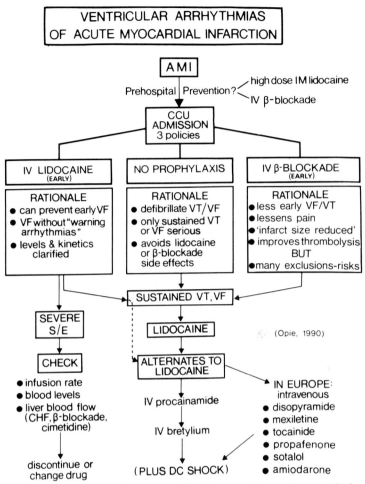

FIGURE 8–6. Schematic and provisional approach to serious ventricular arrhythmias in patients with acute myocardial infarction. (Compiled by LH Opie, DC Harrison, and T Mabin.)

tantly, Class IA agents are tried (especially procainamide) before resorting to Class III agents, such as bretylium or amiodarone.

Clinical Use. **Should lidocaine be administered routinely to all patients with AMI?** The question has been asked for at least 12 years[36] and is still not fully resolved (Fig. 8-6). In the pre-hospital phase, evidence for high-dose intramuscular lidocaine (400 mg) is good[57] but 250 patients with suspected AMI must be treated to save one from VF. Intramuscular administration of a large volume of liquid is far from ideal. In the Coronary Care Unit (CCU), data obtained by pooling of several studies suggest that lidocaine should be used,[21] as does one well-conducted double-blind trial, when patients seen within 6 hours of the onset of myocardial infarction were given a 100 mg bolus followed by an infusion of lidocaine 3 mg/min for 48 hours.[62] However, death in the untreated group did not occur and all patients could be resuscitated. Furthermore, since the incidence of primary VF is now so low (probably less than 5%), it is uncertain whether prophylactic lidocaine is cost-effective if given to all patients sustaining AMI. Many well-run CCUs in the USA and Europe have abandoned the routine use of lidocaine and consider prophylaxis only for selected patients.

Recommendations. Despite the controversy, it appears prudent to use lidocaine in patients admitted to CCUs within 6 hours of the onset of symptoms,[62] when the risk of VF is highest, unless another antiarrhythmic drug such as IV β-blockade is used. Lidocaine should also not be given when there is bradycardia or bradycardia plus ventricular tachyarrhythmias, when atropine (or pacing) and not lidocaine is required. Combination of early lidocaine with β-blockade is not a contraindication, although there is no reported experience. The obvious precaution is that bradyarrhythmias may also become more common because β-blockade reduces liver blood flow so that a standard dose of lidocaine has potentially more side-effects, including inhibition of the sinus node. The aimed rate of infusion of lidocaine after the initial loading dose should be 3 mg/kg, except in elderly patients, those with heart failure, or those receiving cimetidine or β-blockade, all of whom require reduced doses. The advantage of prophylactic lidocaine is that the prevention of VF even in a small number of patients facilitates management and makes for easier nursing, while the risk of serious side-effects is reasonably low.

Tocainide

Tocainide (Tonocard) is an oral analog of lidocaine. Intravenous use is not approved in the USA. Like lidocaine, it has little negative inotropic effect and is unlikely to aggravate CHF. Another advantage is shortening of the QT-interval (Class IB effect). The major side-effects are neurologic; GI side-effects are also frequent. Serious blood dyscrasias, though rare, limit use. For potentially lethal arrhythmias, the drug is about as effective as quinidine but has a different side-effect profile.[75]

Pharmacokinetics. The bioavailability of tocainide is virtually complete because of the absence of first-pass metabolism.[76] Peak plasma levels occur 2 hours after oral administration; optimal plasma levels appear to be 4 to 10 μg/ml.[76] Nearly half an oral dose is recovered unchanged in the urine. There are no active metabolites. The plasma half-life is about 14 hours which is virtually unaltered in the presence of AMI, but prolonged in severe renal disease.

Dose. The usual oral dose is 300 to 600 mg 3x daily; 2x daily administration may be effective. The dose should be decreased in renal failure (renal excretion), as well as in the elderly (low glomerular filtration rate). The IV dose (not approved in the USA) is 250 mg over 2 minutes, 500 mg over 15 minutes, and then 500 mg every 6 hours, for 48 hours.[145]

Indications. The approved indication in the USA is treatment of symptomatic ventricular arrhythmias. That includes those refractory to conventional antiarrhythmic agents, such as quinidine, procainamide, and propranolol.[88] As in the case of other antiarrhythmics, it is much more likely to be effective when used as a first-line agent than when used in patients with arrhythmias already resistant to more conventional drugs. In AMI, serious ventricular arrhythmias are reduced by combined IV and oral tocainide, but VF is not prevented.[13]

Contraindications. Hypersensitivity can cause second- or third-degree heart block in the absence of an artificial pacemaker. Like lidocaine, tocainide appears to have no significant direct negative inotropic effect, although occasional adverse reactions have been described in patients with complex cardiovascular disease. In the package insert, non-digitalized atrial flutter or fibrillation is mentioned as a relative contraindication because of the danger of ventricular acceleration (unexpected effect on atrial tissue).

Side-effects. Tocainide frequently causes dose-dependent nervous system (28%) and GI (11%) reactions, including lightheadedness or dizziness, paresthesia or numbness in the extremities, tremor, nausea, vomiting, or diarrhea.[43] When tremor develops, that is a useful clinical indication that the maximum dose is being approached. Such side-effects cause discontinuation in about one-fifth of patients. Serious immune-based side-effects, such as pulmonary fibrosis, may occur. Polyarthritis and increased antinuclear factors are infrequent. Serious blood dyscrasias, such as leukopenia and thrombocytopenia, occur in about 0.2% of patients treated with this drug. Therefore, it should be limited for use in life-threatening ventricular arrhythmias or carefully selected patients with less severe arrhythmias. Pro-arrhythmic effects may occur. CHF may be aggravated.[135]

Precautions. Weekly blood counts are required for the first 3 months, with periodic counts thereafter. Patients should report bruising or bleeding or symptoms of infection (throat, chest).

Drug Interactions and Combinations. Tocainide may be used freely in digitalized patients with no change in digoxin levels. It has also been used in combination with β-blockers, other antiarrhythmic agents (without controlled studies), anticoagulants, and diuretics without evidence, as yet, of clinically significant interactions.[76]

Mexiletine

Mexiletine (Mexitil), like lidocaine, is used chiefly against ventricular arrhythmias. Unlike lidocaine, it can be given orally. There are several arguments favoring it as one of several reasonable choices as a first-line agent in ventricular arrhythmias requiring therapy: (1) its comparable efficacy to quinidine; (2) little or no hemodynamic depression unless combined with disopyramide or β-blockade; (3) no QT-prolongation; and (4) no vagolytic effects. However, frequent GI and central nervous side-effects limit the dose and possible therapeutic benefit.

Pharmacokinetics. Mexiletine is well absorbed with a high bioavailability and reaches peak plasma levels in 2 to 4 hours. The therapeutic blood level is 1 to 2 μ g/ml. Ninety percent is metabolized in the liver to inactive metabolites and the rest is excreted in the urine as unchanged mexiletine.[16] The half-life is 10 to 17 hours in normals. Higher than normal plasma levels are found in chronic liver disease, but not in renal failure. Mexiletine is lipophilic and enters the brain (central nervous system side-effects).

Dose. The oral loading dose is 400 mg, if high initial levels are required, followed by 300 to 1200 mg (given with food or antacid) in three divided daily doses, starting 2 to 6 hours after the loading dose. In the USA, the highest approved dose is 900 mg daily. The IV dose (not in the USA) is 100 to 250 mg (2.5 mg/kg) at 12.5 mg/min, then 2.0 mg/kg/hr for 3.5 hours, then 0.5 mg/kg/hr as long as needed. In Europe, sustained release capsules (Perlongets) have a usual dose of 360 mg 2x daily. The dose of mexiletine should be reduced in severe liver disease and in CHF. In pregnant women, the drug seems safe, although it crosses the placental barrier. In the elderly, the dose must be reduced because of possible central nervous system side-effects and because of lower hepatic blood flow.

Indications. The major approved indication is treatment of symptomatic ventricular arrhythmias. In Europe, it is especially used in early myocardial infarction and post-infarction, as well as in digitalis-induced arrhythmias. In the chronic oral prophylaxis of ventricular arrhythmias post-infarction, mexiletine 300 mg 8-hourly is as effective as procainamide.[12] A similar dose of mexiletine can be combined with quinidine (about 1 g daily) with a lower incidence of side-effects and better antiarrhythmic action than with higher doses of either agent alone.[23] In VT resistant to more conventional drugs, mexiletine alone gives only modest benefit.[114] In a major clinical trial on post-infarct patients, mexiletine reduced Holter-monitored arrhythmias in the first 6 months without improved mortality over 1 year; in fact, mortality tended to increase.[48]

Side-effects. The major problem is a narrow therapeutic-toxic margin,[86] so that in patients with ventricular arrhythmias resistant to conventional agents, an adequate antiarrhythmic effect is only obtained in 25% or fewer of patients without significant side-effects. Dizziness and mild disorientation may result from a single oral dose of 400 mg. During chronic therapy, side-effects include indigestion in 40%; tremor or nystagmus (10%, higher in some series); and confusional states in less than 10%. Severe side-effects occur in about 35% of patients receiving 1 g or more per day.[10,11] Nausea may be decreased by giving the drug with food. In about 5% of patients, bradycardia and hypotension may occur.[10,11] There may be a pro-arrhythmic effect, but torsades de pointes is rare. Liver damage occasionally occurs. Prochlorperazine 12.5 mg IV can be given 5 minutes before mexiletine injection to lessen dizziness and vomiting.

Contraindications. Cardiogenic shock or second- or third-degree heart block without a pacemaker. Relative contraindications are bradycardia, conduction defects in the presence of a pacemaker, hypotension, hepatic failure, and severe renal or myocardial failure. Caution in patients with liver damage or seizures.

Drug Interactions and Combination Therapy. Narcotics delay the GI absorption of mexiletine. Hepatic enzyme inducers decrease plasma levels of mexiletine. Concurrent disopyramide or β-blocker therapy predisposes to a negative inotropic effect.[7] Mexiletine elevates plasma levels of theophylline.[165] The drug may be combined with quinidine[23,34] and amiodarone,[113] provided contraindications are observed and appropriate dose regimens of the two drugs are chosen.

Phenytoin (Diphenylhydantoin)

Phenytoin (Dilantin, Epanutin) has four specific uses. First, in digitalis-toxic arrhythmias, it maintains conduction or even enhances it, especially in the presence of hypokalemia; it also inhibits delayed afterdepolarizations.[119] Second, phenytoin is effective against the ventricular arrhythmias occurring after congenital heart surgery.[116] Third, phenytoin is used in the congenital prolonged QT-syndrome when β-blockade alone has failed; here, reliable comparable studies have not been done. Why phenytoin is so effective in the ventricular arrhythmias of young children is not known. Fourth, occasionally in patients with epilepsy and arrhythmias this dual action comes to the fore.

The IV dose is 10 to 15 mg/kg over 1 hour, followed by oral maintenance of 400 to 600 mg/day (2–4 mg/kg/day in children). The long half-life allows once daily dosage with, however, the risk of serious side-effects, including dysarthria, pulmonary infiltrates, lupus, gingivitis, and macrocytic anemia.

Phenytoin is an inducer of hepatic enzymes and therefore alters the dose requirements of many other drugs used in cardiology, including quinidine, lidocaine and mexiletine.

Moricizine

Moricizine (Ethmozine) is a phenothiazine derivative originally from the USSR and recently approved in the USA for management of documented ventricular arrhythmias that the physician judges to be life-threatening. Electrophysiologically, it has both lidocaine-like Class IB properties and also prolongs the PR and QRS times, while leaving the QT-interval unchanged. Therefore **ethmozine may represent a "mixed" Class IB/IC agent**. The phenothiazine-like structure (which could perhaps predispose to QT-prolongation) also suggests a third antiarrhythmic mechanism through a central nervous system effect. Clinically, it is effective for the treatment of both ventricular and supraventricular arrhythmias. In patients with AV nodal re-entrant tachycardia, the drug acts by slowing retrograde conduction. In patients with tachycardias complicating the WPW syndrome, the drug increases anterograde and retrograde refractoriness in the re-entry limbs.[14,15] Ethmozine is rapidly and extensively metabolized in the liver with a half-life of approximately 2–5 hours that is prolonged in renal insufficiency. The usual dose for adults is 600–900 mg in 3 divided doses 8-hourly. Neurologic side-effects, most evident during IV infusion (not available in USA), include nervousness, dizziness, and vertigo. Generally, during oral therapy, side-effects are slight and include dizziness, paresthesia, headache, and nausea. A pro-arrhythmic effect has been found.[47] Ethmozine has only mildly depressant effects on LV function, yet further studies on side-effects are required to see whether the drug really is so well tolerated as often supposed. Whether ethmozine is as powerfully antiarrhythmic as its properties theoretically suggest also remains to be evaluated. Ethmozine is still under evaluation for possible benefit in post-infarct ventricular premature systoles, in the same trial in which the flecainide and encainide arms were stopped,[126] so that it can safely be stated that it does not have identical fatal proarrhythmic qualities.

CLASS IC AGENTS

These agents have recently come under the spotlight because of their pro-arrhythmic effects in the CAST study,[126] in which death was increased in post-infarct patients with more than 6 VPBs per minute given flecainide or encainide. As a group, they have three major electrophysiologic effects. First, they are powerful inhibitors of the fast sodium channel causing a marked depression of the upstroke of the cardiac action potential. Second, they have a marked inhibitory effect on His-Purkinje conduction with QRS widening. Third, they markedly shorten the action potential duration of only Purkinje fibers leaving unaltered that of the surrounding myocardium.[141] Class IC agents are all potent antiarrhythmics used largely in the control of ventricular tachyarrhythmias resistant to other drugs. Their markedly depressant effect on conduction may explain their significant pro-arrhythmic action, to which the discrepancies in the action potential duration between Purkinje and ventricular tissue may contribute by promoting inhomogeneity.[141] Recently atrial pro-arrhythmic effects have been described that limit the use of this category of agents in supraventricular tachycardias, particularly in the case of recurrent atrial fibrillation or flutter.[132]

Flecainide

Flecainide (Tambocor) is a powerful new drug, effective for the treatment of both supraventricular and ventricular arrhythmias. However, it prolongs the PR and QRS times. The negative inotropic effect limits its use in ischemic heart disease or dilated cardiomyopathy. In patients with life-threatening arrhythmias, the potentially serious pro-arrhythmic effect requires that this drug should only be started under careful observation, preferably in the hospital, using a gradually increasing low oral dose with checks of serum levels. In an emergency, IV flecainide (not in the USA) can be very effective for supraventricular or ventricular tachycardia. Thus, with care, flecainide may be very effective in some selected patients with severe ventricular arrhythmias but without LV failure[47] and is still sometimes chosen in supraventricular arrhythmias.

Electrophysiology. Besides powerful inhibition of the fast sodium current, there is strong inhibition of His-Purkinje conduction and prolongation of the QRS-interval.

Pharmacokinetics. Flecainide is well absorbed with a bioavailability as high as 95% and peak plasma levels at 2 to 4 hours. When feasible, plasma levels should be monitored and kept below 1.0 μ g/ml (trough levels) to avoid myocardial depression.[93] The plasma half-life is 13 to 19 hours. Flecainide is two-thirds metabolized by the liver to inactive metabolites whereas about one-third is excreted unchanged by the kidneys and a small amount (5%) in the feces.

Dose. The oral dose of flecainide is 100 to 400 mg 2x daily; the IV dose (not approved in the USA) is 1 to 2 mg/kg over 10 minutes, followed by an infusion of 0.15 to 0.25 mg/kg/hr. Lower doses are required for patients with poor LV function or severe renal failure; an initial dose of 100 mg 2x daily is increased at about 4-day intervals to 200 mg 2x daily (flecainide plasma levels should be checked if possible, particularly in the presence of CHF).

Indications. Flecainide is used in symptomatic, life-threatening VT.[1] It is also effective in WPW arrhythmias[85] and in AV nodal re-entrant arrhythmias.[41]

Contraindications. Flecainide is contraindicated in the absence of life-threatening VT or SVT; with significant conduction delay, sick sinus syndrome,[26] and myocardial depression; and in the post-infarct state. A relative contraindication is renal disease.

Side-effects. Cardiac side-effects include aggravation of ventricular arrhythmias in 5 to 12%[28,73,83,93] or possibly even more in the presence of pre-existing LV failure, and threat of sudden death as in the CAST study.[126] The pro-arrhythmic effect is related to non-uniform slowing of conduction.[141,169] Monitoring the QRS-interval is logical,[53] but safe limits are not established. Furthermore, as shown in the CAST study, late pro-arrhythmic effects can occur. In patients with pre-existing sinus node or AV conduction problems, there may be worsening. Clinical heart failure may be precipitated by IV flecainide.[49]

Atrial pro-arrhythmic effects are now coming to the fore. It will be recalled that when patients with rapid supraventricular arrhythmias are given quinidine, digitalis co-administration has been traditional to avoid the decrease in atrial rate being reflected in accelerated AV conduction and ventricular arrhythmias. A similar danger may occur during administration of flecainide, so that as the atrial rate falls the ventricular rate might rise.[130] Therefore, although type IC drugs are effective for the treatment of supraventricular tachycardia, they should be used with great caution and under close supervision for the first days of therapy although, again, late pro-arrhythmia may occur. If prescribed for prevention of atrial flutter or fibrillation, they should probably be co-administered with digitalis, a β-blocker, or verapamil to avoid accelerated AV conduction.

Extracardiac side-effects are related to the central nervous system (blurred vision, dizziness, headache, nausea, paresthesias, fatigue, tremor, and nervousness). Yet in one trial they were uncommon and no different from placebo.[125]

Drug Interactions and Combinations. Additive inhibitory effects require great care when flecainide is combined with other agents inhibiting sinus or AV nodal function (β-blockers, verapamil, diltiazem, digitalis), when there are additive negative inotropic effects (β-blockers, verapamil, disopyramide), or when there may be combined effects on His-Purkinje conduction (quinidine, procainamide, and, to a lesser extent, disopyramide). Amiodarone increases flecainide plasma levels (decrease flecainide dose by one-third).[104]

Encainide

Encainide (Enkaid®) has a spectrum of action and electrophysiologic effects similar to flecainide. Encainide has relatively little negative inotropic effect[109] and may be given with care to patients with poor LV function;[100] nevertheless, severe CHF may be worsened.[135] The clinical indications, electrophysiologic effects and pro-arrhythmic hazards of encainide closely resemble those of flecainide.

There are two phenotypes for metabolism; normal metabolizers (over 90%) produce two active metabolites, ODE and MODE, with a much longer half-life than the parent compound, whereas in poor metabolizers the half-life of encainide itself is prolonged. The dose of encainide in both phenotypes is, however, 25 to 75 mg 3x daily (4x daily doses sometimes given). Such doses do not depress LV function in patients without pre-existing LV failure.[24,109] In patients with moderate to severe renal failure, the dose should be reduced to about one-third of normal.[157] Slowly accumulating metabolites may be important in the antiarrhythmic activity of encainide so that the oral route is more effective than the IV. Cimetidine increases plasma concentrations of encainide. Enzyme inducers should decrease the level. Routine measurements of plasma levels are not available.

Side-effects. These include vertigo, visual disturbances, and headache as well as lengthening of the PR and QRS intervals.[24] Minor side-effects may limit the use of encainide before a therapeutic effect is reached.[3] CHF may be worsened.[135]

Encainide has pro-arrhythmic effects,[118] especially in patients with potentially lethal or lethal arrhythmias and cardiomyopathy (17% pro-arrhythmic events according to package insert). Initial low doses, increasing upwards only every 4 days to a limit of 200 mg daily, and careful monitoring are required in such patients. Nonetheless, as shown in the CAST study,[126] elimination of patients with obvious early pro-arrhythmia does not exclude later fatal pro-arrhythmia. **The full spectrum of drug interactions of encainide is not yet known, but may come to resemble those of flecainide.**

Propafenone

Propafenone (Rytmonorm in Europe, Arytmol in the USA and UK) is a new antiarrhythmic drug, widely used in Europe, of predominant Class IC properties. Usually well tolerated, the spectrum of activity and some of the side-effects resemble those of other Class IC agents, including a pro-arrhythmic effect. Marked interindividual variations in its metabolism mean that dose must be individualized. Propafenone is regarded as relatively safe in suppressing ventricular and supraventricular arrhythmias, including those of the WPW syndrome, although not licensed for this indication in the USA, where it is approved only for life-threatening ventricular arrhythmias such as sustained VT.[134]

Electrophysiology. In keeping with its Class IC effects, propafenone blocks the fast inward sodium channel, has a potent membrane stabilizing activity, and increases PR and QRS times without effect on the QT-interval. It also has mild β-blocking and calcium antagonist properties.

Pharmacokinetics. Oral propafenone is rapidly absorbed, with a bioavailability of about 50%, reaching peak blood levels within 2 hours.[47] Therapeutic plasma concentrations are highly variable, being 0.2 to 3.0 µg/ml[19] and of little practical use. Unexpectedly, steady-state plasma levels of parent drug and metabolites are approached in 3 to 4 days irrespective of hepatic metabolic phenotype.[134] There is variable and sometimes almost complete liver metabolism to 5-hydroxypropafenone and *N*-desalkyl propafenone, both also antiarrhythmic. The variable plasma levels and plasma half-life (2–10 hours in normals, 12–32 hours in poor metabolizers) may be explained by genetic variations in hepatic metabolism; in 7% of whites, the hepatic cytochrome, P-450, is genetically absent, so that propafenone breakdown is much slower.[134]

Dose. Oral: 150 to 300 mg 3x daily, up to 1200 mg daily. Some patients may need 4x daily dose and some only twice. IV: 2 mg/kg followed by an infusion of 2 mg/min (not approved in the USA).

Indications. In the USA, propafenone is limited to use in life-threatening ventricular arrhythmias; elsewhere it is also used for supraventricular arrhythmias. In ventricular arrhythmias, propafenone inhibits PVCs, couplets, VT, and induced VT.[134] Failure to prevent induced VT does not preclude long-term benefit, unless the induction is done after oral dosage, when active metabolites accumulate.[134] In supraventricular tachycardias with AV nodal or bypass re-entry, propafenone is fully effective in almost 40% or more of patients. In the WPW syndrome, it inhibits conduction in both directions.[134] Data from open studies suggest benefit in prevention of recurrent atrial fibrillation.

Contraindications. Pre-existing sinus, AV or bundle branch abnormalities, or depressed LV function are relative contraindications. Asthma is a relative contraindication, especially when the propafenone dose exceeds 450 mg daily,[139] probably the side-effect of the mild β-blocking qualities of the drug.

Side-effects. These are dose-related. Cardiac side-effects (in about 13%) include PR- and QRS-prolongation and conduction block, as well as sinus node dysfunction. In nearly 5%, CHF may be precipitated by a modest negative inotropic effect,[159] so that close monitoring of LV function is required soon after starting the drug. Pro-arrhythmia manifests as incessant wide complex VT, typical of Class I agents,[84] but may not be as frequent as with flecainide or encainide.[134,156]

Extracardiac side-effects (in about 14%) are relatively uncommon and are chiefly gastrointestinal, including abdominal discomfort and alteration in taste or smell;[89] blurred vision also occurs. Hepatitis is rare.[8,19]

Drug Interactions and Combinations. Like other Class IC agents, propafenone is likely to interact adversely with drugs depressing nodal function, intraventricular conduction, or the inotropic state. Propafenone has been combined with quinidine or procainamide at reduced doses of both drugs in the treatment of PVCs.[54] Propafenone substantially increases serum digoxin levels[42] and increases the anticoagulant effect of warfarin.[144]

Other Class IC Agents

Lorcainide, not yet approved for use in the USA, has been widely used in Europe. Like flecainide, it has the advantages of both IV and oral administration. An American trial showed that IV lorcainide (loading dose 2 mg/kg at 2 mg/min followed by 8 mg/hr) compared well with a standard lidocaine infusion.[2] The use of lorcainide is limited by severe neurologic side-effects.

Indecainide likewise is investigational.

CLASS II AGENTS: β-ADRENERGIC ANTAGONISTS

β-Blockade is used especially for inappropriate or unwanted sinus tachycardia, for paroxysmal atrial tachycardia provoked by emotion or exercise, for exercise-induced ventricular arrhythmias, in the arrhythmias of pheochromocytoma (combined with α-blockade to avoid hypertensive crises), in the hereditary prolonged QT-syndrome, and sometimes in the arrhythmias of mitral valve prolapse. In AMI, the cardiodepressant effects argue against the use of β-blockers as antiarrhythmic agents of choice, but, in appropriate dosage and in patients without manifest heart failure, β-blockade may be used to prevent and control supraventricular and ventricular arrhythmias. A common denominator to most of these indications is increased sympathetic β-adrenergic activity. β-Blockers are also effective as monotherapy in severe recurrent VT not obviously ischemic in origin.[124] They are especially used as antiarrhythmic agents when there is an added indication such as angina or hypertension. The mechanism of benefit of β-blockade in post-infarct patients is uncertain, likely to be multifactorial, and probably antiarrhythmic in part.[31]

The antiarrhythmic activity of the various β-blockers is reasonably uniform, the critical property being that of β-adrenergic blockade, without any major role for associated properties such as membrane depression (local anesthetic action), cardioselectivity, and intrinsic sympathomimetic activity having no major influence on the antiarrhythmic potency. There is one exception: the additional Class III effect of sotalol.

CLASS III AGENTS: AMIODARONE, SOTALOL, AND BRETYLIUM

Class III compounds act by lengthening the action potential duration and hence the effective refractory period, and must inevitably prolong the QT-interval to be effective.[108] In the presence of added hypokalemia or other specific factors (see Fig. 8–5), QT-prolongation may predispose to torsades de pointes. This may especially occur with agents causing a simultaneous bradycardia, when agents such as sotalol become more effective in prolonging action potential duration—a "reverse use-dependency."[140] By acting only on the repolarization phase of the action potential, Class III agents should leave conduction unchanged. However, amiodarone, sotalol, and bretylium all have additional properties that modify conduction—amiodarone being a significant sodium channel inhibitor, sotalol a β-blocker, and bretylium initially releasing catecholamines besides blocking adrenergic neurons.

Class III agents make more uniform the action potential pattern throughout the myocardium, thereby opposing electrophysiologic heterogeneity that underlies some serious ventricular arrhythmias. Furthermore, as a group these compounds have little or no negative inotropic effect (sotalol, a β-blocker, is by definition negatively inotropic). The efficacy of amiodarone is generally thought to exceed that of other antiarrhythmic compounds.

Despite these common electrophysiologic features, Class III agents are structurally, pharmacokinetically, and electrophysiologically dissimilar, so that neither the antiarrhythmic effects nor the clinical indications are interchangeable. In the USA, IV bretylium has long been available, and oral amiodarone is approved for use for refractory ventricular arrhythmias. Extensive investigational studies with sotalol are under way, and this drug is likely to be approved in the USA in the near future. In Europe, amiodarone is the drug of choice for severe refractory arrhythmias, with sotalol increasingly being seen as a safe, albeit probably less powerful, agent.

Amiodarone

Amiodarone (Cordarone) is a "wide-spectrum" antiarrhythmic agent acting through multiple mechanisms. Its benefits need to be balanced against, first, the slow onset of action of oral therapy, which may in turn require large oral loading doses. IV use (not in the USA) in truly urgent life-threatening arrhythmias does not give a full effect rapidly. Second, the serious side-effects, especially pulmonary infiltrates, mean that there must be a fine balance between the maximum antiarrhythmic effect of the drug and the potential for the side-effects caused by high doses and prolonged therapy. Third, there are a large number of potentially serious drug interactions, some of which predispose to torsades de pointes, which is nonetheless rare when amiodarone is used as a single agent. In recurrent supraventricular arrhythmias, low-dose amiodarone may be strikingly effective with little risk of side-effects. Otherwise, the use of amiodarone in as low a dose as possible should be restricted to patients with refractory ventricular arrhythmias failing to respond to other less toxic agents, only after careful evaluation, and with an adequate knowledge of its side-effect profile.

Electrophysiology. Amiodarone lengthens the effective refractory period by prolonging the action potential duration in all cardiac tissues, including the bypass tract. It also has a powerful Class I antiarrhythmic effect inhibiting inactivated sodium channels at high stimulation frequencies.[68] Amiodarone also non-competitively blocks α and β-adrenergic receptors. A calcium antagonist effect might explain bradycardia and AV nodal inhibition[33] and the relatively low incidence of torsades de pointes.[162] Furthermore, there are coronary and peripheral vasodilator actions. Amiodarone is therefore a complex antiarrhythmic agent that shares at least some of the properties of each of the four electrophysiologic classes of antiarrhythmics.

Pharmacokinetics. After variable (30–50%) and slow GI absorption, amiodarone is slowly eliminated, with a half-life of about 25 to 110 days.[45] The onset of action after oral administration is delayed and a steady-state drug effect (amiodaronization) may not be established for several months unless large loading doses are used. Even when given intravenously, its full electrophysiologic effect is delayed. Amiodarone is lipid-soluble and extensively distributed in the body and highly concentrated in many tissues, especially in the liver and lungs. It undergoes extensive hepatic metabolism to the pharmacologically active metabolite, desethylamiodarone. A correlation between the clinical effects and serum concentrations of the drug or its metabolite has not been clearly shown, although there is a direct relation between the oral dose and the plasma concentration[105] and between metabolite concentration and some late effects, such as that on the ventricular functional refractory period.[150] The therapeutic level, not well defined, may be between 1.0 and 2.5 μg/ml, almost all of which (95%) is protein bound. Amiodarone is not excreted by the kidneys, but rather by the lacrimal glands, the skin, and the biliary tract.

Dose. When reasonably rapid control of an arrhythmia is needed, the initial loading regimen is 1200 to 1600 mg in two divided doses usually given for 7 to 14 days, which is then reduced to 400 to 800 mg/day for a further 1 to 3 weeks, and thereafter to a maintenance dose that rarely needs to exceed 200 to 400 mg/day, given as a single dose. The loading dose is essential because of the slow onset of full action, with a delay of about 10 days.[105] Downward dose adjustment may be required during prolonged therapy to avoid development of side-effects while maintaining optimal antiarrhythmic effect. Maintenance doses for supraventricular arrhythmias are generally lower (200 mg daily or less) than those needed for serious ventricular arrhythmias. IV administration (not in the USA) may be used for intractable arrhythmias or for atrial fibrillation in AMI (5 mg/kg over 20 minutes, 1000 mg over 24 hours, then orally[161]); comparative studies are lacking. When thus given IV, the anti-adrenergic properties could be of importance[63] and there is still a latent period to the onset of full action.

Indications. In the prophylactic control of life-threatening ventricular tachyarrhythmias and in recurrent cardiac arrest,[40,79] amiodarone is one of the most effective agents available. Amiodarone is highly effective in preventing recurrences of paroxysmal atrial fibrillation or flutter, of paroxysmal supraventricular tachycardias,[46,67,87] and in WPW arrhythmias.[96] Amiodarone may be tried for variant angina[98] complicated by severe ventricular arrhythmias.

Serious Side-effects. In higher doses there is an unusual spectrum of toxicity, the most serious being pneumonitis,[97] potentially leading to pulmonary fibrosis and occurring in up to 10% of some series, although in only 1 to 5% in others. Pulmonary complications usually regress if recognized early, and if amiodarone is discontinued and the patient is kept alive by symptomatic therapy, which may include steroids. Pulmonary toxicity may be dose-related.[18,99] Torsades de pointes effect may result from QT-prolongation plus hypokalemia (see Drug Interactions).

Cardiac Side-effects. Inhibition of SA or AV node.

CNS Side-effects. Proximal muscle weakness, peripheral neuropathy, and neural symptoms (headache, ataxia, tremors, impaired memory, insomnia, dreams) occur with variable incidence.[29,122]

Thyroid Side-effects. Amiodarone also has a complex effect on the metabolism of thyroid hormones (it contains iodine and shares a structural similarity to thyroxine), the main action being to inhibit the peripheral conversion of T_4 to T_3, with a rise in the serum level of T_4 and a small fall in the level of T_3; serum reverse T_3 is increased as a function of the dose and duration of amiodarone therapy.[80] In most patients, thyroid function is not altered by amiodarone; in about 3 to 5% hypothyroidism or hyperthyroidism may develop; the exact incidence varies geographically. At a low dose of amiodarone (200–400 mg daily), there may be biochemically documented but clinically silent alterations in thyroid function in 10% of patients.[18]

GI Side-effects. Nausea can occur in 50% of patients with CHF, even at a dose of only 200 mg daily.[137] Increased plasma levels of liver function enzymes may occur in 10 to 20% of all patients.[99] These effects usually resolve with dose reduction.

Less Serious Side-effects. Corneal microdeposits develop in nearly all adult patients given prolonged amiodarone. Symptoms and impairment of visual acuity are rare and respond to reduced dosage. Macular degeneration rarely occurs. In over 10% of patients a photosensitive slate-gray or bluish skin discoloration develops after prolonged therapy, usually exceeding 18 months. The pigmentation regresses slowly on drug withdrawal.

Long-term Use. In one series, at 12 months of therapy the incidence of success against VT or VF was just over 50%, which however fell to 30% at 2 years, whereas at 4 years the chances of a patient being alive and still on amiodarone were only about 20%.[121] On the other hand, (1) discontinuation of amiodarone leads to an even worse prognosis,[149] and (2) other investigators show that amiodarone is effective in nearly 60% of patients unresponsive to other antiarrhythmic drugs, even after 5 years.[138]

Drug Interactions. The most serious interaction[66] is an additive **proarrhythmic effect** with other drugs prolonging the QT-interval, such as Class IA antiarrhythmic agents, phenothiazines, tricyclic antidepressants, thiazide diuretics, and sotalol (Fig. 8–7). Amiodarone prolongs the prothrombin time and may cause bleeding in patients on **warfarin**, perhaps by a hepatic interaction;[35] decrease warfarin by about one-third and retest the INR (See p 228). Amiodarone increases the plasma digoxin concentration,[81] predisposing to digitalis toxic effects (not arrhythmias, because amiodarone protects); decrease **digoxin** by about half and remeasure digoxin levels. Amiodarone, by virtue of its weak β-blocking and calcium antagonist effect, tends to inhibit nodal activity and may therefore interact adversely with β-blocking agents and calcium antagonists.[66]

Precautions. To initiate therapy, the patient may require hospitalization, especially for life-threatening VT/VF. Otherwise therapy can be initiated on an out-patient basis. Plasma electrolytes should be normal and drug interactions considered. During chronic therapy the ECG and Holter recordings are monitored and periodic lung functions, chest x-rays, and thyroid tests are required. Keep the dose as low as possible.

Comparative Studies. Post-infarct, amiodarone 400 mg daily was better than propranolol 160 mg daily.[133] In refractory VT or VF, in non-infarct patients, amiodarone seemed similar to sotalol although initially with less dropouts;[121] this study needs confirmation.

Sotalol

Although still not available in the USA except in investigational centers, sotalol (Sotacor) is now widely used in Europe for control of

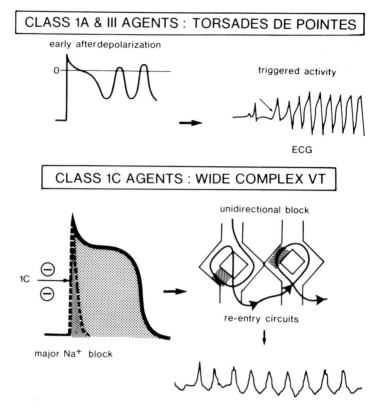

FIGURE 8–7. Major pro-arrhythmic mechanisms.[169] Class IA and Class III agents widen the action potential duration and, in the presence of an early afterdepolarization, through complex mechanisms can give rise to triggered activity of the variety known as torsades de pointes. Note major role of QT-prolongation (see Fig. 8–8). Class IC agents have as their major pro-arrhythmic mechanism a powerful inhibition of the sodium channel, particularly in conduction tissue. Increasing heterogeneity together with unidirectional block sets the stage for re-entry circuits and monomorphic wide complex ventricular tachycardia. Figure copyright L.H. Opie.

ventricular arrhythmias resistant to other measures, especially when amiodarone toxicity is feared. Sotalol seems safer than amiodarone, although probably less effective. Sotalol has combined Class II and III activities; only the latter is found with the d-isomer.[50,64] The chief hazard is torsades de pointes in 4 to 5% of patients, so that it is important that sotalol should only be given cautiously with thiazide diuretics[69] or with any other agent prolonging the QT-interval. The major indication for sotalol is for its antiarrhythmic capacity, rather than for its β-blocking antihypertensive effect (it is the only β-blocker with risk of torsades). On the other hand, it is the only Class III antiarrhythmic with simple pharmacokinetics, being totally lipid-insoluble and not subject to hepatic metabolism. Sotalol should be especially effective when a combined β-blocking and antiarrhythmic potency is required, as in some post-infarct patients, hypertrophic cardiomyopathy, and hypertension with symptomatic arrhythmias. All these possibilities require testing. A limited number of studies have shown the superiority of sotalol to other β-blockers in inducible VT[95] and its efficacy in patients with recurrent VT/VF.[82] The oral antiarrhythmic dose is 160 to 480 mg 2x daily (i.e., higher than the β-blocking doses). **The usual contraindications to β-blockade** (see Table

1-1) apply, but are joined by hypokalemia and co-therapy with other agents likely to produce QT-prolongation. Furthermore, the high antiarrhythmic doses may produce severe β-blocking side-effects. There is some suggestion that sotalol may not be as negatively inotropic as other β-blockers,[121] although heart failure can nonetheless be precipitated.[160]

Dose. Theoretically a much higher dose of sotalol is required to achieve Class III activity than the β-blocking effects.[152] In a double-blind trial, preliminary data show that sotalol 640 mg daily was more effective on chronic ventricular arrhythmias than was 320 mg daily, and both were much better than placebo.[122] In ventricular arrhythmias refractory to other drugs, dose-titration showed an average sotalol requirement of 340 mg daily.[160] In the amiodarone-sotalol study, a mean sotalol dose of 490 mg equalled amiodarone 400 mg daily.[121] However, in other studies lower doses have been effective, for example, a mean dose of 250 mg daily against monomorphic ventricular tachycardia.[142] The problem is to know whether these lower effective doses are acting through the β-blocking or through the Class III activity.

Side-effects. The three most common side-effects are bradycardia, increased CHF, and torsades de pointes.[160] In addition, β-blocker side-effects include drowsiness and fatigue.[121]

Bretylium Tosylate

Bretylium (Bretylol) is generally limited to recurrent VF or VT after lidocaine and DC cardioversion have failed in the setting of AMI. It differs from all other antiarrhythmics in being concentrated in the terminal sympathetic neurons, where it accumulates initially to release stored norepinephrine (NE) and then to inhibit further release of NE with a "chemical" sympathectomy.[101]

Electrophysiology. The antiarrhythmic effect may be due only in part to the chemical sympathectomy because bretylium has Class III activity in Purkinje fibers, but less in ventricular muscle, and none in atrial tissue. There is little inhibitory effect on nodal or conduction tissue.[22]

Pharmacokinetics. After IV administration, bretylium is widely distributed to various tissues and then excreted almost entirely by the kidneys by active tubular secretion. There is no liver metabolism and the elimination half-life is 7 to 9 hours (much prolonged in renal failure).

Dose. The initial dose of 5 mg/kg can be increased to 10 mg/kg in the absence of hypotension (major problem). It should be diluted 1:4 to a minimum of 50 ml with 5% dextrose or sodium chloride and infused over 10 to 30 minutes to minimize nausea and vomiting.[47] However, in emergencies, it is given undiluted by rapid IV injection. After loading, a constant infusion of 1-2 mg/min may be given, or the loading dose may be repeated at 1 to 2 hour intervals.

Indications. Bretylium may have a special use in patients subject to defibrillation and external cardiac massage. In seven patients with VF after AMI,[101] bretylium 5 to 10 mg/kg was given intravenously with the patient's arm raised above the heart, and resuscitation was continued. In five patients, defibrillation ensued without DC shock. In a series of 27 patients treated by a hospital cardiac arrest team, VF was resistant to 30 minutes of conventional electric and pharmacologic procedures (lidocaine plus one or more of the following: procainamide, propranolol, and phenytoin),[44] yet after a single IV bolus of bretylium tosylate (5 mg/kg), 20 patients were successfully defibrillated by DC shock. A randomized clinical trial of 147 patients compared bretylium and lidocaine in VF occurring outside the hospital; the two drugs were equieffective.[39]

Side-effects. The major side-effect is drug-induced hypotension, which can be treated by vasopressor catecholamines or by protriptyline (5 mg every 6 hours), which pharmacologically antagonizes the hypotensive effect.[92] With bretylium, initial sympathomimetic effects (transient hypertension and increased arrhythmias) probably result from transient discharge of NE from the terminal neurons. Nausea and vomiting are common after rapid IV bolus injection.

CLASS IV AGENTS: VERAPAMIL, DILTIAZEM, AND ADENOSINE

Verapamil and diltiazem inhibit slow channel dependent conduction through the AV node. Verapamil has been a major advance in the acute therapy of supraventricular arrhythmias (see Chapter 3). Diltiazem is of similar value to verapamil, but neither is available in the IV form nor licensed for an antiarrhythmic effect in the USA. Nifedipine is devoid of antiarrhythmic effects.

The potassium channel openers are indirect calcium antagonists. These agents hyperpolarize the cell membrane thereby moving the polarity away from that required for "opening" of the slow calcium channel, so that they are particularly useful in supraventricular tachycardias with re-entrant circuits utilizing the AV node. Adenosine and ATP given intravenously are increasingly used to inhibit the AV node in supraventricular re-entrant tachycardias with the same locus of action in the middle of the AV node as has verapamil.

Adenosine

Adenosine (Adenocard), an agent with multiple cellular effects, including potassium channel opening, inhibits the sinus and especially the AV node. Its **chief indication** is **PSVT** (AV nodal re-entrant tachycardia, AV tachycardia in WPW). In **broad complex tachycardia**, which can either be VT or SVT (with aberrant conduction), the use of verapamil can be fatal if the arrhythmia is VT, because the drug causes long-lasting myocardial depression. However, the action of adenosine is so fleeting that it can stop broad complex SVT without too much adverse effect in VT, thereby providing a combined therapeutic and diagnostic test.[136] Very occasionally adenosine is effective in certain types of VT, such as those induced by exercise in a normal heart. Adenosine has no effect on the basic atrial arrhythmia, such as an ectopic focus or flutter. It has an extremely short half-life of 10 to 30 seconds, and side-effects are likewise transient, including dyspnea, flushing, and chest pain.

Dose. To minimize side-effects and to lessen excess AV nodal depression, the drug is given as an initial rapid IV bolus of 6 mg; if it does not work within 1 to 2 minutes, a 12 mg bolus is given that may be repeated once. At the appropriate dose, the antiarrhythmic effect occurs as soon as the drug reaches the AV node.[127]

Side-effects. Side-effects of adenosine include dyspnea in many[166] because it is a bronchoconstrictor, flushing (18%) and headache (2%) because it is a vasodilator, and chest pain (occasionally) because it is thought to be involved in the genesis of anginal pain. Excess sinus or nodal inhibition may occur. Transient new arrhythmias at the time of chemical cardioversion occur in 65%.

Contraindication. Asthma, second or third degree AV block, sick sinus syndrome.

Drug Interactions. Dipyridamole inhibits the breakdown of adenosine and therefore the dose should be reduced in patients on dipyridamole therapy.[147,166] Methylxanthines (caffeine, theophylline) competitively antagonize adenosine so that it becomes less effective. In patients pre-treated with β-blocking agents or with myocardial failure, adenosine is preferred to verapamil in the treatment of PSVT to avoid combined depressant effects. It is likely that adenosine may replace IV verapamil for the rapid termination of narrow QRS complex PSVT, in which there is anterograde conduction over the AV node during the tachycardia.

ATP (Adenovine Triphosphate)

ATP probably acts by conversion to adenosine and is likewise used in supraventricular arrhythmias. ATP 10 to 20 mg IV was somewhat more effective than verapamil 5 to 10 mg IV in terminating PSVT[123] at the cost of more side-effects (AV block, new arrhythmias, non-cardiac side-effects of adenosine). Hence the authors recommend ATP only if verapamil up to 10 mg has failed.

By inference, adenosine itself should also be limited to similar indications unless used diagnostically in broad complex tachycardias.

METABOLIC AGENTS

Hypokalemia predisposes to ventricular arrhythmias, especially in the context of AMI and during the use of agents prolonging the action potential duration when torsades becomes a risk. In such situations, **potassium infusions** may be required. It is prudent always to check plasma potassium during antiarrhythmic therapy, during digoxin therapy, or at the start of AMI.

Magnesium salts are reported to be of benefit in the therapy of torsad)es[164] and also in the arrhythmias of early AMI.[91]

COMBINATION THERAPY

A combination of antiarrhythmic agents is increasingly used with the supposition that added antiarrhythmic potency may be achieved while side-effects are minimized. A useful guide is not to combine agents of the same class or subclasses or agents with potentially additive side-effects, such as the extra-risk arrhythmias with Class IA and Class IC agents[37] or the added QT-prolongation with Class IA drugs and amiodarone. However, the addition of sotalol to Class I drugs that have increased VT cycle length by more than 50 msec may prevent inducibility of VT in nearly 50% of patients.[128] A logical combination is that of a Class I drug that preferentially binds to inactivated sodium channels (Class IB) with a drug binding preferentially to activated channels, such as a Class IA drug,[171] thus explaining the benefits of mexiletine combined with quinidine[129] or mexiletine with procainamide.[34] Other useful combinations are quinidine and procainamide,[52] mexiletine plus propranolol,[59] quinidine plus verapamil (with the risk of added hypotension[65]), verapamil and disopyramide (in experimental animals[60]), and propafenone with quinidine or procainamide.[54] Drug interactions merit careful attention (see Table 8-4). "Rules," although helpful, do not always apply because of the complex mode of action of many antiarrhythmic agents.[120] When amiodarone has failed as maximal therapy, a useful and not easily explicable combination may be that with xamoterol, a cardioselective β-blocker with a high degree of ISA (see Chap. 1).[154] Of all the combinations, the one most often used is a β-blocker with a membrane-active Class I drug.[170]

PRO-ARRHYTHMIC EFFECTS OF ANTIARRHYTHMIC COMPOUNDS

Traditional concepts of pro-arrhythmia have been challenged by the results of the CAST study,[126] in which an initial test period of encainide or flecainide was used to show antiarrhythmic benefit without any early pro-arrhythmic effect, and yet during the actual prolonged study period these drugs caused an increased mortality. Besides encainide and flecainide, virtually all antiarrhythmics have been reported to have a pro-arrhythmic effect, varying between 5% and 15%.[111] There are two basic mechanisms for pro-arrhythmia:[169] prolongation of the action potential duration and QT-interval, particularly when combined with diuretic-induced hypokalemia or when there is bradycardia (next section), and, secondly, incessant wide complex tachycardia often terminating in VF (see Fig. 8–7). The former typically occurs with Class IA and Class III agents, the latter with Class IC agents. In addition, incessant VT can complicate therapy with any Class I agent when conduction is sufficiently severely depressed. Of the Class III agents, sotalol may be particularly prone to cause torsades de pointes because of its reverse-use dependency[140] so that the action potential duration is prolonged more in the presence of bradycardia. A third type of pro-arrhythmia is when the patient's own tachycardia, previously paroxysmal, becomes incessant—the result of either Class IA or IC agents.[143] Whereas early vigilance is required with the institution of therapy with antiarrhythmics of the Class IA, IC, and III types, continuous vigilance is required throughout therapy. Furthermore, the CAST study[126] shows that pro-arrhythmic sudden death can occur even when ventricular premature complexes are apparently eliminated. Solutions to this problem include (1) avoiding the use of Class I, and especially Class IC, agents, (2) not treating unless the overall effect will clearly be beneficial, and (3) ultimately defining better those subjects at high risk for pro-arrhythmia and arrhythmic death.[143]

A new proposal is the potential reversal of the pro-arrhythmic effects of Class IC agents by β-blockade;[151] however, in the CAST study,[126] β-blocked patients had the same incidence of sudden death as the others.

QT-PROLONGATION AND TORSADES DE POINTES

Delayed repolarization is a mechanism for controlling arrhythmias (Class IA and III agents) that at the same time predisposes to potentially life-threatening arrhythmias. It is clinically recognized by a prolonged QT (500–600 msec[51,74]) or QTU interval (QTc, corrected for heart rate) exceeding 440 msec.[77] The prolonged QT-syndrome may either be acquired or be a congenital abnormality (Romano-Ward and related conditions). The realization that quinidine, disopyramide, procainamide, and related Class IA agents, Class III agents, and others (see Fig. 8–8) can all prolong the QT-interval has led to a reassessment of the mode of use of such agents in antiarrhythmic therapy. Prolongation of the QT-interval is an essential part of the antiarrhythmic effect of amiodarone,[108] without being the complete explanation, because antiarrhythmic properties of a variety of compounds do not simply correlate with their effect on QT-prolongation.[162] Serious problems may arise when antiarrhythmic QT-prolongation is combined with any other factor increasing the QT-interval or QTU, such as bradycardia, hypokalemia, hypomagnesemia, hypocalcemia, intense or prolonged diuretic therapy, or combined Class IA and Class III therapy. A number of non-cardiac drugs prolong the QT-interval (mechanism unclear), including tricyclic antidepressants, phenothiazines, and erythromycin. When amiodarone is given to patients not receiving diuretics or other drugs who are not hypokalemic and without pre-existing QT-prolongation, torsades is very rare.

Prevention. Probably the most effective way to avoid the drug-induced QT-syndrome is by regular monitoring of the ECG for the appearance of ventricular pauses, post-pause T-wave changes, and late cycle PVCs,[5] as well as QT-prolongation, while checking blood potassium and magnesium, and using a potassium-sparing diuretic whenever possible.

Treatment. Torsades de pointes is best treated by agents that shorten the QT-interval, such as isoproterenol or temporary cardiac pacing. Isoproterenol is contraindicated in ischemic heart disease and the congenital prolonged QT-syndrome. A recent report stresses the value of IV magnesium sulfate.[164] If the QT-interval is not markedly prolonged, torsades de pointes is excluded and therapy with conventional ventricular antiarrhythmic agents is acceptable.[30] For **congenital QT-prolongation**, the underlying cause may be an imbalance of the sympathetic drive coming from the left and right sympathetic chains. The therapy now becomes full-dose β-blockade, with added phenytoin if needed,[77] or left stellate ganglionectomy.

ARRHYTHMIAS IN CONGESTIVE HEART FAILURE

Prophylactic antiarrhythmic therapy is contraindicated in CHF, especially in view of the high incidence of bradyarrhythmic deaths.[148] In **symptomatic arrhythmias**, it is first essential to pinpoint precipitating factors such as hypokalemia or use of sympathomimetics or phosphodiesterase inhibitors or digoxin. The hemodynamic status of the myocardium must be made optimal. Antiarrhythmics are only given after documentation of benefit by electrophysiologic studies in patients presenting with sustained VT or VF. At present it is not certain that the suppression of asymptomatic PVCs, no matter how complex, leads to a decrease in arrhythmia mortality.

A Paradox: Antiarrhythmics May Worsen CHF. Here is the paradox: Ventricular arrhythmias can be a fatal event in CHF, yet antiarrhythmic agents can precipitate CHF. Besides β-blockers and calcium antagonists, Class I agents[135,159] and sotalol may all precipitate CHF. A large VA co-operative trial, far advanced, suggests that amiodarone is well tolerated in CHF. However, in another trial, amiodarone 400 mg daily was as likely as sotalol to precipitate CHF, but when 200 mg was used, it increased the ejection fraction from 19% to 29% and had a borderline effect on VT (p=0.06).[121] There are no controlled studies on the effects of antiarrhythmics on mortality in CHF. The realization that the mechanism of sudden cardiac arrest in patients with CHF sufficiently severe to warrant transplantation is often severe bradyarrhythmia or electromechanical dissociation rather than VF,[148] and that most antiarrhythmics depress the sinus node, should cool enthusiasm for the use of such agents in CHF.

Pharmacokinetics of Antiarrhythmics in CHF. In CHF, diverse factors can influence antiarrhythmic drug kinetics. For example, the volume of distribution is decreased by about 50%, so that the loading dose should be lower, yet liver blood flow is decreased so that the maintenance dose may need to be higher. The elimination half-life is prolonged, which tends to decrease the dose. Furthermore, antiarrhythmics may increase the severity of CHF[135] so that therapy needs to be started at low doses in hospitalized patients and side-effects, as well as the hemodynamic and metabolic status of the patients, need to be carefully monitored.[167]

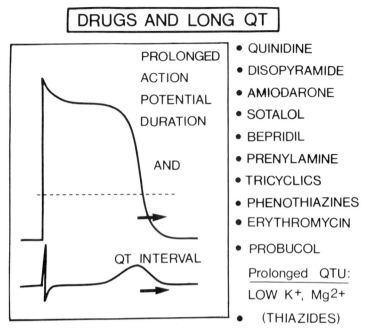

FIGURE 8–8. Therapeutic agents, including antiarrhythmics, that may cause QT-prolongation. Hypokalemia causes QTU, not QT-prolongation. Some antiarrhythmic agents, such as amiodarone and sotalol, act, at least in part, by prolonging the action potential duration. QT-prolongation is therefore an integral part of their therapeutic benefit. On the other hand, QT-prolongation, especially in the presence of hypokalemia and other electrolyte disturbances, or when there is co-therapy with one of the other agents prolonging the QT-interval, may precipitate torsades de pointes. Figure copyright L.H. Opie.

PRINCIPLES OF TREATMENT OF VENTRICULAR TACHYCARDIA

First, full work-up and optimal cardiac and electrolyte status are required. There is no unanimity of cardiologic opinion on the principles and indication for antiarrhythmic therapy or on the relative merits of non-invasive or invasive monitoring in drug selection.[170] Nonetheless, some guidelines are given in Figure 8–9. Logically, only one compound of one category should be tried (e.g., only one Class IA agent, either quinidine *or* disopyramide *or* procainamide). In reality, side-effects may limit the effective dose with one drug (e.g., GI effects of quinidine) to allow another drug of the same class to be effective unless also limited by side-effects (e.g., disopyramide and vagolytic side-effects). Furthermore, many antiarrhythmic mechanisms are complex and not simply explained by effects on the action potential.[120] Also, the experience of many cardiologists not specializing in arrhythmia therapy is likely to be limited to a small number of drugs. Hence the progression in Figure 8–9 is highly hypothetical. For each category of agent, the profile of electrophysiologic and hemodynamic side-effects needs to be matched against the clinical situation in the individual patient. The potential for pro-arrhythmic events and the lack of firm evidence for prevention of sudden death by antiarrhythmics need stressing. Exceptions to these statements appear to be (1) post-infarct β-blockade that prolongs life and reduces sudden death; (2) therapy of truly life-threatening, serious symptomatic ventricular arrhythmias; and (3) the prevention of recurrent cardiac arrest. Note that in early AMI, VF but not mortality has been shown to be reduced by pre-hospital lidocaine or very early IV propranolol. IV β-blockade followed by oral β-blockade has been shown to prolong life.

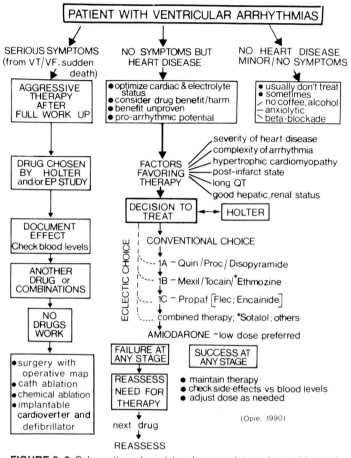

FIGURE 8–9. Schematic and provisional approach to patients with ventricular arrhythmias. Note that considerable controversy exists and there is no unanimity of opinion. Suppression of premature ventricular complexes in post-myocardial infarction patients by any Class I agent may cause some excess mortality. Specific individual consideration is required for each patient, because the exact nature of the ventricular arrhythmia and its significance may be different in each. (Compiled by LH Opie and DC Harrison.)
* = Not in the USA.

SUMMARY

The complexity of the numerous agents available and the ever-increasing problems with side-effects and pro-arrhythmic events underline the requirement for careful cardiologic evaluation and monitoring in patients receiving such drugs. In terms of drug effects, the therapy of supraventricular arrhythmias is assuming an increasingly rational basis with a prominent role for verapamil and adenosine in supraventricular tachycardia with AV nodal re-entry. Sodium blockers can inhibit the bypass tract or retrograde fast AV nodal fibers. The therapy of ventricular arrhythmias remains a controversial and constantly evolving area of development, and antiarrhythmic drug therapy may be only one avenue of overall management. A distinction must be made between suppression of premature ventricular complexes and the control of VT/VF. In AMI, IV lidocaine remains the agent of choice while prophylaxis of VF by very early β-blockade is not yet fully established. In other patients, whether or not ventricular arrhythmias should be treated largely depends on the nature and severity of the underlying heart disease and the nature of the arrhythmia. All seriously symptomatic arrhythmias need therapy; whether asymptomatic arrhythmias should be treated is a moot point, even if they look "premalignant" and "life-threatening." Not only has there been no definite proof that treatment of asymptomatic arrhythmias improves mortality, but rather the CAST study[126] showed a definite pro-arrhythmic risk for the use of flecainide or encainide in post-myocardial infarction patients. To varying degrees; this may apply to most class I agents.

REFERENCES

References from Previous Editions

1. Anderson JL, Lutz JL, Allison SB: J Am Coll Cardiol 2:105–114, 1983
2. Anderson JL, Anastasiou-Nana M, Lutz JR, et al: J Am Cardiol 5:333–341, 1985
3. Berchtold-Kanz E, Schwarz G, Hust M, et al: Clin Cardiol 7:493–497, 1984
4. Bexton RS, Hellestrand KG, Cory-Pearce R, et al: Circulation 67:38–44, 1983
5. Bhandari AK, Scheinman M: Mod Concepts Cardiovasc Dis 54:45–49, 1985
6. Birkhead S, Vaughan Williams EM: Br Heart J 39:657–660, 1977
7. Breithardt G, Selpel L, Abendroth RR: Circulation 62(suppl III):III-153, 1980
8. Breithardt G, Borggrefe M, Wiebringhaus E, et al: Am J Cardiol 54:29D–39D, 1984
9. Burton JR, Mathew MT, Armstrong PW: Am J Med 61:215–219, 1976
10. Campbell NPS, Pantridge JF, Adgey AAJ: Eur J Cardiol 6:245–258, 1978
11. Campbell NPS, Kelly JG, Adgey AJ et al: Br Heart J 40:1371–1375, 1978
12. Campbell RWF, Dolder MA, Prescott LF, et al: Lancet 1:1257–1260, 1975
13. Campbell RWF, Hutton I, Elton RA, et al: Br Heart J 49: 557-563, 1983
14. Chazov EI, Shugushev KK, Rosenshtraukh LV: Am Heart J 108:475–482, 1984
15. Chazov EI, Rosenshtraukh LV, Shugushev KK: Am Heart J 108:483–489, 1984
16. Chew CYC, Collett J, Singh BN: Drugs 17:161–181, 1979
17. Christian CO Jr, Meredith CG, Speeg KV, Jr: Clin Pharmacol Ther 36:221–227, 1984
18. Collaborative Group for Amiodarone Evaluation: Am J Cardiol 53:1564–1569, 1984
19. Connolly SJ, Kates RE, Lebsack CS, et al: Circulation 68:589–596, 1983
20. Desai JM, Scheinman M, Roberts RW, et al: Circulation 59:215–225, 1979
21. De Silva RA, Hennekens CH, Lown B, et al: Lancet 2:855–858, 1981
22. Dhurandhar RW, Bakersmith D: In Gould LA (ed): Drug Treatment of Cardiac Arrhythmias. Mount Kisco, NY, Futura Publishing, 1983, pp 299–324
23. Duff HJ, Roben D, Primm RK, et al: Circulation 67:1124–1128, 1983
24. Dumoulin P, Jaillon P, Kher A, et al: Am Heart J 110:575–581, 1985
25. Ellrodt AG, Murata GH, Riedinger MS, et al: Ann Intern Med 100:197–201, 1984
26. Estes NAM, Garan H, Ruskin JN: Am J Cardiol 53:26B–29B, 1984
27. Farringer JA, McWay-Hess K, Clementi WA: Clin Pharmacol 3:81–83, 1984
28. Flecainide Ventricular Tachycardia Study Group: Am J Cardiol 57:1299–1304, 1986
29. Fogoros RN, Anderson KP, Winkle RA, et al: Circulation 68:88–94, 1983
30. Fontaine G, Frank R, Grosgogeat Y: Mod Concepts Cardiovasc Dis 51:103–108, 1982
31. Friedman LM, Byington RP, Capone RJ, et al: J Am Coll Cardiol 7:1-8, 1986
32. Gerstenblith G, Scherlag BJ, Hope RR, et al: Am J Cardiol 42:587–591, 1978
33. Gloor HO, Urthaler F, James TN: J Clin Invest 71:1457–1466, 1983
34. Greenspan AM, Spielman SR, Webb CR, et al: Am J Cardiol 56:277–284, 1985
35. Hamer A, Peter T, Mandel WJ, et al: Circulation 65:1025–1029, 1982
36. Harrison DC: Circulation 58:581–583, 1978

37. Harrison DC: Am J Cardiol 56:185–187, 1985
38. Hartel G, Louhija A, Konttinen A: Clin Pharmacol Ther 15:551–555, 1974
39. Haynes RE, Chinn TL, Copass MK, et al: Am J Cardiol 48:353-360, 1981
40. Heger J, Prystowsky EN, Jackman WM, et al: N Engl J Med 305:539–546, 1981
41. Hellestrand KJ, Nathan AW, Bexton RS, et al: Am J Cardiol 51:770–776, 1983
42. Hodges M, Salerno D, Granrud G: Am J Cardiol 54:45D–50D, 1984
43. Hohnloser SH, Lange HW, Raeder EA, et al: Circulation 73:143–149, 1986
44. Holder DA, Smiderman AD, Fraser G, et al: Circulation 55:541–544, 1977
45. Holt DW, Tucker GT, Jackson PR, et al: Am Heart J 106:840–847, 1983
46. Horowitz LN, Spielman SR, Greenspan AM, et al: J Am Coll Cardiol 6:1402–1407, 1985
47. Huang SK, Marcus FI: Curr Problems Cardiol 11:179–240, 1986
48. IMPACT Research Group: J Am Coll Cardiol 4:1148–1163, 1984
49. Josephson MA, Kaul S, Hopkins J, et al: Am Heart J 109:41–45, 1985
50. Kato R, Ikeda N, Yabek SM, et al: J Am Coll Cardiol 7:116–125, 1986
51. Keren A, Tzivoni D, Gavish D, et al: Circulation 64:1167–1174, 1981
52. Kim SG, Seiden SW, Matos JA, et al: Am J Cardiol 56:84–88, 1985
53. Kjekshus J, Bathen J, Orning OM, et al: Am J Cardiol 53:72B–78B, 1984
54. Klein R, Huang SK, Southwest Cardiology Research Group (abstract): J Am Coll Cardiol 5:423, 1985
55. Koch-Weser J, Klein SW, Foo-Canto LL, et al: N Engl J Med 281:1253–1260, 1969
56. Kosowsky BD, Taylor J, Lown B, et al: Circulation 47:1204–1210, 1973
57. Koster RW, Dunning AJ: N Engl J Med 313:1105–1110, 1985
58. LaBarre A, Strauss HC, Scheinman MM, et al: Circulation 59:226–235, 1979
59. Leahey EB, Heissenbuttel RH, Giardina EGV, et al: Br Med J 2:357–358, 1980
60. Lee JT, Davy J-M, Kates RE: J Cardiovasc Pharmacol 7:501–507, 1985
61. Lerman BB, Waxman HL, Buxton AE, et al: Am J Cardiol 51:759–764, 1983
62. Lie KI, Wellens HJ, Van Capelle FJ, et al: N Engl J Med 291:1324–1326, 1974
63. Lubbe WF, McFadyen ML, Muller CA, et al: Am J Cardiol 43:533–540, 1979
64. Lynch JJ, Coskey LA, Montgomery DG, et al: Am Heart J 109:949–958, 1985
65. Maisel AS, Motulsky HJ, Insel PA: N Engl J Med 312:167–171, 1985
66. Marcus FI: Am Heart J 106:924–930, 1983
67. Marcus FI, Fontaine GH, Frank R, et al: Am Heart J 101:480–493, 1981
68. Mason JW, Hondeghem LM, Katzung BG: Circ Res 55:277–285, 1984
69. McKibbin JK, Pocock WA, Barlow JB, et al: Br Heart J 51:157–162, 1984
70. Meltzer RS, Robert EW, McMorrow M, et al: Am J Cardiol 42:1049–1056, 1978
71. Mirro MJ, Manalan AS, Bailey JC: Circ Res 47:855-865, 1980
72. Morganroth J, Panadis I, Lee G, et al: Circulation 67:1117–1123, 1983
73. Morganroth J, Horowitz LN: Am J Cardiol 53:89B–94B, 1984
74. Morganroth J, Horowitz LN: Am J Cardiol 56:585–587, 1985
75. Morganroth J, Oshrain C, Steele PP: Am J Cardiol 56:581–585, 1985
76. Morganroth J, Nestico PF, Horowitz LN: Am Heart J 110:856–863, 1985
77. Moss AJ, Schwartz PJ: Mod Concepts Cardiovasc Dis 51:85–90, 1982
78. Motulsky HJ, Maisel AS, Snavely MD, et al: Circ Res 55:376–381, 1984
79. Nademanee K, Hendrickson JA, Cannom DS, et al: Am Heart J 101:759–768, 1981
80. Nademanee K, Singh BN, Hendrickson JA, et al: Ann Intern Med 98:577–587, 1983
81. Nademanee K, Kannan R, Hendrickson J, et al: J Am Coll Cardiol 4:111–116, 1984
82. Nademanee K, Feld G, Hendrickson J, et al: Circulation 72:555–564, 1985
83. Nathan AW, Hellestrand KJ, Bexton RS, et al: Am Heart J 107:222–228, 1984
84. Nathan AW, Bexton RS, Hellestrand KJ, et al: Postgrad Med J 60:155–156, 1984
85. Neuss H, Buss J, Schlepper M, et al: Eur Heart J 4:347–353, 1983
86. Palileo EV, Welch W, Hoff J, et al: Am J Cardiol 50:1075–1081, 1982
87. Podrid PJ, Lown B: Am Heart J 101:374–379, 1981
88. Podrid PJ, Lown B: Am J Cardiol 49:1279–1286, 1982
89. Podrid PJ, Cytryn R, Lown B: Am J Cardiol 54: 53D-59D, 1984
90. Pollick C, Detsky A, Ogilvie RI, et al: Circulation 72(suppl III):III-155, 1985

91. Rasmussen HS, McNair P, Norregard P, et al: Lancet 1:234–236, 1986
92. Reele S, Woosley RL, Oates JA: Circulation 58(suppl II):II-962, 1978
93. Reid PR, Griffith LSC, Platia EV, et al: Am J Cardiol 53:108B–111B, 1984
94. Reidenberg MM, Campcho M, Kluger J, et al: Clin Pharmacol Ther 28:732–735, 1980
95. Rizos I, Senges J, Jauernig R, et al: Am J Cardiol 53:1022–1027, 1984
96. Rosenbaum MB, Chiale PA, Halpern MS, et al: Am J Cardiol 38:934–944, 1976
97. Rotmensch HH, Liron M, Tupilski M, et al: Am Heart J 100:412–413, 1980
98. Rutitzky B, Girotti AL, Rosenbaum MB: Am Heart J 103:38–43, 1982
99. Salerno JA, Bressan MA, Vigano M, et al: Eur Heart J 6:1054–1062, 1985
100. Sami MH, Derbekyan VA, Lisbona R: Am J Cardiol 52:507–512, 1983
101. Sanna G, Arcidiancono R: Am J Cardiol 32:982–987, 1973
102. Sbarbaro JA, Rawling DA, Fozzard HA: Am J Cardiol 44:513–520, 1979
103. Selzer A, Wray HW: Circulation 30:17–26, 1964
104. Shea P, Lal R, Kim SS, et al: J Am Coll Cardiol 7:1127–1130, 1986
105. Siddoway LA, McAllister CB, Wilkinson GR, et al: Am Heart J 106:951–956, 1983
106. Spurrell RAJ, Thorburn CW, Camm J, et al: Br Heart J 37:861–867, 1975
107. Strathman I, Schubert EN, Cohen A, et al: Drug Intell Clin Pharm 17:635–638, 1983
108. Torres V, Tepper D, Flowers D, et al: J Am Coll Cardiol 7:142–147, 1986
109. Tucker CR, Winkle RA, Peters FA, et al: Am Heart J 104:209–215, 1982
110. Ueda CT, Dzindzio BS, Vosik WM: Clin Pharmacol Ther 36:326–336, 1984
111. Velebit V, Podrid P, Lown B, et al: Circulation 65:886–894, 1982
112. Vismara LA, Vera Z, Miller RR, et al: Am J Cardiol 39:1027–1034, 1977
113. Waleffe A, Mary-Rabine L, Legrand V, et al: Am Heart J 100:788–793, 1980
114. Waspe L, Waxman HL, Buxton AE, et al: Am J Cardiol 51:1175–1181, 1983
115. Waxman HL, Buxton AE, Sadowski LM, et al: Circulation 67:30-37.
116. Webb Kavey RE, Blackman MS, Sondheimer HM: Am Heart J 104:794–798, 1982
117. Wigle ED, Sasson Z, Henderson MA, et al: Prog Cardiovasc Dis 28:1-83, 1985
118. Winkle RA, Mason JW, Griffin JC, et al: Am Heart J 102:857–864, 1981
119. Wit AL, Rosen MR, Hoffman BF: Am Heart J 90:397–404, 1975
120. Zipes DP: Circulation 72:949–956, 1985

New References

121. Amiodarone vs Sotalol Study Group: Multicentre randomized trial of sotalol vs amiodarone for chronic malignant ventricular tachyarrhythmias. Eur Heart J 10:685–694, 1989
122. Anastasiou-Nana MI, Anderson JL, Gilbert EM, et al: Suppression of chronic ventricular arrhythmias with d,l-sotalol: Final report of a multicenter randomized, double-blind, placebo-controlled trial (abstract). Circulation 80(suppl II):II-651, 1989
123. Belhassen B, Glick A, Laniado S: Comparative clinical and electrophysiologic effects of adenosine triphosphate and verapamil on paroxysmal reciprocating junctional tachycardia. Circulation 77:795–805, 1988
124. Brodsky MA, Allen BJ, Luckett CR, et al: Antiarrhythmic efficacy of solitary β-adrenergic blockade for patients with sustained ventricular tachyarrhythmias. Am Heart J 118:272–280, 1989
125. Cardiac Arrhythmia Pilot Study (CAPS) Investigators: Effects of encainide, flecainide, imipramine and moricizine on ventricular arrhythmias during the year after acute myocardial infarction: The CAPS. Am J Cardiol 61:501–509, 1988
126. CAST Investigators (Cardiac Arrhythmia Suppression Trial): Preliminary report: Effect of encainide and flecainide on mortality in a randomized trial of arrhythmia suppression after myocardial infarction. N Engl J Med 321:406–412, 1989
126a. Coplen SE, Antman EM, Berlin JE et al: Prevention of recurrent atrial fibrillation by quinidine. A meta-analysis of randomized trials. Circulation 80(Suppl II):II-633, 1989
127. DiMarco JP, Sellers TD, Lerman BB, et al: Diagnostic and therapeutic use of adenosine in patients with supraventricular tachyarrhythmias. J Am Coll Cardiol 6:417–425, 1985

128. Dorian P, Berman ND: Sotalol-Type IA combination prevents sustained ventricular tachycardia recurrence (abstract). Circulation 80(suppl II):II-651, 1989

129. Duff HJ, Mitchell B, Manyari D, Wyse DG: Mexilitine-quinidine combination: Electrophysiologic correlates of a favorable antiarrhythmic interaction in humans. J Am Coll Cardiol 10:1149–1156, 1987

130. Epstein M, Jardine RM, Obel IWP: Flecainide acetate in the treatment of resistant supraventricular arrhythmias. SA Med J 74:559–562, 1988

131. Euler DE, Wedel VA, Scanlon PJ: Adrenergic influences on ischemic and reperfusion arrhythmias in a canine model with diminished collateral blood flow. J Cardiovasc Pharmacol 14:430–437, 1989

132. Falk RH: Flecainide-induced ventricular tachycardia and fibrillation in patients treated for atrial fibrillation. Ann Intern Med 111:107–111, 1989

133. Fournier C, Brunet M, Bah M, et al: Comparison of the efficacy of propranolol and amiodarone in suppressing ventricular arrhythmias following myocardial infarction. Eur Heart J 10:1090–1100, 1989

134. Funck-Brentano C, Kroemer HK, Lee JT, Roden DM: Propafenone. N Engl J Med 322:518–525, 1990

135. Gottlieb SS, Kukin ML, Medina N, et al: Comparative hemodynamic effects of procainamide, tocainide, and encainide in severe chronic heart failure. Circulation 81:860–864, 1990

136. Griffith MJ, Linker NJ, Ward DE, Camm AJ: Adenosine in the diagnosis of broad complex tachycardia. Lancet 1:672–675, 1988

137. Hamer AWF, Arkles B, Johns JA: Beneficial effects of low-dose amiodarone in patients with congestive cardiac failure: A placebo-controlled trial. J Am Coll Cardiol 14:1768–1774, 1989

138. Herre JM, Sauve MJ, Malone P, et al: Long-term results of amiodarone therapy in patients with recurrent sustained ventricular tachycardia or ventricular fibrillation. J Am Coll Cardiol 13:442–449, 1989

139. Hill MR, Gotz VP, Harman E, et al: Evaluation of the asthmogenicity of propafenone, a new antiarrhythmic drug. Chest 90:698–702, 1986

140. Hondeghem LM, Snyders DJ: Class III antiarrhythmic agents have a lot of potential but a long way to go: Reduced effectiveness and dangers of reverse use dependence. Circulation 81:686–690, 1990

141. Ikeda N, Singh BN, Davis LD, Hauswirth O: Effects of flecainide on the electrophysiologic properties of isolated canine and rabbit myocardial fibers. J Am Coll Cardiol 5:303–310, 1985

142. Jordaens LJ, Palmer A, Clement DL: Low-dose oral sotalol for monomorphic ventricular tachycardia: Effects during programmed electrical stimulation and follow-up. Eur Heart J 10:218–226, 1989

143. Josephson ME: Antiarrhythmic agents and the danger of proarrhythmic events. Ann Intern Med 111:101–103, 1989

144. Kates RE, Yee Y-G, Kirsten EB: Interaction between warfarin and propafenone in healthy volunteer subjects. Clin Pharmacol Ther 42:305–311, 1987

145. Keefe DL, Williams S, Torres V, et al: Prophylactic tocainide or lidocaine in acute myocardial infarction. Am J Cardiol 57:527–531, 1986

146. Langenfeld H, Weirich J, Kohler C, Kochsiek K: Comparative analysis of the action of Class I antiarrhythmic drugs (lidocaine, quinidine, and prajmaline) in rabbit atrial and ventricular myocardium. J Cardiovasc Pharmacol 15:338–345, 1990

147. Lerman BB, Wesley RC, Belardinelli L: Electrophysiologic effects of dipyridamole on atrioventricular nodal conduction and supraventricular tachycardia. Role of endogenous adenosine. Circulation 80:1536–1543, 1989

148. Luu M, Stevenson WG, Stevenson LW, et al: Diverse mechanisms of unexpected cardiac arrest in advanced heart failure. Circulation 80:1675–1680, 1989

149. Marks ML, Graham EL, Powell JL, et al: Mortality and arrhythmia recurrence following amiodarone discontinuation (abstract). Circulation 80(suppl II):II-651, 1989

150. Mitchell LB, Wyse G, Gillis AM, et al: Electropharmacology of amiodarone therapy initiation. Time courses of onset of electrophysiologic and antiarrhythmic effects. Circulation 80:34–42, 1989

151. Myerburg RJ, Kessler KM, Cox MM, et al: Reversal of proarrhythmic effects of flecainide acetate and encainide hydrochloride by propranolol. Circulation 80:1571–1579, 1989

152. Nattel S, Feder-Elituv R, Matthews C, et al: Concentration dependence of Class III and β-adrenergic blocking effects of sotalol in anesthetized dogs. J Am Coll Cardiol 13:1190–1194, 1989

153. Opie LH. Adverse cardiovascular drug interactions. In Hurst JW, Schlant RC, et al (eds): The Heart, 7th ed. New York, McGraw-Hill Information Services, 1990, pp 1803–1816
154. Paul V, Griffith M, Ward DE, Camm AJ: Adjuvant xamoterol or metoprolol in patients with malignant ventricular arrhythmia resistant to amiodarone. Lancet 2:302–305, 1989
155. Pollick C: Disopyramide in hypertrophic cardiomyopathy. II: Noninvasive assessment after oral administration. Am J Cardiol 62:1252–1255, 1988
156. Puech P, Gagnol JP: Class IC drugs: Propafenone and flecainide. Cardiovasc Drugs Ther 4:549–553, 1990
157. Quart BD, Gallo DG, Sami MH, Wood AJJ: Drug interaction studies and encainide use in renal and hepatic impairment. Am J Cardiol 58:104C–113C, 1986
158. Ragosta M, Weihl AC, Rosenfeld LE: Potentially fatal interaction between erythromycin and disopyramide. Am J Med 86:465–466, 1989
159. Ravid S, Podrid PJ, Lampert S, Lown B: Congestive heart failure induced by six of the newer antiarrhythmic drugs. J Am Coll Cardiol 14:1326–1330, 1989
160. Ruder MA, Ellis T, Lebsack C, et al: Clinical experience with sotalol in patients with drug-refractory ventricular arrhythmias. J Am Coll Cardiol 13:145–152, 1989
161. Schutzenberger W, Leisch F, Kerschner K, et al: Clinical efficacy of intravenous amiodarone in the short term treatment of recurrent sustained ventricular tachycardia and ventricular fibrillation. Br Heart J 62:367–371, 1989
162. Singh BN: When is QT-prolongation antiarrhythmic and when is it proarrhythmic (editorial)? Am J Cardiol 63:867–869, 1989
163. Singh BN, Nademanee K: Control of arrhythmias by selective lengthening of cardiac repolarization: Theoretical considerations and clinical observations. Am Heart J 109:421–430, 1985
164. Tzivoni D, Banai S, Schuger C, et al: Treatment of torsade de pointes with magnesium sulfate. Circulation 77:392–397, 1988
165. Vacek JL, Sztern MI, Botteron GW, et al: Mexiletine-theophylline interaction. J Am Coll Cardiol 15:39A, 1990
166. Watt AH, Bernard MS, Webster J, et al: Intravenous adenosine in the treatment of supraventricular tachycardia: A dose-ranging study and interaction with dipyridamole. Br J Clin Pharmacol 21:227–230, 1986
167. Woosley RL: Pharmacokinetics and pharmacodynamics of antiarrhythmic agents in patients with congestive heart failure. Am Heart J 114:1280–1290, 1987

Reviews

168. Akhtar M, Breithardt G, Camm AJ, et al: CAST and beyond: Implications of the cardiac arrhythmia suppression trial. Circulation 81:1123–1127, 1990
169. Levine JH, Morganroth J, Kadish AH: Mechanisms and risk factors for proarrhythmia with Type IA compared with IC antiarrhythmic drug therapy. Circulation 80:1063–1069, 1989
170. Podrid J: Antiarrhythmic drug selection. Ann Rev Med 38:1–17, 1987
171. Woosley RL: Antiarrhythmic agents. In Hurst JW, Schlant RC, et al (eds): The Heart, 7th ed. McGraw-Hill Information Services, New York, 1990, pp 1682–1711

B.J. Gersh
L.H. Opie

9

Antithrombotic Agents: Platelet Inhibitors, Anticoagulants, and Fibrinolytics

MECHANISMS OF THROMBOSIS

To form a thrombus, the three steps are (1) exposure of the circulating blood to a thrombogenic surface, such as a damaged vascular endothelium; (2) a sequence of platelet-related events, involving first platelet adhesion, platelet aggregation, and release of agents further promoting aggregation and causing vasoconstriction; and (3) activation of the clotting mechanism with an important role for thrombin in the formation of fibrin. Thrombin is in itself a very powerful stimulator of platelet aggregation and adhesion (Fig. 9–1). Once formed, the clot may be broken down by plasmin-stimulated fibrinolysis. Current antithrombotic medications include those inhibiting platelets (antiplatelet agents), anticoagulants, and fibrinolytics. The typical arterial thrombus at the site of a coronary stenosis has a white head due to platelet aggregation at the site of arterial injury and shear stress, and a red tail due to stasis beyond the lesion.

The above sequence relates to the three main types of agents considered in this chapter. First, platelet inhibitors may be expected to act on arterial thrombi and to help prevent their consequences, such as transient ischemic attacks (TIAs) and myocardial infarction. Furthermore, the apparent efficacy of aspirin in atrial fibrillation suggests that platelets, among other elements in the blood, may also play a role in stasis-induced thrombosis. Second, anticoagulants may be expected to benefit thromboembolism derived from veins, such as those in the legs, or from a dilated left atrium. Third, fibrinolytics will be most useful in clinical syndromes of acute arterial thrombosis and occlusion, typified by acute myocardial infarction (AMI), but also including peripheral arterial thrombosis. Different sites of action mean that combination therapy can be logical, for example using thrombolytic agents with antiplatelet agents and anticoagulants.

In addition to their potential for acting against arterial thrombosis, it may be predicted that platelet inhibitors should also protect against other proposed consequences of platelet malfunction, such as excessive vasoconstriction, because platelets release powerful vasoconstricting agents, such as serotonin. Platelets, perhaps by release of platelet derived growth factor (PDGF), may also stimulate smooth muscle cell proliferation and migration into the subintimal layer with subsequent synthesis of connective tissue and intimal hyperplasia, thereby promoting the development of atheroma.

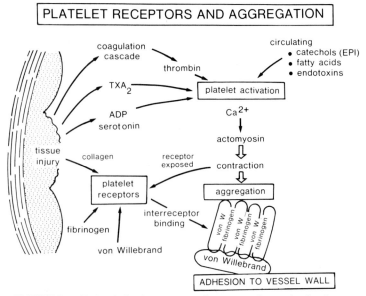

FIGURE 9–1. Role of platelet receptors in aggregation and adhesion. von Willebrand = von Willebrand factor. Figure copyright L.H. Opie.

The processes of platelet adhesion and aggregation are intimately involved with the pathways of prostaglandin synthesis, having two chief end-products with opposing effects: thromboxane A_2, which is pro-aggregatory and vasoconstrictive, and prostacyclin, which is anti-aggregatory and vasodilating.

Platelet Adhesion. This is the first of the three steps in the development of an arterial thrombus, typically occurring in relation to a damaged arterial endothelium at the site of an atherosclerotic plaque or on an artificial surface, such as a prosthetic heart valve, or on the arteriovenous shunt used for renal dialysis. Microfibrils of collagen from the deeper layers of the vessel wall become exposed as a result of endothelial injury and appear to promote platelet adhesion. Superficial injury activates **platelet receptors**,[159] which are membrane glycoproteins (GP) that allow binding to the platelets of the von Willebrand factor (receptor GPIb), subendothelial collagen (receptor GPIa), or fibrinogen (receptors GPIIb and IIIa). These receptors have a twofold function. They help to activate the platelet by releasing calcium from the endoplasmic reticulum (probably by a system coupled to IP_3) and they allow macromolecules such as the von Willebrand factor to "chain" receptors together and thereby to promote platelet adhesion (Fig. 9-1). Von Willebrand factor also binds to the IIb-IIIa receptor, thus contributing to both processes, namely adhesion and platelet aggregation.

Platelet Aggregation. The critical but not yet fully explained event causing aggregation of platelets is a rise in intracellular platelet calcium, in response to several mediators, including collagen from deep injury to the vessel, thrombin, ADP from platelets or tissue injury, and serotonin from hemolyzed red cells, as well as thromboxane A_2 synthesized by the prostaglandin pathway in the damaged vessel wall. All these agonists can initiate the release of arachidonic acid to start the pathway to thromboxane, yet all can activate platelets directly even if this pathway is blocked. An enhanced platelet calcium has several consequences, including (1) stimulation of the pathways breaking down the platelet phospholipids eventually to form thromboxane (Fig. 9–2) and (2) activation of platelet actin and myosin to

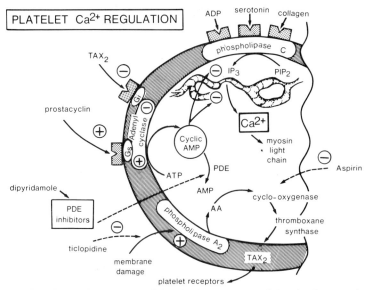

FIGURE 9–2. Role of intracellular platelet systems and sites for therapeutic control. Figure copyright L.H. Opie.

cause contraction and promote platelet aggregation. Contraction of the platelets exposes the glycoprotein receptors GPIIb/IIIa, which, in turn, allows a greater rate of interaction with various macromolecules, including the von Willebrand factor, fibrinogen, and thrombin, thereby causing more aggregation of platelets to each other and adhesion to the vessel wall.[146]

Activation of Clotting Mechanisms. The **intrinsic coagulation pathway** involves the generation of thrombin during activation of the platelet membrane (Fig. 1[146]). The **extrinsic coagulation pathway** involves thromboplastin generated by the vessel wall, which then converts prothrombin to thrombin. Prothrombin is one of several vitamin K–dependent clotting factors; the oral anticoagulants such as warfarin are vitamin K–antagonists. Thrombin from either source enhances platelet membrane activation further to promote platelet aggregation and to convert fibrinogen to fibrin, which adheres to platelet surfaces to stabilize and fix the arterial thrombus. Fibrinolytic mechanisms, involving the conversion of plasminogen to plasmin, act to limit the size of the clot and eventually to dissolve it at least in part.

Platelets and Vascular Contraction. During and after platelet aggregation, platelets release 5-hydroxytryptamine (serotonin) and other potentially important products such as platelet factor 4 and β-thromboglobulin that may help in the formation of the hemostatic plug. Serotonin normally causes vasodilation in the presence of an intact vascular endothelium. In contrast, when the endothelium is damaged, serotonin causes vasoconstriction[75] that may promote vascular stasis and thrombosis. Hence platelets are suspected of a role in vasoconstrictive diseases such as coronary spasm or Raynaud's disease. This vasoconstrictive effect of platelets may be aided by leukotrienes.

Leukotrienes are prostaglandin-like agents released from white cells and tissue macrophages to act as powerful vasoconstrictors. Because they are prostaglandin derivatives and also eventually derived from arachidonic acid, aspirin and other inhibitors of cyclo-oxygenase may act by leukotriene inhibition. Such concepts are still being explored.

PLATELET INHIBITION BY ASPIRIN

The major mechanism whereby aspirin acts is inactivation of cyclo-oxygenase, especially in platelets and in vascular endothelium (see Fig. 9–2); other mechanisms of action may also operate.[30,41] Aspirin irreversibly acetylates cyclo-oxygenase, and activity is not restored until new platelets are formed. Platelets, being very primitive cells, cannot synthesize new proteins, so that aspirin removes all the platelet cyclo-oxygenase activity for the lifespan of the platelet.[80] Therefore, aspirin stops the production of the pro-aggregatory thromboxane A_2 and eventually acts as an antithrombotic agent.[49] On the other hand, aspirin also has important non-platelet effects and in the vascular endothelium likewise inactivates cyclo-oxygenase that could diminish formation of anti-aggregatory prostacyclin. The difference is that vascular cyclo-oxygenase can be resynthesized within hours. Theoretically, aspirin has both antithrombotic and prothrombotic effects. The overwhelming clinical message is that the antithrombotic effects predominate.[112] The net result is that platelet inhibition is achieved by both high- and low-dose aspirin.

Aspirin Kinetics. Aspirin undergoes substantial presystemic hydrolysis to form salicylic acid, which is only a weak inactivator of cyclo-oxygenase with, however, a longer half-life of 2 to 3 hours, versus 15 to 20 minutes for aspirin.[61] Because the concentration of the parent compound is highest in the splanchnic circulation, the platelets circulating in that region will be exposed to a higher dose of aspirin than those in the systemic vascular bed. This difference may explain why ultra-low doses of aspirin (20 mg) could have a greater platelet inhibitory than vascular inhibitory effect.[60]

Clinical Indications for Aspirin

Aspirin in association with thrombolytic therapy will be dealt with later.

Unstable Angina. In a large trial on the acute phase, 650 mg aspirin was given, followed immediately by 325 mg 2x daily; it reduced the incidence of myocardial infarction from 12% in controls to 3%, being nearly as good as heparin.[148] However, aspirin did not decrease anginal pain in this study or in that of Neri Serneri and colleagues,[125] nor was aspirin effective against silent ST-segment shifts.[125] Two trials on the follow-up after unstable angina have also shown benefit for aspirin: 325 mg daily in men[45] and 1300 mg daily in either sex.[10] Aspirin was started within 2 to 8 days of hospitalization and continued for up to 2 years.

Threatened Stroke. In TIAs, aspirin 1300 mg daily (650 mg 2x daily or 325 mg 4x daily) benefitted only men, with stroke and death occurring in unsuccessfully treated patients.[11,20] In the UK-TIA trial,[153] aspirin 300 mg 1x daily was as good as aspirin 1200 mg daily and less gastrotoxic. When considering the occurrence of TIAs, women also seem to benefit.[7,20]

Post-infarction Follow-up. There have been nine randomized trials.[88] Pooled data show that vascular mortality is decreased by 13%, non-fatal myocardial infarction by 31%, non-fatal stroke by 42%, and all vascular events by 25%. Aspirin 300 to 325 mg daily is a reasonable recommendation accepting that absolutely definitive data are not available. No additional benefit is derived from co-therapy with dipyridamole.

Post-coronary Bypass Surgery. This is another firm indication for aspirin, with the aims of avoiding graft closure and lessening long-term chronic graft arteriosclerosis. In a large series, aspirin 325 mg given 12 hours before surgery and maintained thereafter was as good as aspirin 1000 mg daily plus dipyridamole or sulfinpyrazone.[107] Very low-dose aspirin (50 mg daily) combined with dipyridamole helped to prevent graft closure in a prospective randomized trial,[134] and it was recommended that the treatment should be continued for 1 year. In view of the definitely increased risk of bleeding with **pre-operative aspirin**, there are two policies: (1) to replace pre-operative aspirin by pre-operative dipyridamole and then to stop the dipyridamole soon after the operation while continuing aspirin started 7 hours after the operation,[13] or (2) to give low-dose aspirin such as 1 mg/kg.[139]

Others. Less firm indications for aspirin are (1) **artificial heart valves** to prevent emboli,[15] although warfarin is superior to aspirin alone and the combination warfarin-dipyridamole is preferred to warfarin-aspirin; (2) **arteriovenous shunts**—aspirin 160 mg daily decreases thrombosis[31] although there are reservations concerning this conclusion;[47] (3) **preceding balloon dilation** by percutaneous transluminal coronary angioplasty (PTCA), because aspirin plus dipyridamole may reduce acute re-occlusion without preventing stenosis;[89] (4) **chronic atrial fibrillation**—although the Danish trial[132] speaks strongly in favor of warfarin rather than of aspirin to prevent recurrent thromboemboli, the issue is by no means solved as there are many defects in the Danish trial (in a more recent trial,[143] aspirin and anti-coagulants appeared to be similar in their benefit although the trial is still ongoing); (5) **peripheral vascular disease**—prophylactic aspirin is logical to reduce stroke and myocardial infarction although the data are inferential; (6) **renovascular hypertension**—the blood pressure falls in this specific type of hypertension, suggesting that prostaglandins are involved in renin release;[115] and (7) **prevention of pregnancy-induced hypertension** by aspirin 60 mg daily.[77]

Side-effects

High-dose aspirin causes GI side-effects in about half the patients, whereas low-dose (about 300 mg daily) lessens the incidence to about 40% compared with about 30% in placebo.[153] Side-effects (dyspepsia, nausea, vomiting) may be dose-limiting in about 10 to 20% of patients. GI bleeding may occur in about 5%, with frank melena only in about 1% of patients per year and hematemesis in about 0.1% per year. Uncommonly, gout may be aggravated (by impaired urate secretion). GI side-effects may be reduced by **buffered aspirin** (Bufferin 325 mg in the USA; in the UK, Disprin contains 300 mg aspirin, 90 mg calcium carbonate) or **enteric-coated aspirin** (Ecotrin 3–5 mg; Cosprin 325–650 mg),[54] by Alka-Seltzer (with, however, 567 mg sodium per tablet), or by dose-reduction or intermittent therapy.

Side-effects of High-dose Aspirin. A truly high dose of aspirin (4000 mg/day) can aggravate angina in patients with Prinzmetal's variant angina, possibly by promotion of coronary artery spasm;[55] this dose also increases fibrinolytic activity,[57] and GI side-effects are much more likely. Clinically, however, similar high doses have been used in rheumatoid arthritis for an average period of 10 years without any increase in angina, sudden death, or stroke; rather, there was a reduction of myocardial infarction in men.[46]

Contraindications

Aspirin intolerance, hemophilia, history of GI bleeds or peptic ulcer, or other potential sources of GI or genito-urinary bleeding. Congestive heart failure (CHF) is a contraindication to Alka-Seltzer (sodium content) as are renal failure or stones or hepatic cirrhosis.[19] *Relative contraindications* include potentially dangerous drug interactions, dyspepsia, iron deficiency anemia, gout, and the possibility of enhanced peri-operative bleeding[74] unless the dose is 20 mg daily.[80] Common sense says that retinal hemorrhages are probably a contraindication unless very low-dose aspirin is used, yet data are lacking.

Besides checking for contraindications and drug interactions, patients chronically receiving aspirin should have their hemoglobin checked periodically in case of occult GI bleeding. Blood sugar and urate may need periodic checks.

Drug Interactions

Generally, nonsteroidal anti-inflammatory drugs (NSAIDs) attenuate the efficacy of **antihypertensive therapy** by complex mechanisms;[78] aspirin appears not to share this interaction. Aspirin may decrease the urinary excretion of uric acid, the plasma levels of which need monitoring in patients also receiving thiazides or in patients with a family history of gout.[28] Aspirin may interfere with the uricosuric effect of sulfinpyrazone and probenecid and reduce the natriuretic effect of spironolactone. Aspirin may rarely precipitate gout, so there is a potential indirect interaction with thiazides. The **risk of aspirin-induced GI bleeding** is increased by alcohol, corticosteroid therapy, and other NSAIDs. Enteric-coated preparations may have their efficacy reduced by antacids by altering the pH of the stomach. Phenobarbital, phenytoin, and rifampin decrease aspirin efficacy by hepatic enzyme induction. The effect of oral hypoglycemic agents and insulin might be enhanced. Aspirin, especially in high doses, **may exaggerate a bleeding tendency** and anticoagulant-induced bleeding,[57] which may explain why disopyramide-warfarin causes less bleeding than aspirin-warfarin in patients with prosthetic heart valves.[14]

High versus Low-dose Aspirin

Knowledge that aspirin 300 mg daily is as good as 1200 mg for TIA prevention[153] means that a dose of approximately 300 mg is now becoming standard. Furthermore, the use of 160 mg daily for 1 month in the ISIS-2 myocardial infarct trial[116] means that this lower dose is now widely accepted as having prophylactic efficacy. There are as yet no trials showing benefit of even lower doses of aspirin although, theoretically, cyclo-oxygenase inhibition can be obtained with only 20 mg aspirin.

Primary Prevention by Aspirin—Is it Worth It?

Two primary prevention trials of aspirin have been reported. In the US Physicians Health Study, 325 mg aspirin on alternate days reduced the risk of non-fatal myocardial infarction in volunteers over the age of 50. Nonetheless, there was a trend toward an increase in hemorrhagic stroke, and overall cardiovascular mortality was unchanged.[145] In the smaller British primary prevention study (500 mg aspirin daily), there was also a reduction in the incidence of myocardial infarction, but once again mortality was unchanged.[133]

Our recommendation is that aspirin should not be used prophylactically in the general population, especially in the elderly.[130] When a comprehensive attack on risk factors is being mounted, however, low-dose aspirin appears a useful adjunct to other measures.[111] Thus, in patients with established coronary artery disease or peripheral vascular disease, 160 to 325 mg aspirin daily is reasonable.[98,105] Diabetic retinopathy and uncontrolled hypertension are presumed contraindications.

Aspirin—Summary

Aspirin is now of proven value in unstable angina to prevent myocardial infarction and in TIAs to prevent strokes (men only) and recurrent attacks. In post-infarct patients, its protective effects are recognized by the FDA although the statistics involve trial combinations. Aspirin is used (combined with pre-operative dipyridamole) to reduce the incidence of early graft closure following bypass surgery. Aspirin is also used in selected patients with artificial heart valves or arteriovenous shunts. Aspirin may reduce thromboembolism in atrial fibrillation. The optimal dose remains unsure, but most trials showing beneficial outcome have used 160 to 300 mg daily with a few trials on TIAs using 1300 mg daily. For post-infarct prophylaxis, 325 mg daily is recommended by the FDA, but 160 mg seems equally reasonable. In patients intolerant to aspirin, lower doses may be used down to a minimum of 20 mg daily.

PLATELET INHIBITION BY SULFINPYRAZONE

Sulfinpyrazone (Anturane) also inhibits cyclo-oxygenase and has ultimate effects similar to those of aspirin, decreasing the production of the prostanoids, prostacyclin, and thromboxane A_2. The mechanism of action on the cyclo-oxygenase is different from aspirin's in that sulfinpyrazone competitively and reversibly *inhibits* the enzyme, whereas aspirin *inactivates* it, so that sulfinpyrazone is much weaker.[61] Sulfinpyrazone also limits platelet adhesion to collagen, an action not shared by aspirin. The critical questions are (1) whether sulfinpyrazone, which is more expensive and needs multiple daily doses, gives any added protection to patients already taking aspirin; and (2) whether sulfinpyrazone might be used as an alternative to aspirin. On first principles, these two agents should be closely similar in their effects. However, for two of the major indications for aspirin, namely unstable angina and threatened stroke in males, sulfinpyrazone (200 mg 4x daily) is not effective.

In the USA, the only licensed **indication** is gouty arthritis, chronic or intermittent. In mitral stenosis, however, a 4-year prospective blinded study showed that sulfinpyrazone (200 mg 4x daily) decreased thromboembolism and reverted the shortened platelet survival time toward normal.[68] Benefitted patients appeared to include those with mitral valve replacement during the trial. Data from this highly specific trial may not be extrapolated to other situations where there is risk of cardiovascular thromboembolism, as in patients with artificial valves, even though sulfinpyrazone does shorten platelet survival times in such patients.

"The **dose** most commonly used, 800 mg/day.....is at the lower end of the dose-response curve and close to the maximum tolerable level."[61]

Contraindications. Peptic ulcer, renal impairment, renal stones.[81] Early after AMI, sulfinpyrazone may cause temporary renal failure.[6]

Drug Interactions. Sulfinpyrazone, being highly bound (98–99%) to plasma proteins, may displace warfarin to precipitate bleeding. Sulfinpyrazone may potentiate the effects of sulfa drugs, sulfonylureas, and insulin.

Problems in Post-infarct Prophylaxis. Much confusion has been created by the results of a large post-infarct trial reported in 1980, which appeared to show a dramatic reduction in sudden death.[4] Subsequently, careful dissection of the data by the FDA led to a rejection of the claim for benefit,[71] chiefly because sudden death was imprecisely defined and certain patients were retrospectively excluded from the study. **No amount of subsequent re-analysis and attempted re-instatement of the data has been able to elicit enthusiasm for the use of sulfinpyrazone in post-infarct patients.** It remains to be seen whether interest in post-infarct sulfinpyrazone can be revived by the results of the Anturan Reinfarction Italian Study,[3] in which sulfinpyrazone 400 mg 2x daily (started as 200 mg daily to avoid a sudden uricosuric effect) reduced re-infarction in the 19-month post-infarct follow-up period. There was no effect on mortality, possibly the result of selection of patients with no signs of heart failure. Sulfinpyrazone should not be given in high dose (800 mg daily) in the acute phase of myocardial infarction, when it substantially elevates serum urea and creatinine, even though decreasing urate levels.[81]

Except in gout, when aspirin impairs urate excretion, aspirin is a better platelet-inhibitor than sulfinpyrazone.

PLATELET INHIBITION BY DIPYRIDAMOLE

Dipyridamole (Persantine) has five effects. First, there are the well-known coronary vasodilator effects mediated by the inhibition of adenosine deaminase, which is the basis of the dipyridamole-thallium stress test. Second, it inhibits platelet adhesion to the damaged vessel. Third, dipyridamole may potentiate the anti-aggregatory effect of prostacyclin.[52] Fourth, at high and supraclinical doses,[52,61] dipyridamole inhibits phosphodiesterase in platelets, thereby enhancing cyclic AMP formation and lowering platelet calcium (see Fig. 9–2). Fifth, dipyridamole indirectly increases cyclic AMP by inhibiting the breakdown of adenosine, thereby inhibiting platelet aggregation.[29,30] In comparison with aspirin, dipyridamole has far more inhibitory effects on **platelet adhesion** to the vessel wall and much less on **platelet aggregation**. There have been few clinical trials using dipyridamole alone; usually combination with aspirin is undertaken, and in almost all trials there is no convincing evidence that dipyridamole adds anything to the benefits obtained by aspirin alone.

Indications. Therapy by dipyridamole plus anticoagulation is licensed for patients with prosthetic valves on the basis of five trials showing that the combination is superior to placebo.[131] Dipyridamole is classified as possibly effective for long-term therapy of angina pectoris. There is no evidence that dipyridamole alone decreases myocardial re-infarction.

Dose. Most trials have used 75 mg 3x daily. The manufacturers recommend 50 mg 3x daily, taken at least 1 hour before meals.

Side-effects. GI irritation; vasodilatory and hypotensive effects such as dizziness, flushing, syncope, occasional angina pectoris ("coronary steal").

Combination Dipyridamole with Aspirin

Dipyridamole dramatically increases the antithrombotic effect of aspirin on artificial surfaces.[30] Hence the combination makes most sense when dealing with prosthetic valves or prosthetic bypasses. In a comprehensive review of 31 trials on 29,000 patients studying prophylactic antiplatelet therapy of TIAs, stroke, unstable angina, or acute myocardial infarction, the Antiplatelet Trialists' Collaboration[88] concluded that there is no benefit to be gained by combining dipyridamole with aspirin; aspirin alone is appropriate for almost all conditions. There are two exceptions: in the case of prosthetic heart valves,[146] and in the case of saphenous vein bypass grafts. In the latter case, the large Goldman study[107] showed no better patency for the combination dipyridamole-aspirin; however, aspirin was started 12 hours pre-operatively and increased the risk of bleeding. Therefore, the previous Mayo Clinic study[13] is usually taken to justify the practice of initiating dipyridamole 2 days pre-operatively (100 mg 4x daily) plus aspirin (325 mg 3x daily) started 7 hours post-operatively; extrapolation of data suggests that aspirin 325 mg daily is an appropriate dose and that dipyridamole should be discontinued after 1 week.[147]

In **unstable angina**, there is no case for adding dipyridamole to aspirin. Likewise, in the long-term therapy of patients with unstable angina, aspirin is of definite value, but the addition of dipyridamole confers no proven added benefit.

In **threatened stroke**, dipyridamole 75 mg 3x daily with aspirin 325 mg 3x daily improved survival and decreased both non-fatal and fatal strokes.[103]

In **post-infarct patients**, the combination dipyridamole 75 mg 3x daily with aspirin 324 mg 3x daily was no different from the results with aspirin alone. Neither agent showed a statistically significant effect by the study criteria, although total mortality and coronary mortality fell by about 20%.[62] In another colossal follow-up trial (PARIS II[37]), aspirin-dipyridamole reduced coronary "incidence" (definite non-fatal re-infarction, plus all cardiac deaths) by about 30%, without any change in total mortality. The combination appeared particularly effective in patients with non-Q-wave infarction, probably because of higher risk of re-infarction in this group. It seems doubtful that this result is better than that obtained with aspirin alone although more strict comparisons are required.

In **peripheral vascular disease**, dipyridamole 75 mg with aspirin 330 mg 3x daily may limit the progress of the disease, especially in smokers and hypertensives.[32] Aspirin alone is effective, but less so.

In **renal disease** (type 1 membranoproliferative glomerulo-nephritis[17]), dipyridamole helps to prevent deterioration.

In **patients with prosthetic valves**, the combination of dipyridamole with warfarin seems more effective than warfarin alone in controlling thromboembolism[70] and is less likely than aspirin to provoke bleeding when given with warfarin.[14] The dose is 75 mg 3x daily with meals and 150 mg at bedtime.[131]

Dipyridamole—Summary

Dipyridamole theoretically differs from aspirin in its site of antiplatelet action, so that combination therapy with aspirin is logical. Nevertheless little hard data substantiate the presumed superiority of combination dipyridamole-aspirin over aspirin, especially for the major indications for aspirin, namely unstable angina, post-infarction prophylaxis, and TIAs. In the specific case of patients with coronary artery bypass grafts, dipyridamole may be given pre-operatively, and a long-term dipyridamole-aspirin regimen is of proven use, but aspirin is probably just as good. In patients with prosthetic valves, dipyridamole-warfarin may be better than warfarin alone, but the data are inconclusive.

OTHER PLATELET INHIBITORS

Ticlopidine. This agent inhibits platelet aggregation without acting on cyclo-oxygenase or on phosphodiesterase. Perhaps it acts on membrane receptors to inhibit phospholipase-C and hence the rise of intraplatelet calcium (Fig. 9–2). In the Canadian-American Ticlopidine Study (CATS) on 1072 patients with recent thromboembolic stroke, in a dose of 250 mg 2x daily, ticlopidine reduced stroke, myocardial infarction, and vascular death, although disappointingly the overall death rate was unchanged.[106] Side-effects included neutropenia (1%), skin rash (2%), and diarrhea (2%)—all were reversible. The neutropenia occurred within the first 3 months of treatment. Other proposed benefits of ticlopidine are management of unstable angina,[88a] management of the post-angioplasty state, and reduction of vein graft closure.[146]

Indomethacin. Besides inhibiting cyclo-oxygenase, indomethacin is anti-inflammatory. Indomethacin is seldom used as a specific antiplatelet agent in patients with cardiovascular diseases, because it seems to inhibit the formation of vasodilatory prostaglandins. The vasoconstrictive action is likely to be worse in the presence of endo-thelial damage.[42] Thus, indomethacin may (1) promote coronary vasoconstriction;[22] (2) attenuate the effects of antihypertensive agents such as β-blockers and diuretics;[78] and (3) cause clinical deterioration in patients with CHF and hyponatremia.[18]

Thromboxane Synthetase Inhibitors. Clinical tests are being carried out on new synthetase inhibitors, which have two important theoretical advantages: (1) They might divert precursors from formation of thromboxane to that of prostacyclin by the so-called endoperoxide steal,[53] although this mechanism does not operate in all models;[65] (2) they specifically inhibit the formation of thromboxane, but not that of prostacyclin. The prototype agent is **dazoxiben**. The major problem with this group of agents is the short half-life of their effect on the synthetase.[21]

Other Platelet Inhibitors. These include β-blockers, calcium antagonists, α-receptor antagonists, ketanserin, and nafazatrom.

ANTICOAGULANTS: HEPARIN

Anticoagulation, when given in an acute situation, such as myocardial infarction, acute venous thrombosis, or acute pulmonary embolism, is usually initiated by IV heparin while awaiting the effect of oral warfarin. Alternatively, in uncomplicated AMI, only heparin may be used until the patient is mobile.[25] Either heparin sodium or heparin calcium may be used. Heparin may be given by infusion, by intermittent injection, or subcutaneously, but not orally. Fixed-dose regimens are now popular, although strictly speaking the effects of IV heparin should be monitored by the activated partial thromboplastin time and kept at 2 to 3 times the pretherapy value. In patients with bleeding disorders or in whom the effects of bleeding could be serious (subacute bacterial endocarditis, GI or genito-urinary lesions), ultra-low dose heparin should be considered.

Administration

IV Heparin. The standard IV schedule is usually a 5,000 unit IV injection loading dose, followed by 20,000 to 40,000 units/day given by an infusion pump. United States Pharmacopeia units may be about 10 to 15% more potent than the international units used in other countries. The heparin may be diluted either in isotonic saline or in dextrose water (which may be better in AMI). **Intermittent injection** may be preferred in AMI to avoid fluid overload; the schedule is 10,000 units given as an initial dose, followed by 5,000 to 10,000 units every 4 to 6 hours. **Ultra-low dose IV heparin** (1 unit/kg/hr for 3–5 days, about 17,000 units/day) seems as effective as other methods in preventing post-operative deep vein thrombosis.[58]

Subcutaneous Heparin. After the initial IV loading dose, heparin may be given as a deep subcutaneous injection 10,000 units 8-hourly or 15,000 12-hourly, using a different site at each rotation. This procedure is as effective as IV heparin in reducing venous thrombosis. The best documented use of subcutaneous heparin is in the prophylaxis of surgical thromboembolism, where the schedule is 5,000 units subcutaneously 2 to 8 hours pre-operation and every 8 hours for 7 days.[36]

Precautions and Side-effects

An increased danger of heparin-induced hemorrhage exists in patients with subacute bacterial endocarditis, hematologic disorders including hemophilia, and GI or genito-urinary ulcerative lesions. Platelet plugs are the main hemostatic defense of heparinized patients, and the co-administration of aspirin, sulfinpyrazone, dipyridamole, or indomethacin may predispose to bleeding, as may **heparin-induced thrombocytopenia** (in about 10% of patients after heparin for 5 days or more,[2] usually reversible upon heparin withdrawal). **Heparin hemorrhage** may occur in clinically inapparent sites such as the adrenal glands, which can be life-threatening, and demands immediate cortisol replacement therapy. Some patients have **heparin resistance**, and monitoring by coagulation tests every 4 hours during early therapy with full-dose heparin is advised. Heparin is derived from animal tissue and occasionally causes **allergy**; a trial dose of 100 to 1,000 units is required in allergic patients. Patients with severe hepatic disease may be predisposed to bleeding disorders. In renal disease, the dose of heparin is controversial. In AMI, heparin mildly elevates blood free fatty acids that could be potentially harmful; however, the magnitude of this effect may be overestimated.[63]

Heparin overdosage is treated by stopping the drug and, if clinically required, giving protamine sulfate (1% solution), at no more than 50 mg, very slowly in any 10-minute period as a slow infusion.

Indications

Heparin in Acute Myocardial Infarction. The urgent use of an **IV bolus** dose of heparin is logical and is strongly recommended to initiate protection against venous thrombosis, possibly to help prevent further coronary artery thrombosis, and to prevent mural thrombosis and systemic embolism. Thereafter it is conventional to give high-dose IV infusions, although subcutaneous heparin in high doses may be equally effective.[16,152] In the SCATI Italian Study,[138] a randomized trial of 711 patients, 12,500 units of calcium-heparin subcutaneously given within 24 hours of the onset of symptoms was better than placebo because mortality was lower and there was a decreased prevalence of mural thrombosis in patients with anterior infarcts. It is important to note that anticoagulation was initiated with 2,000 units of calcium-heparin given intravenously, followed 9 hours later by 12,500 units subcutaneously.

There are no studies on the possible disadvantage of giving sodium, either in the forms of **sodium heparin** or of isotonic saline used as the diluent. In patients with borderline heart failure, sodium loading can be avoided by the use of calcium heparin (Calciparine, 5,000 to 20,000 USP units/ampoule) and by diluting heparin in dextrose water. Heparin is usually given until the patient is mobile or until oral anticoagulants take effect. In uncomplicated AMI, the present trend is to give only heparin. When acute thrombolysis is achieved in AMI, heparin is given thereafter in the hope of preventing rethrombosis (see discussion of poststreptokinase policy, p 240). Meticulous laboratory control of the heparin dose is required (activated partial thromboplastin time 1.5–2.0x normal).

Prevention of Re-infarction. Low-dose heparin 12,500 units given daily over 9 months to patients with a Q-wave myocardial infarction 6 to 18 months previously reduced the rate of re-infarction and overall mortality.[124]

Heparin in Unstable Angina. Heparin is highly effective in preventing myocardial infarction[148] and in decreasing anginal pain and electrocardiographic features of ischemia.[125] An IV bolus of 5,000 units is followed by an infusion of 10,000 units per hour[148] and, in the study of Neri Serneri and colleagues,[125] the dose is adjusted to a partial thromboplastin time (PTT) of 1.5 to 2x baseline. Stopping heparin acutely without concomitant aspirin exposes the patient to the risk of rebound of unstable angina.[128]

ORAL ANTICOAGULANTS: WARFARIN

Warfarin (coumarin, Coumadin, Panwarfin) is the most commonly used oral anticoagulant, because a single dose causes a stable anticoagulation as a result of the excellent oral absorption and a circulating half-life of about 36 hours; warfarin also has remarkably few side-effects apart from bleeding.[25] As a group, the oral anticoagulants inactivate vitamin K in the liver, thereby interfering with the vitamin-K-dependent clotting factors including prothrombin.

Dose. The usual initial dose of warfarin is 10 to 15 mg daily; the maintenance dose, 1 to 20 mg daily; this wide range means that doses must be individualized. Another standard procedure is to give warfarin 5 mg/day for 5 days and then to check the prothrombin time. Avoiding a large primary dose may also avoid an excess fall of prothrombin and may decrease the risk of skin necrosis. Patients with heart failure or liver disease require lower doses. The effect is monitored by reporting the INR (international normalized ratio), which is based on a theoretical international reference thromboplastin and is approved by the World Health Organization. For almost all indications for anticoagulation including prosthetic heart valves,[137] an INR of 2.5 to 4.5 (prothrombin ratio is 1.5–2.0) is usually adequate; even lower doses of warfarin might be as effective and are safer.

Dose reduction of anticoagulants is required in the presence of CHF and liver damage from any source, including alcohol, malnutrition, renal impairment, and thyrotoxicosis. The presence of interacting drugs needs to be considered.

Drug Interactions. Warfarin may be subject to approximately 80 drug interactions.[69] These include drugs such as cholestyramine that may reduce absorption of vitamin K or of warfarin; drugs that displace warfarin from its albumin binding sites, such as sulfinpyrazone and the previously used agent phenylbutazone; drugs such as barbiturates or phenytoin that accelerate warfarin degradation and decrease the anticoagulant effect; and drugs that decrease warfarin degradation and increase the anticoagulant effect, such as a variety of antibiotics including metronidazole (Flagyl), co-trimoxazole (Bactrim), and cimetidine. Clofibrate increases the anticoagulant effect by unknown means.

Potentiating drugs include the cardiovascular agents allopurinol, quinidine,[38] and amiodarone.[50] Antiplatelet drugs such as aspirin may act by potentiating the risk of bleeding with a large interindividual variation.[59] High doses of aspirin (6–8 tablets/day) may act by a different mechanism to potentiate the anticoagulant effect, because synthesis of clotting factors becomes impaired. Sulfinpyrazone powerfully displaces warfarin from blood proteins, to reduce the dose of warfarin required down to 1 mg in some patients.[5] **The safest rule is to tell patients on oral anticoagulation not to take any over-the-counter drugs without consultation, and for the physician to check any new drug used.** If in doubt, more frequent measurements of the prothrombin ratio are required. Otherwise, once the warfarin requirement is known, the prothrombin ratio is checked only once every 4 to 6 weeks.

Contraindications. Stroke, uncontrolled hypertension, hepatic cirrhosis, and potential GI and genito-urinary bleeding points, such as hiatus hernia, peptic ulcer, gastritis, colitis, proctitis, and cystitis.[19] If anticoagulation is deemed essential, the risk-benefit ratio must be evaluated carefully. Old age is not of itself a contraindication to anticoagulation.[109] Heparin should not be given to older patients unsteady on their feet or those with syncope. Warfarin in early pregnancy predisposes to spontaneous abortion.[44]

Warfarin-Associated Skin Necrosis. Phenindione has been recommended for this rare but potentially serious hemorrhagic skin condition. The cause of the necrosis is ill-understood, but a protein-C deficiency may predispose,[35] especially when high-dose warfarin is initiated. Phenindione carries a much higher risk of renal or hepatic toxicity, and may also cause necrosis, so it is not frequently the agent of choice. Awareness of protein-C deficiency as in cardiopulmonary bypass operations, together with a low initial dose of warfarin, should avoid skin necrosis.

Warfarin Overdose. Excess prothrombinemia without bleeding or with only minor bleeding can be remedied by discontinuation of the warfarin. If bleeding becomes significant, oral or parenteral **vitamin K_1** 2 to 5 mg may be required. In patients with prosthetic valves, vitamin K should be strictly avoided because of the risk of valve thrombosis, unless there is a life-threatening intracerebral bleed. In patients unresponsive to vitamin K, plasma 15 ml/kg or fresh, whole blood transfusions are given.

CLINICAL INDICATIONS FOR ORAL ANTICOAGULATION

Myocardial Infarction

In the acute stage, the use of full-dose IV heparin followed by standard anticoagulant therapy has been the norm during the hospital phase of myocardial infarction,[12] provided that relative or absolute contraindications are absent. Oral anticoagulation is started 4 to 5 days before heparin therapy is discontinued. A trial aimed at un-equivocally documenting the efficiency of this regimen in reducing mortality is unlikely to be undertaken. An alternative procedure, usually chosen in uncomplicated AMI, is to use only heparin until the patient is mobile.[25]

Early Post-infarct Anticoagulation. Accumulating evidence sug-gests that, within the first 3 to 6 months, mural thrombosis and the subsequent incidence of systemic thromboembolism is more frequent in patients with large anterior Q-wave infarctions, apical dyskinetic areas identifiable echocardiographically (even before any intraven-tricular thrombus is present), severe left ventricular (LV) dysfunction, congestive heart failure, and atrial fibrillation. Furthermore, the like-lihood of systemic thromboembolism is greatest in the first 3 months post-discharge. Although definitive data are unavailable, fairly good evidence supports the use of oral warfarin for a 3- to 6-month period in these specific post-infarct patients,[136] aiming at an INR of 2.0 to 3.0.

Prolonged Oral Anticoagulation. Chronic post-infarct therapy, previously given for years, has now lost its popularity. However, a new large-scale trial in Scandinavia shows a decisive advantage for warfarin in patients not receiving aspirin.[142a] Dogmatic decisions or rules cannot be made. **Successful anticoagulation therapy requires a co-operative patient, meticulous medical supervision, and an excel-lent laboratory. There must be a constant guard against the use of additional drugs and their interactions. The risks of warfarin therapy are appreciable and must be weighed against the potential benefits for every individual patient.** For most, neither the risk-benefit ratio nor the cost-benefit ratio favors prolonged oral anticoagulation.[136] Even the presence of an LV aneurysm is not an indication for prolonged anticoagulation[43] unless there is a history of systemic embolism. Therefore, although selected compliant groups of elderly patients appear to benefit from prolonged anticoagulation,[67] the benefit is only modest and the effort immense.

Post-infarct Anticoagulation Versus Aspirin. A French trial[19] compared high-dose aspirin (500 mg 3x daily) with oral anticoagulation; results were similar with an almost identical total mortality with, however, different side-effects. The incidence of bleeding was 6x higher in the anticoagulant group and the GI problems 5x higher in the aspirin group. The excess bleeding in the anticoagu-lant group was in non–GI tract bleeding; the incidence of the latter was similar in the two treatment groups. Aspirin may be given with considerably less risk of hemorrhagic complications and without the same degree of supervision. In the case of both agents, however, possible benefits shown by the pooled data are rather similar.[19,25,40] Neither agent has shown clear benefit in good trials. For a prolonged antithrombotic effect post-infarct, aspirin is much simpler and is recommended by the FDA. **We do not advise routine post-infarct oral anticoagulation, but rather a careful evaluation of the needs of each individual patient.**

Unstable Angina at Rest: Role of Warfarin

In unstable angina (intermediate coronary syndrome), an intracoronary thrombus is found in approximately 40% of patients undergoing angiography, thereby focusing on the role of anticoagulation and platelet inhibitor therapy in patients with rest angina.[9] The benefit of heparin is real[148] and the arguments for aspirin are strong. However, the combination is no better than either agent alone. Generally, heparin is given for 4 to 5 days and aspirin started just before the heparin is stopped. **Oral anticoagulation is generally not undertaken,** especially because such patients may come to coronary artery surgery or balloon angioplasty. Thrombolytic therapy has a place in some patients but the overall results are not impressive.[125,131]

In patients with severe repetitive attacks of variant angina, there is a risk of secondary coronary thrombosis following severe coronary artery spasm, and oral anticoagulation becomes logical although unproven. In others, low-dose aspirin remains the pragmatic albeit unproven approach to the prevention of spasm-induced platelet stasis and thrombosis.

Warfarin for Venous Thromboembolism

In deep venous thrombosis, warfarin is initiated concurrently with IV heparin as standard therapy for acute episodes. Thereafter, oral anticoagulation alone is continued for at least 3 months.[114] In patients with recurrent venous thrombosis, risk factors such as antithrombin-III deficiency, protein-C or -S deficiency, or malignancy should be evaluated for indefinite treatment.

For objectively documented **pulmonary embolism**, heparin followed by oral warfarin is used. Warfarin is continued for approximately 6 months in the absence of recurrences; when the latter occur, indefinite therapy is considered.

Atrial Fibrillation: Indications for Warfarin

Atrial fibrillation in the presence of heart disease is strongly associated with thromboembolism.[82] **Cardioversion** in patients with atrial fibrillation probably increases the risk of an embolus. After 3 days of atrial fibrillation, anticoagulation for 3 weeks is strongly recommended prior to elective cardioversion, provided this is logistically feasible, followed by another 2 to 4 weeks.[101] In patients with dilated left atria, even earlier anticoagulation makes sense to prevent thromboembolism at the onset of atrial fibrillation, even though scientific support for this view is absent.

Mitral Stenosis or Regurgitation. In patients with mitral valve disease, the risk of thromboembolism is greatest in those with atrial fibrillation, marked left atrial enlargement, and previous embolic episodes. Anticoagulation is strongly indicated in this setting. In contrast, in patients with mitral stenosis with sinus rhythm, anticoagulation is usually reserved for secondary prevention after the first episode of systemic embolism.[27] An argument can be made for earlier anticoagulation if the left atrium is dilated.

Hypertensive Heart Disease. This condition is an indication for anticoagulation only if there is marked left atrial or LV enlargement, or in the presence of atrial fibrillation. These are not, however, firm indications.

Ischemic Heart Disease. In the presence of good LV function, atrial fibrillation is an unsettled indication for anticoagulation. LV failure strengthens the argument for anticoagulation.[39] However, chronic LV aneurysm is not an indication for oral anticoagulation.[43]

Dilated Cardiomyopathy. There is a substantial risk of systemic embolism, particularly if there is atrial fibrillation; anticoagulants substantially reduce thromboembolism.[23] Even in the absence of atrial fibrillation, dilated cardiomyopathy may predispose to mural thrombi, and oral anticoagulation with or without platelet inhibitors may be considered, even though statistical evidence for this procedure is lacking.

The Tachycardia/Bradycardia Syndrome. This syndrome complicated by atrial fibrillation may cause thromboembolism. Anticoagulation may require consideration, especially if there is underlying organic heart disease (ischemic heart disease, hypertension, cardiomyopathy). Once again the evidence is unproven.

Atrial Septal Defects. In older patients with atrial septal defects and pulmonary hypertension, anticoagulation is strongly recommended as prophylaxis against in situ pulmonary arterial thromboses or, rarely, paradoxical emboli. Anticoagulation is also required for those with repaired septal defects later developing atrial fibrillation.

Thyrotoxic Heart Disease. In patients with atrial fibrillation and thyrotoxicosis, the first aim is to render the patient euthyroid, which reverts the atrial fibrillation in the majority.[101] In the others, cardioversion should be performed at about the 16th week after the patient becomes euthyroid, as further spontaneous reversion then becomes unlikely. Anticoagulation cover is required and should be maintained for 4 weeks after the conversion.[101]

"Lone" Atrial Fibrillation. In the absence of any other cardiac or precipitating condition, including thyrotoxicosis, atrial fibrillation may be rare.[8] In patients younger than 60, it has a risk of thromboembolism no greater than that in any age- and sex-matched population, so that the morbidity of anticoagulant therapy outweighs the potential advantages.[118] Elderly patients with "lone" atrial fibrillation have a somewhat increased risk of TIAs or stroke without any increased mortality or risk of AMI, so that anticoagulation needs consideration.[119]

In summary, in **chronic non-valvular atrial fibrillation**, there are reasonable arguments favoring anticoagulation (exception young "lone" fibrillators). However, the Danish trial[132] has not settled the issue, in part because it was not blinded and in part because the excess events in the aspirin group were largely non-disabling stroke, TIAs, and the like. A more recent trial suggests aspirin as a reasonable alternative.[143] It is reasonable to anticoagulate, especially if there is some structural underlying heart disease; however, it may be almost as reasonable to give aspirin. At present there are four independent randomized trials in the USA and Canada evaluating anticoagulation in atrial fibrillation in non-valvular heart disease.

Prosthetic Heart Valves: Use of Warfarin

In patients with **mechanical prosthetic heart valves**, warfarin is standard and preferred to aspirin alone, to dipyridamole-aspirin, or to pentoxifylline-aspirin.[24,56] The intensity of anticoagulation can be relatively low, with a prothrombin time ratio of about 1.5 (INR about 2.5–3.0) without losing benefit but with less bleeding;[137] these data need confirmation. Adding an antiplatelet agent to warfarin is logical in the hope of further reducing the risk of systemic embolism. Because added aspirin increases the risk of bleeding, dipyridamole is chosen

TABLE 9–1 ANTITHROMBOTIC THERAPY FOR PROSTHETIC HEART VALVES: CURRENT RECOMMENDATIONS

Valve	Situation	Therapy
Mechanical	Routine	Warfarin + D 400 mg/day
	D side-effects	Warfarin + sulf 800 mg/day
	Problems such as bleeding	1. Decreased warfarin + D 400 mg/day
		2. D 400 mg/day + sulf 800 mg/day
	Recurrent embolism	Consider re-operation
Bioprosthetic	AVR routine	SC heparin for 7–10 days, then ASA 80 mg/day
	MVR routine	SC heparin, warfarin for 3 mo, then ASA 80 mg/day
	If LA > 55 mm or AF	Warfarin long-term

AF = atrial fibrillation; ASA = aspirin; AVR = aortic valve replacement; D = dipyridamole; LA = left atrium; MVR = mitral valve replacement; sulf = sulfinpyrazone; SC = subcutaneous.
From Chesebro, et al,[97] with permission.

instead.[14] When there are relative contraindications to warfarin or platelet inhibitors, patients with a history of thromboembolism, marked left atrial enlargement, or atrial fibrillation are those most in need of treatment. In children or others in whom warfarin is difficult to manage, aspirin is a reasonable alternative.[79] In patients with **porcine valves**,[1] the risk of thromboembolism is highest in the first 3 months and then falls. The ideal agent is not yet clear; aspirin may be a reasonable alternative to warfarin. Arguments for warfarin are strong when mitral porcine valves are combined with atrial fibrillation or a large left atrium or LV failure (Table 9-1).

Marginal or Possible Indications for Warfarin

Cerebral Vascular Disease. Anticoagulation in cerebrovascular disease remains a source of fierce debate. Certainly in patients who have had a complete stroke, there is no evidence to support anticoagulation. In patients with TIAs of less than 2 months' duration (who do not undergo surgery), warfarin for a period of 3 months has been advised, followed by aspirin 1300 mg (approximately) per day. In males with TIAs in whom the last attack was within 2 to 12 months, treatment with aspirin until the patient has been free of symptoms for at least a year seems reasonable.[64]

Primary Pulmonary Hypertension. This entity includes a variety of histologic appearances and, probably, pathogenic mechanisms. Diffuse pulmonary thromboembolism or pulmonary arteriolar thrombosis calls for anticoagulation. When the pathogenesis cannot be established, long-term anticoagulation is usually chosen.

Mitral Valve Prolapse. In patients with marked mitral valve prolapse and suggestive evidence of thrombotic or thromboembolic events, there might be an indication for warfarin or platelet inhibitors, but this remains a moot issue.

Oral Anticoagulants—Summary

In AMI, anticoagulants during the hospital phase are now standard, although many other centers give only heparin, limited to the duration of bed rest, for uncomplicated AMI. Only a minority of patients qualify for limited anticoagulation for 3 to 6 months, whereas only a very few require prolonged anticoagulation. Oral anticoagulants are frequently used to prevent systemic embolism, especially in selected patients with atrial fibrillation and those with prosthetic heart valves

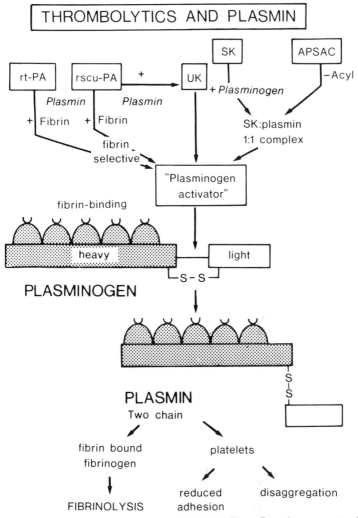

Figure 9–3. Plasminogen activators and their effects. Based on concepts of Marder VJ, Sherry S: Thrombolytic therapy. N Engl J Med 318:1512–1520, 1988; Handin RI, Loscalzo J: Hemostasis, thrombosis, fibrinolysis, and cardiovascular disease. In Braunwald E(ed): Heart Disease, 3rd ed. Philadelphia, WB Saunders, 1988, pp 1758–1781.

or dilated cardiomyopathy. They are used in both treatment and prevention of venous thrombosis and pulmonary embolism. Long-term anticoagulation requires obsessive patient compliance and a careful consideration of the risk-benefit ratio for the individual patient. For example, although benefit could well be achieved in a patient with chronic atrial fibrillation by meticulous anticoagulation, in a relatively non-compliant patient or in a patient with a vigorous physical lifestyle it may be safer to use aspirin.

FIBRINOLYTIC (THROMBOLYTIC) THERAPY

"All of these agents when used early and in the proper dosage can effect rapid reperfusion of most infarct-related arteries, a requirement for reducing irreversible myocardial damage during evolving infarction."[140]

TABLE 9–2 ADVANTAGES AND DISADVANTAGES OF VARIOUS THROMBOLYTIC AGENTS IN ACUTE EVOLVING MYOCARDIAL INFARCTION

Agent	Advantages	Disadvantages
Streptokinase	Effective Least expensive Proven value	Severe hemostatic defect Antigenic Occasional allergic reaction Hypotensive when given too rapidly Least clot selective
rtPA	Effective Non-antigenic Highly clot selective Proven value	Moderate hemostatic defect Simultaneous heparin treatment required Short half-life Very expensive
Anistreplase (APSAC)	Effective Rapid injection Prolonged action Proven value	Severe hemostatic defect Antigenic Occasional allergic reaction Moderately expensive
Pro-urokinase	Effective Non-antigenic Highly clot selective	Mild hemostatic defect Simultaneous heparin treatment required Very short half-life Antigenic Very expensive
Urokinase	Effective Modest clot selectivity Non-antigenic Bolus injection	Moderately severe hemostatic defect Expensive

Modified with permission from Sherry.[141]

Initial expectations that acute reperfusion would salvage myocardium and reduce the mortality of patients with evolving myocardial infarction have been met. Numerous randomized trials have demonstrated a striking reduction in mortality with the use of streptokinase, tissue plasminogen activator (tPA), and anisoylated plasminogen streptokinase activator complex (APSAC), all of which activate plasminogen (Fig. 9–3). There have been consistent but small improvements in global and regional left ventricular function. The maximum benefit from acute reperfusion is seen with treatment started soon after the onset of symptoms but the ISIS-2 trial documented efficacy also in patients treated by streptokinase and aspirin within 6 to 24 hours after the onset of symptoms.[116]

The reperfusion era has revolutionized the management of acute myocardial infarction, and many initial questions have been answered, although new issues have emerged. These are currently the objective of numerous ongoing trials.

Which Drug or Combinations Thereof?

In randomized trials,[149,154] tPA was distinctly superior to streptokinase using early patency of the infarct-related artery as an end-point. Likewise, the use of pro-urokinase as in the PRIMI trial[135] led to more rapid reperfusion and fewer bleeding complications than did IV streptokinase (Table 9-2). Whether such differences in arterial patency will be translated into a reduction of mortality must await the results of large ongoing randomized trials such as GISSI-II and ISIS-3. Preliminary data from the GISSI-II trial, presented at the American College of Cardiology in March, 1990, showed that streptokinase and tPA were equally effective in reducing mortality and had somewhat similar incidences of serious side-effects (see Table 9-4). Arterial patency was not measured, although it is widely accepted that tPA achieves better rates of early recanalization (see Table 9-3). Three interpretations of these data are possible. First, the explanation most

TABLE 9–3 CHARACTERISTICS OF THROMBOLYTIC AGENTS

	SK	APSAC	tPA 2 chain	scu-PA	UK
Fibrin selective	No	No	Yes	Yes	No
Plasminogen binding	Indirect	Indirect	Direct	Direct	Direct
Duration of infusion (min)	60	2–5	90–180	90–180	5–15
Half-life (min)	23	90	8	7	16
Fibrinogen breakdown	4+	3+	1–2+	2+	3+
Early heparin required	No	No	Yes	No	Yes
Hypotension	Yes	Yes	No	No	No
Allergic reactions	Yes	Yes	No	No	No
Approximate cost/dose	$200/ 1.5 MU	$1200/ 30 U	$2200/ 100 mg	High	$2200/ 3 MU
Patency at 90 min	53[1]–65[5] (53)[6]	55[1]–65[2]	69[4]–79[3] (75)[6]	71[5]	66[4]
Patency at 24 hours	81[1]–88[5]	88[1]–92[2]	78[4]–85	85[5]	73[4]

Abbreviations: APSAC = Anisoylated plasminogen streptokinase activator complex (anistreplase); PUK = pro-urokinase; SK = streptokinase; tPA = tissue plasminogen activator; UK = urokinase; scu-PA = single chain urokinase (pro-urokinase) plasminogen activator; MU = million units; U = units.

1 = Hogg et al.[113]
2 = Pacouret et al.[129]
3 = Topol et al.[150]
4 = Neuhaus et al.[126]
5 = PRIMI Trial Study Group.[135]
6 = Mean value of 11 trials for streptokinase and 13 for tPA.[158]
For other data sources, see Marder and Sherry.[161]

favored in the USA is that the protocol used in the GISSI-II study was not optimal for testing tPA because of the delayed administration of heparin, with risk of re-occlusion, which occurs more frequently with tPA.[92, 110] (A small preliminary study suggests that early heparin can also improve results with streptokinase.[123]) Second, factors other than the degree of early arterial patency may determine mortality during thrombolytic therapy. For example, a more rapid patency could be balanced by a greater degree of reperfusion damage; this possibility could be tested by measurements of free radical formation during thrombolysis with various agents.[100] Third, the enhanced velocity of reperfusion achieved by tPA in other studies has not directly correlated with improved clinical status.[151] In an increasingly cost-conscious era, the far greater expense of tPA and the results of the GISSI-II study are likely to favor the use of streptokinase (Table 9-3), although a protocol with the early use of heparin is going to be required to assess what the best possible patency results with tPA can produce. Furthermore, new tPA regimens favoring "front-loading"[94] with "ultrathrombosis"[151] will also need to be taken into consideration in such comparisons, as will combinations such as tPA and streptokinase.[108]

SPECIFIC THROMBOLYTIC AGENTS

Streptokinase

The earlier IV streptokinase is given, the better the result.[34] Very early thrombolysis (within 1 hour) is much more effective at reducing enzymatic infarct size than thrombolysis 1 to 2 hours later.[66] Yusuf and co-workers[83] advocate a simple 1 hour high-dose (dose not stated) IV streptokinase infusion, without anticoagulation, which will successfully convert virtually all of the available plasminogen into plasmin and will also cause a major degradation of circulating fibrinogen, a co-factor for platelet aggregation (see Fig. 9–1). As a result of the GISSI and ISIS-2 trials, intravenous administration of streptokinase has completely supplanted intracoronary use except in certain selected circumstances.

TABLE 9–4 SIDE-EFFECTS OF STREPTOKINASE AND tPA IN THE GISSI-II TRIAL

	Streptokinase	tPA
Mortality	8.5%	8.9%
Overall stroke	1.0%	1.3%*
Hemorrhagic stroke	0.3%	0.4%
Major bleeds	0.9%	0.6%*
Allergic reactions	1.7%	0.2%*
Hypotension	3.8%	1.7%*

*Statistically significant; however, in the absence of CT scanning, data for stroke are not firm.
See ref. 106a.

Dose and Rate of Infusion of Streptokinase. In the first GISSI Italian trial,[26] the rate was 1.5 million units of streptokinase in 100 ml of physiologic saline in 1 hour. However, a higher dose (3 million units) can achieve a patency rate of 82%,[142] which is as good as any results reported with any other agent.

Recognition of Reperfusion. In the absence of early or simultaneous coronary angiography, the criteria are (1) rapid relief of chest pain; (2) accelerated ECG evolution; (3) very high peak blood creatine kinase values as enzyme is washed out from the infarcting myocardium; and (4) reperfusion arrhythmias that are common but usually minor.[48] However, these criteria are relatively ineffective,[95] highlighting the use of more sophisticated techniques such as the rapid rise of plasma myoglobin.

Indications for Streptokinase Other Than AMI. Indications are venous thrombosis, pulmonary embolism, and thrombosed arteriovenous shunts. Infusion dose: 250,000 to 600,000 units over 30 minutes, then 100,000 units every hour for up to 1 week.

Contraindications. Contraindications are recent hemorrhage or cerebrovascular accident, advancing age with fear of intracranial hemorrhage, coagulation defects, severe uncontrolled hypertension, recent streptococcal infections (bacterial toxins induce resistance to streptokinase), hemorrhagic retinopathy, and high risk of left heart thrombus as in mitral stenosis with fibrillation or subacute bacterial endocarditis. Potential sources of microemboli such as enlarged left atrium and ventricular or aortic aneurysm[144] are also contraindications as are recent peptic ulcer, pregnancy or menstruation, and previous treatment within 1 year by streptokinase (allergic risk).[113]

Precautions. Ideally check blood count and clotting factors before use. Discontinue heparin. Sometimes **hydrocortisone** 100 to 250 mg IV is given before streptokinase to prevent allergic reactions (not in GISSI study).

Side-effects and Complications. Allergic reactions (Table 9-4) include fever and rashes and, rarely (0.1%), anaphylactoid reactions. Minor bleeding requires local measures, not cessation of lytic therapy (danger of rebound excess lytic state). Major bleeding requires cessation of streptokinase and administration of fresh frozen plasma or whole blood. Poststreptokinase bleeding diathesis is a risk especially with combined heparin therapy.

Poststreptokinase Policy. This has not yet been clarified. Prolonged heparin treatment beyond 24 hours was no more effective than brief heparin in preventing rethrombosis.[117] The use of aspirin is routine in view of the ISIS-2 study. It is not known whether additional dipyridamole confers any added benefit. If rethrombosis occurs, urokinase or tPA should be the agent of choice to avoid allergic problems with streptokinase.

Combination with Coronary Vasodilators. In a preliminary trial, the combination of early streptokinase with IV nitrates and verapamil gave improved patency of the infarct-related artery[91] without proof of clinical benefit.

Tissue-type Plasminogen Activator (tPA) = Alteplase (Activase)

Tissue-type plasminogen activator (tPA) binds to fibrin with a greater affinity than does streptokinase or urokinase; once bound, it is activated and converts plasminogen to plasmin on the fibrin surface. Experimentally, even in equivalent thrombolytic doses, tPA produces less bleeding than streptokinase and has the further advantage of being non-antigenic. The dose of tPA required to produce nearly complete clot lysis (85%) can, however, produce some delayed bleeding. Human tPA is now produced by modern recombinant-DNA techniques and is becoming more freely available. In several large trials, IV tPA has been very effective, achieving recanalization in about 75% of patients with symptoms of myocardial infarction of less than 6 hours.

Dose. Standard IV doses are 80 to 100 mg tPA spread over 3 hours. "Front-loading," over 90 minutes with an initial bolus of 15 mg, then 50 mg over 30 minutes, then 35 mg over 1 hour, may give even better patency rates.[94,127] A higher total dose (150 mg) leads to no greater benefit and more cerebral hemorrhage.[149] Although an initial heparin bolus of 500 units is standard, the heparin can be delayed for at least 20 minutes after the start of tPA.[150] Thereafter IV heparin is continued until day 6, when subcutaneous heparin is substituted until hospital discharge. Aspirin is started on day 1.

Contraindications. These are similar in principle to those for streptokinase; gentamicin sensitivity is an exclusion, because gentamicin is used in the preparation of tPA; previous streptokinase is an indication, not a contraindication.

Comparisons with Placebo. In the European Co-operative Study,[154] 366 patients were given 250 mg aspirin and a bolus injection of 5,000 units of heparin before the start of the trial and 355 patients in the treatment group were also given 100 mg tPA over 3 hours as a 10 mg IV bolus, 50 mg infused during the next hour, and 40 mg over the next 2 hours. Three-month mortality rates of patients treated within 3 hours of the onset of symptoms were 59% lower in the tPA group. In the Anglo-Scandinavian Study of Early Thrombosis (ASSET) in 5,000 patients, tPA was given by a similar protocol, heparin 5,000 units was given initially, and then infused as 1,000 units per hour over the next 21 hours.[157] The 1-month mortality was 7.2% in the treated and 9.8% in the control groups, a reduction of 26%.

Comparisons with Streptokinase. In the European trial, tPA was infused at 0.75 mg/kg over 90 minutes and was superior to 1,500,000 units of streptokinase given IV over 60 minutes.[76] In the American National Heart, Lung and Blood Institute TIMI trial,[73] 80 mg tPA was infused over 3 hours and streptokinase for only 90 minutes. Ninety minutes after the onset of therapy, patency was achieved in 66% of patients versus 36% in the streptokinase group. Regarding long-term follow-up, despite the much higher patency rate with tPA in the TIMI trial, the mortality rate at 1 year was no different in the tPA and streptokinase groups (10.5% tPA, 11.6% streptokinase). The frequency of recurrent AMI, coronary bypass grafting, and PTCA was similar in the two groups.[99] In another comparison between tPA and streptokinase, using somewhat different dose regimens for the tPA, arterial patency was identical in both groups 3 weeks after the infarction, and LV ejection fraction was exactly the same.[156] The major comparison between tPA and streptokinase has been in the large GISSI-II trial, thus far not published in detail, in which the agents were virtually equieffective with some small differences in side-effects (see Table 9-4). It should be noted that early heparin is held to be essential for the full benefit of tPA, which has the disadvantage of more ready re-occlusion than with streptokinase. On the other hand, preliminary data suggest that early heparin may also improve results with streptokinase.[123]

Side-effects. The GISSI-II trial showed that the incidence of hemor-rhagic stroke was similar with tPA and streptokinase with the overall stroke rate lower in streptokinase, which was compensated for by an increased incidence of major bleeds, allergic reactions, and hypotension in the streptokinase group (see Table 9-4). Preliminary analysis sug-gests that co-administration with IV β-blockade can substantially re-duce stroke as a complication of tPA.[151]

New Types of tPA. The standard tPA consists predominantly of two chain molecules. Previously a predominantly single chain type was used and was somewhat more effective than streptokinase.[121] In development are mutant or chimeric tPAs, which may have longer half-lives, may be resistant to the effects of plasminogen activator inhibition, and may have increased thrombolytic efficacy.

Urokinase

This agent has similar indications, contraindications, and effects to streptokinase. However, being prepared from cultured human renal cells, allergic effects are minimal. Furthermore, a shorter half-life than streptokinase causes less systemic fibrinolysis, and is a safer drug if early coronary bypass is the aim.[72] Logically rethrombosis after early clot lysis in AMI should respond better to urokinase than streptoki-nase (blocking antibodies to streptokinase may persist for 3 to 6 months). A specific indication is for intraocular clot lysis (chosen because of absence of allergic properties). The defect of urokinase is great expense. The **dose** for intracoronary use is 3x that of streptoki-nase.[72] For IV use, high-dose urokinase (3 million units over 45–60 minutes) gives a patency rate of 62% with a low incidence of bleeding and re-occlusion.[155]

Anistreplase (Anisoylated Plasminogen Streptokinase Activator Complex [APSAC]; Eminase)

Anistreplase is a stoichiometric combination of streptokinase and plasminogen with an anisoyl group bound to the catalytic center of the plasminogen moiety; despite this structural modification the mol-ecule still has fibrin-binding capacity. Anistreplase is deacylated at a controlled rate so that it has a relatively long half-life and can be given as a single intravenous injection. The latter point is its major advan-tage, so that pre-hospital use is feasible,[96] although absolute proof of its benefit at that stage awaits the results of ongoing European studies.

Compared with streptokinase, anistreplase offers a higher early patency rate in some studies,[87,129] although a recent large randomized trial in which patency was assessed at 90 minutes and 24 hours did not show such a difference.[113] Mortality, cardiogenic shock, and asystole are all reduced when compared with heparin;[122] furthermore, infarct size measured by single photon emission computed tomography falls by about 31%.[90] In a definitive large-scale study versus placebo,[85] anistreplase given within 6 hours of the onset of symptoms reduced mortality at 1 month from 12% to 6% and at 1 year from 18% to 11%. Complications of AMI were also reduced. Hemorrhage was increased; the tendency to more strokes just avoided being statistically signifi-cant. Hypotension, the probable result of bradykinin activation by increased levels of plasmin, might theoretically be beneficial or harm-ful. The mortality data from existing trials cannot directly be com-pared with those attained by streptokinase or by tPA, so that a proper prospective controlled trial is required (ISIS-3).

Dose. In the AIMS Study, 30 units anistreplase were given as a single IV injection over 5 minutes with IV heparin 6 hours thereafter and warfarin for at least 3 months.[85] There was no co-therapy with aspirin.

Contraindications. These are similar to those for streptokinase, except for the prior administration of streptokinase.

Co-therapy. Although it is likely that co-therapy with aspirin will further reduce mortality, data are not available, nor is the general question of co-therapy with antiplatelet agents analyzed.

Combination of Fibrinolytic Agents

Combination therapy is logical, because different agents act in different ways. Thus the combination of low-dose tPA (50 mg) and 1.5 million units of streptokinase had a re-occlusion rate of only 6%.[108] Theoretically, fibrinogen degradation products resulting from the breakdown of fibrin by streptokinase could help prevent platelet aggregation and thereby reduce rethrombosis (see Fig. 9–1). Another combination therapy is that of low-dose (12 mg) tPA over 30 minutes and pro-urokinase 48 mg over 40 minutes, with a patency rate of 61% (not remarkable), the induction of a highly specific coagulation defect, and the absence of any bleeding sufficiently severe to require transfusion.[93] An important aspect is that these two lytic agents, at fibrin-specific doses, activate distinctly different portions of the available fibrin-bound plasminogen. Such therapy must be combined with high-dose heparin (12,500 units) to prevent cleavage of pro-urokinase by thrombin.

Combination Thrombolytic β-Blockade Therapy

In view of the benefits of early β-blockade in myocardial infarction, and also of early thrombolysis, it is logical to consider a combination. There has, however, been no formal trial of β-blocker versus tPA versus combination therapy. In the TIMI-II trial, there were less re-infarctions and recurrent ischemic episodes in patients receiving IV metoprolol, although there were few other overall long-term benefits.[149] An unexpected bonus of β-blockade may be the ability to reduce the incidence of cerebral bleeds.[151] In the GISSI-II trial, IV atenolol was used whenever possible, which was in about half the patients.

Fibrinolytic Therapy: Recommendations

There is a growing consensus that the early administration (less than 6 hours after the onset of symptoms, ideally within 2 hours[51]) of any of the standard fibrinolytic agents improves ventricular function and limits infarct size. The reduction in mortality is best shown when fibrinolysis is really early;[34,66] even at 6 hours benefits are modest.[33] Nonetheless, later administration may still achieve some benefits. IV fibrinolysis has now become standard practice in the management of early myocardial infarction. Co-administration of aspirin is standard but only proven for the combination with streptokinase. While awaiting the results of the giant ISIS-3 study, which will compare tPA, streptokinase, and anistreplase, a reasonable hypothesis is that the differences in early mortality between these agents may not be as large as expected, as suggested by the results of the GISSI-II trial showing a comparable mortality for streptokinase and tPA. A crucial unresolved question at this stage is whether different results would be found if early IV heparin were added to tPA, as is standard practice in the USA. Nonetheless, tPA appears to achieve greater early patency rates than does streptokinase; whether such patency confers additional benefits remains to be evaluated.[95,151]

SPECIFIC THROMBOLYTIC PROBLEMS

Lytic Failure

Some degree of resistance of thrombi to lysis can be expected in perhaps 10 to 15% of patients; the cause may include deep fissuring or rupture of the plaque with exposure of platelet-rich thrombus, which is very resistant to lysis.[151]

Re-occlusion

Re-occlusion remains the "Achilles heel" of successful thrombolysis. It occurs in 5 to 20% of patients[104,141] and can be lessened by early heparin.[92,110] Major contributory factors to restenosis include the presence of a residual luminal **stenosis**, and the persistence of residual thrombus (the latter is a powerful thrombogenic surface). It should be remembered that successful lysis re-exposes the site of the original thrombus, namely the plaque fissure. The potential for re-thrombosis is easily understandable.

The role of **heparin following thrombolysis** is under evaluation (see p 264). Pending the results of more trials, it is highly prudent to give heparin as a bolus, 100 units per kg, **after lysis**, followed by maintenance infusion of approximately 1,000 units/hr, for approximately 5 days[122a] (adjust to maintain APTT II-2.5 x the control value) in addition to aspirin 80 mg/day. An alternate regimen is an early IV bolus of heparin of only 2000 units followed 9 hours later by subcutaneous heparin 12,500 units.[138] If coronary revascularization is not contemplated, the patient can be discharged on aspirin 160–325 mg/day.[104] A bolus of heparin at the initiation of lytic therapy rather than after lysis may be unnecessary.[150]

New approaches to preventing re-occlusion will probably involve the use of monoclonal antiplatelet glycoprotein IIb-IIIa antibody; monoclonal antibodies against the von Willebrand factor; hirudin (obtained from leeches and new recombinant techniques), which is a very powerful antithrombin agent; inhibitors of the thromboxane and serotonin pathways; and prostacyclin derivatives.

Thrombolysis in the Elderly

Early reports described major side-effects in patients over the age of 75 years undergoing thrombolytic therapy, so that almost all trials have imposed an upper age limit. Nonetheless, the ISIS-2 trial documented a substantial mortality benefit in patients over the age of 70 years, and similar results for a survival benefit among patients over the age of 65 or 70 years were shown in the ASSET trial of tPA.[84,157] However, in elderly patients it would be prudent to exclude hypertension with end-organ damage and even transient hypertension with values exceeding 180 mm Hg systolic or 120 mm Hg diastolic.[86] Also those already taking aspirin are more likely to bleed.

PTCA after Thrombolysis

Three trials have shown that after apparently successful thrombolytic therapy, emergency PTCA was not beneficial but probably harmful and as such is contraindicated. In the TIMI IIB trial in which patients were randomized to either routine angioplasty 18 to 48 hours following thrombolytic therapy or conservative therapy with the option to perform angioplasty in the event of symptomatic ischemia, there was no difference in mortality at 42 days.[149] Thus a policy of "watchful waiting" following successful thrombolysis is favored. The role of "primary" angioplasty without thrombolytic therapy in hospitals with suitable facilities requires further evaluation, but in patients with cardiogenic shock, it is probably the best option.[120] "Rescue" PTCA after failed thrombolytic therapy is a rational and logical approach, but its efficacy is limited by the current inability to detect non-invasively the failure to achieve patency with thrombolytic therapy.

The "Achilles heel" of PTCA (like that of thrombolysis) is restenosis. There appears to be no benefit from aspirin, dipyridamole, or warfarin.[102]

SUMMARY

Antithrombotic agents include platelet inhibitors, anticoagulants, and fibrinolytics. Aspirin irreversibly inhibits the cyclo-oxygenase concerned in the synthesis of prostaglandins with, in practice, a beneficial clinical effect over a wide dose range. Aspirin is now indicated for unstable angina, threatened stroke (TIAs), and post-infarct management. Sulfinpyrazone and dipyridamole are used only in selected patients. In coronary bypass operations, dipyridamole should be started pre-operatively and continued thereafter with the addition of aspirin. When combination of warfarin with an antiplatelet agent is required, dipyridamole is preferred to aspirin (but such combinations are not yet of proven value). Warfarin is now chiefly used in the acute phase of myocardial infarction and in the prevention of venous thromboembolism. In uncomplicated AMI, warfarin may be omitted and only heparin used until the patient is mobile. Prolonged post-infarction anticoagulation is selected for patients at definite risk of thromboembolism or when aspirin is contraindicated. Anticoagulation should be considered for those with prosthetic heart valves and for dilated cardiomyopathy. In atrial fibrillation, anticoagulation must be considered though not necessarily always given. Fibrinolytics such as streptokinase, tissue plasminogen activator, or anistreplase are now standard therapy in the very early stages of AMI, and are combined with oral aspirin.

REFERENCES

References from Previous Editions

1. Angell WW, Angell JD: Prog Cardiovasc Dis 23:141–166, 1980
2. Ansell JE, Price JM, Shah S, et al: Chest 88:878–882, 1985
3. Anturan Reinfarction Italian Study: Lancet 1:237–242, 1982
4. Anturane Reinfarction Trial Research Group: N Engl J Med 302:250–256, 1980
5. Bailey RR, Reddy J: Lancet 1:254, 1980
6. Boelaert J, Lijnen P, Robbens E, et al: J Cardiovasc Pharmacol 8:386–391, 1986
7. Bousser MG, Eschwege E, Haguenau M, et al: Stroke 14:5–14, 1983
8. Brand FN, Abbott RD, Kannel WB, et al: JAMA 254:3449–3453, 1985
9. Bresnahan DR, Davis JL, Holmes DR, et al: J Am Coll Cardiol 6:285–289, 1985
10. Cairns JA, Gent M, Singer J, et al: N Engl J Med 313:1369–1375, 1985
11. Canadian Cooperative Study Group: N Engl J Med 299:53–59, 1978
12. Chalmers TC, Matta RJ, Smith H, et al: N Engl J Med 297:1091–1096, 1977
13. Chesebro JH, Clements IP, Fuster V, et al: N Engl J Med 307:73–78, 1982
14. Chesebro JH, Fuster V, Elveback LR, et al: Am J Cardiol 51:1537–1541, 1983
15. Dale J, Myhre E, Stortstein O, et al: Am Heart J 94:101–111, 1977
16. Davis MJE, Ireland MA: Am J Cardiol 57:1244–1247, 1986
17. Donadio JV, Anderson CF, Mitchell JC, et al: N Engl J Med 310:1421–1426, 1984
18. Dzau VJ, Packer M, Lilly LS, et al: N Engl J Med 310:347–352, 1984
19. EPSIM Research Group: N Engl J Med 307:701–708, 1982
20. Fields WS, Lemak NA, Frankowski RF, et al: Stroke 8:301–314, 1977
21. Fitzgerald GA, Reilly IAG, Pedersen AK: Circulation 72:1194–1201, 1985
22. Friedman PL, Brown EJ, Gunther S, et al: N Engl J Med 305:1171–1175, 1981
23. Fuster V, Gersh BJ, Giuliani ER, et al: Am J Cardiol 47:525–531, 1981
24. Gadboys HL, Litwak RS, Niemetz J, et al: JAMA 202:134–138, 1967
25. Gallus AS: Drugs 26:543–549, 1983
26. GISSI Trial: Lancet 1:397–401, 1986
27. Goodnight SH: Circulation 62:466–468, 1980
28. Grayzel AI, Liddle L, Seegmiller JE: N Engl J Med 265:763–768, 1961
29. Gresele P, Zoja C, Deckmyn H, et al: Thromb Haemost 50:852–856, 1983
30. Hanson SR, Harker LA, Bjornsson TD: J Clin Invest 75:1591–1599, 1985

31. Harter HR, Burch JW, Majerus PW, et al: N Engl J Med 301:577–579, 1979
32. Hess H, Mietaschik A, Deichsel E: Lancet 1:415–419, 1985
33. ISAM Study Group: N Engl J Med 314:1465–1471, 1986
34. Italian Group: Lancet 1:397–401, 1986
35. Kazmier FJ: Mayo Clin Proc 60:673–674, 1985
36. Kiil J, Kiil J, Axelsen F, et al: Lancet 1:1115–1116, 1978
37. Klimt CR, Knatterud GL, Stamler J, et al: J Am Coll Cardiol 7:251–269, 1986
38. Koch-Weser J: Ann Intern Med 68:511–517, 1968
39. Kramer RJ, Zeldis SM, Hamby RI: Br Heart J 47:606–608, 1982
40. Editorial: Lancet 1:1172–1173, 1980
41. Editorial: Lancet 1:592–593, 1986
42. Lane GE, Bove AA: Circulation 72:389–396, 1985
43. Lapeyre AC, Steele PM, Kazmier FJ, et al: J Am Coll Cardiol 6:534–538, 1985
44. Lee P-K, Wang RYC, Chow JSF, et al: J Am Coll Cardiol 8:221–224, 1986
45. Lewis HD, Davis JW, Archibald DG, et al: N Engl J Med 309:396–403, 1983
46. Linos A, Worthington JW, O'Fallon W, et al: Mayo Clin Proc 53:581–586, 1978
47. Livio M, Benigni A, Vigano G, et al: Lancet 1:414–416, 1986
48. MacLennan BA, McMaster A, Webb SW, et al: Br Heart J 55:231–239, 1986
49. Marcus AJ: N Engl J Med 309:1515–1516, 1983
50. Martinowitz U, Rabinovici J, Goldfarb D, et al: N Engl J Med 304:671–672, 1981
51. Mathey DG, Sheehan FH, Schofer J, et al: J Am Coll Cardiol 6:518–525, 1985
52. Mehta J, Mehta P, Pepine CJ, et al: Am J Cardiol 47:1111–1114, 1981
53. Mehta JL, Mehta P, Lopez L, et al: J Am Coll Cardiol 4:806–811, 1984
54. Mielants H, Veys EM, Verbruggen G, et al: J Rheumatol 6:210–218, 1979
55. Miwa K, Kambara H, Kawai C: Am Heart J 105:351–355, 1983
56. Mok CK, Boey J, Wang R, et al: Circulation 72:1059–1063, 1985
57. Moroz L: N Engl J Med 296:525–529, 1977
58. Negus D, Friedgood A, Cox SJ, et al: Lancet 1:891–894, 1980
59. O'Reilly RA, Sahud MA, Aggeler PM: Ann NY Acad Sci 179:173–186, 1971
60. Pedersen AK, Fitzgerald GA: N Engl J Med 311:1206–1211, 1984
61. Pedersen AK, Fitzgerald GA: Circulation 72:1164–1176, 1985
62. Persantine-Aspirin Reinfarction Study (PARIS). Circulation 62:449–461, 1980
63. Riemersma RA, Russel DC, Oliver MF: Lancet 2:471, 1981
64. Sandok BA, Furlan AJ, Whisnant JP, et al: Mayo Clin Proc 53:665–674, 1978
65. Schmitz JM, Apprill PG, Buja LM: Circ Res 57: 223-231, 1985.
66. Simoons ML, Serruys PW, van den Brand M, et al: J Am Coll Cardiol 7:717–728, 1986
67. Sixty-Plus Reinfarction Study Research Group: Lancet 1:64–68, 1982
68. Steele P, Rainwater J: Circulation 62:462–465, 1980
69. Stratton F, Chalmers DG, Flute PT, et al: Br Med J 285:274–275, 1982
70. Sullivan JM, Harken DE, Gorlin R: N Engl J Med 284:1391–1394, 1971
71. Temple R, Pledger GW: N Engl J Med 303:1488–1492, 1980
72. Tennant SN, Dixon J, Venable TC, et al: Circulation 69:756–760, 1984
73. TIMI Study Group: N Engl J Med 312:932–936, 1985
74. Torosian M, Michelson EL, Morganroth J, et al: Ann Intern Med 89:325–328, 1978
75. Vanhoutte PM: In Vanhoutte PM (ed): Serotonin and the Cardiovascular System. New York, Raven Press, 1985, pp 123–133
76. Verstraete M, Bernard R, Bory M, et al: Lancet 1:842, 1985
77. Wallenburg HCS, Dekker GA, Makowitz JW, et al: Lancet 1:1–3, 1986
78. Webster J: Drugs 30:32–41, 1985
79. Weinstein GS, Mavroudis C, Ebert PA: Ann Thorac Surg 33:549–553, 1982
80. Weksler BB, Tack-Goldman K, Subramanian VA, et al: Circulation 71:332–340, 1985
81. Wilcox RG, Richardson D, Hampton JR, et al: Br Med J 3:531–534, 1980
82. Wolf PA, Dawber TR, Thomas HE Jr, et al: Neurology 28:973–977, 1978
83. Yusuf S, Collins R, Peto R, et al: Eur Heart J 6:556–585, 1985

New References

84. AIMS Trial Study Group: Effect of intravenous APSAC on mortality after acute myocardial infarction, preliminary report of a placebo-controlled clinical trial. Lancet 1:545–549, 1988

85. AIMS Trial Study Group: Long-term effects of intravenous anistreplase in acute myocardial infarction: Final report of the AIMS study. Lancet 335:427–431, 1990

86. Althouse R, Maynard C, et al: Risk factors for hemorrhagic and ischemic stroke and myocardial infarct: Patients treated with tissue plasminogen activators (abstract). J Am Coll Cardiol 13:153A, 1989

87. Anderson JL, Hackworthy RA, Sorenson SG, et al: Comparison of intravenous anistreplase (APSAC) and streptokinase in acute myocardial infarction: Interim report of a randomized, double-blind patency study (abstract). Circulation 80(suppl II):II-420, 1989

88. Antiplatelet Trialists' Collaboration: Secondary prevention of vascular disease by prolonged antiplatelet treatment. Br Med J 296:320–331, 1988

88a. Balsano F, Rizzon P, Vroli F, et al: Antiplatelet treatment with ticlopidine in unstable angina. A controlled multicenter trial. Circulation 82:17–26, 1990

89. Barnathan ES, Schwartz S, Taylor L, et al: Aspirin and dipyridamole in the prevention of acute coronary thrombosis complicating coronary angioplasty. Circulation 76:125–134, 1987

90. Bassand J-P, Machecourt J, Cassagnes J, et al: Multicenter trial of intravenous anisoylated plasminogen streptokinase activator complex (APSAC) in acute myocardial infarction: Effects on infarct size and left ventricular function. J Am Coll Cardiol 13:988–997, 1989

91. Better N, Johnson PR, Connoley GL, et al: Coronary vasodilator interactions with outcome of streptokinase therapy (abstract). Circulation 80(suppl II):II-113, 1989

92. Bleich SD, Nichols T, Schumacher R, et al: The role of heparin following coronary thrombolysis with tissue plasminogen activator (tPA)(abstract). Circulation 80(suppl II):II-113, 1989

93. Bode C, Schuler G, Nordt T, et al: Intravenous thrombolytic therapy with a combination of single-chain urokinase-type plasminogen activator and recombinant tissue-type plasminogen activator in acute myocardial infarction. Circulation 81:907–913, 1990

94. Braunwald E: Enhancing thrombolytic efficacy by means of 'front-loaded' administration of tissue plasminogen activator. J Am Coll Cardiol 14:1570–1571, 1989

95. Califf RM, O'Neil W, Stack RS, et al: Failure of simple clinical measurements to predict perfusion status after intravenous thrombolysis. Ann Intern Med 108:658–662, 1988

96. Castaigne AD, Herve C, Duval-Moulin A-M, et al: Prehospital use of APSAC: Results of a placebo-controlled study. Am J Cardiol 64:30A–33A, 1989

97. Chesebro JH, Adams PC, Fuster V: Antithrombotic therapy in patients with valvular heart disease and prosthetic heart valves. J Am Coll Cardiol 8:41B–56B, 1986

98. Clagett GP, Genton E, Salzman EW: Antithrombotic therapy in peripheral vascular disease. Chest 95 (suppl):128C–139S, 1989

99. Dalen JE, Gore JM, Braunwald E, et al: Six- and twelve-month follow-up of the phase I thrombolysis in myocardial infarction (TIMI) trial. Am J Cardiol 62:179–185, 1988

100. Davies SW, Ranjadayalan K, Wickens DG, et al: Lipid peroxidation associated with successful thrombolysis. Lancet 335:741–743, 1990

101. Dunn M, Alexander J, de Silva R, Hildner F: Antithrombotic therapy in atrial fibrillation. Chest 96(suppl):118S–127S, 1989

102. Ellis SG, Shaw RE, Gershony G, et al: Risk factors, time course and treatment effect for restenosis after successful percutaneous transluminal coronary angioplasty of chronic total occlusion. Am J Cardiol 63:897–901, 1989

103. ESPS Group: The European Stroke Prevention Study (ESPS): Principal end-points. Lancet 2:1351–1354, 1987

104. Fuster V, Stein B, Badimon L, et al: Antithrombotic therapy after myocardial reperfusion in acute myocardial infarction. J Am Coll Cardiol 12(suppl A):78A–84A, 1988

105. Fuster V, Cohen M, Halperin J: Aspirin in the prevention of coronary disease. N Engl J Med 321:183–185, 1989

106. Gent M, Blakely JA, Easton JD, et al: The Canadian-American Ticlopidine Study (CATS) in thromboembolic stroke. Lancet 1:1215–1220, 1989

106a. GISSI-II. A factorial randomised trial of alteplase versus streptokinase and heparin versus no heparin among 12,490 patients with acute myocardial infarction. Lancet 336:65–71, 1990

107. Goldman S, Copeland J, Moritz T, et al: Improvement in early saphenous vein graft patency after coronary artery bypass surgery with antiplatelet therapy: Results of a Veterans Administration Cooperative Study. Circulation 77:1324–1332, 1988

108. Grines CL, Nissen SE, Booth DC, et al: A new thrombolytic regimen for acute myocardial infarction using combination half dose tissue-type plasminogen activator with full dose streptokinase: A pilot study. J Am Coll Cardiol 14: 573–580, 1989

109. Gurwitz JH, Goldberg RJ, Holder A, et al: Age-related risks of long-term oral anticoagulant therapy. Arch Intern Med 148: 1733–1736, 1988

110. HART Study: Heparin versus aspirin reperfusion trial. Preliminary data presented by Ross at the American College of Cardiology Meeting, New Orleans, 1990

111. Hennekens CH, Buring JE, Sandercock P, et al: Aspirin and other antiplatelet agents in the secondary and primary prevention of cardiovascular disease. Circulation 80:749–756, 1989

112. Hirsh J, Salzman E, Harker L, et al: Aspirin and other platelet active drugs. Relationship among dose, effectiveness and side-effects. Chest 95(suppl):12S–18S, 1989

113. Hogg KJ, Gemmill JD, Burns JMA, et al: Angiographic patency study of anistreplase versus streptokinase in acute myocardial infarction. Lancet 335:254–258, 1990

114. Hyers TM, Hull RD, Weg JG: Antithrombotic therapy for venous thromboembolic disease. Chest 95(suppl):37S–51S, 1989

115. Imanishi M, Kawamura M, Akabane S, et al: Aspirin lowers blood pressure in patients with renovascular hypertension. Hypertension 14:461–468, 1989

116. ISIS-2 (Second International Study of Infarct Survival) Collaborative Group: Randomized trial of intravenous streptokinase, oral aspirin, both, or neither among 17,187 cases of suspected acute myocardial infarction: ISIS-II. Lancet 2:350–360, 1988

117. Kander NH, Holland KJ, Pitt B, Topol EJ: A randomized pilot trial of brief versus prolonged heparin after successful reperfusion in acute myocardial infarction. Am J Cardiol 65:139–142, 1990

118. Kopecky SL, Gersh BJ, McGoon MD, et al: The natural history of idiopathic "lone" atrial fibrillation: A three decade population-based study. N Engl J Med 317:669–674, 1987

119. Kopecky SL, Gersh BJ, McGoon MD, et al: Lone atrial fibrillation in the elderly: A population-based long-term study (abstract). Circulation 80(suppl II):II-409, 1989

120. Lee L, Bates ER, Pitt B, et al: Percutaneous transluminal coronary angioplasty improves survival in acute myocardial infarction complicated by cardiogenic shock. Circulation 78:1345–1351, 1988

121. Magnani B, for the PAIMS Investigators. Plasminogen Activator Italian Multicenter Study (PAIMS): Comparison of intravenous recombinant single-chain human tissue-type plasminogen activator (rt-PA) with intravenous streptokinase in acute myocardial infarction. J Am Coll Cardiol 13:19–26, 1989

122. Melandri G, Branzi A, Semprini, et al: The simultaneous infusion of streptokinase and heparin leads to quicker reperfusion and smaller infarct size (abstract). Eur Heart J 10:224, 1989

122a. Mahan EF, Chandler JW, Roger WJ, et al: Heparin and infarct coronary artery patency after streptokinase in acute myocardial infarction. Am J Cardiol 85:867–972, 1990

123. Meinertz T, Kasper W, Schumacher M, et al: The German Multicenter Trial of anisoylated plasminogen streptokinase activator complex versus heparin for acute myocardial infarction. Am J Cardiol 62:347-351, 1988

124. Neri Serneri GG, Rovelli F, Gensini GF, et al: Effectiveness of low-dose heparin in prevention of myocardial reinfarction. Lancet 1:937–942, 1987

125. Neri Serneri GG, Gensini GF, Poggesi L, et al: Effect of heparin, aspirin, or alteplase in reduction of myocardial ischaemia in refractory unstable angina. Lancet 335:615–618, 1990

126. Neuhaus K-L, Tebbe U, Gottwik M, et al: Intravenous recombinant tissue plasminogen activator (rt-PA) and urokinase in acute myocardial infarction: Results of the German Activator Urokinase Study (GAUS). J Am Coll Cardiol 12:581–587, 1988

127. Neuhaus K-L, Feuerer W, Jeep-Tebbe S, et al: Improved thrombolysis with a modified dose regimen of recombinant tissue-type plasminogen activator. J Am Coll Cardiol 14:1566–1569, 1989

128. Ouimet H, Theroux P, McCans J, Waters D: Rebound caused by withdrawal of heparin in the acute phase of unstable angina (abstract). Circulation 80(suppl II):II-266, 1989

129. Pacouret G, Charbonnier B for the IRS II Study: Multicentre European Randomized Trial of anistreplase versus streptokinase in acute myocardial infarction (abstract). Circulation 80(suppl II):II-420, 1989

130. Paganini-Hill A, Chao A, Ross RK, Henderson BE: Aspirin use and chronic diseases: A cohort study of the elderly. Br Med J 299:1247–1250, 1989

131. Penny WJ, Chesebro JH, Heras M, Fuster V: Antithrombotic therapy for patients with cardiac disease. Curr Problems Cardiol 13:427–513, 1988

132. Petersen P, Hodtfredsen J, Boysen G, et al: Placebo-controlled, randomised trial of warfarin and aspirin for prevention of thromboembolic complications in chronic atrial fibrillation: The Copenhagen AFASAK Study. Lancet 1:175–179, 1989

133. Peto R, Gray R, Collins R, et al: Randomized trial of prophylactic daily aspirin in British male doctors. Br Med J 296:313–316, 1988

134. Pfisterer M, Burkart F, Jockers G, et al: Trial of low-dose aspirin plus dipyridamole versus anticoagulants for prevention of aortocoronary vein graft occlusion. Lancet 2:1–7, 1989

135. PRIMI Trial Study Group: Randomised double-blind trial of recombinant pro-urokinase against streptokinase in acute myocardial infarction. Lancet 1:863–868, 1989

136. Resnekov L, Chediak J, Hirsch J, Lewis HD: Antithrombotic agents in coronary artery disease. Chest 95:52S–72S, 1989

137. Saour JN, Sieck JO, Mamo LAR, Gallus AS: Trial of different intensities of anticoagulation in patients with prosthetic heart valves. N Engl J Med 322:428–432, 1990

138. SCATI (Studio Sulla Calciparina Nell'Angina e Nella Trombosi Ventricolare Nell'Infarto) Group: Randomised controlled trial of subcutaneous calcium-heparin in acute myocardial infarction. Lancet 2:182–186, 1989

139. Sethi GK, Copeland JG, Goldman S, et al: Implications of preoperative administration of aspirin in patients undergoing coronary artery bypass grafting. J Am Coll Cardiol 15:15–20, 1990

140. Sherry S: Recombinant tissue plasminogen activator (rt-PA): Is it the thrombolytic agent of choice for an evolving acute myocardial infarction. Am J Cardiol 59:984–989, 1987

141. Sherry S: Appraisal of various thrombolytic agents in the treatment of acute myocardial infarction. Am J Med 83:31–46, 1987

142. Six AJ, Louwerenburg HW, Braams R, et al: A double-blind randomized multicenter dose-ranging trial of intravenous streptokinase in acute myocardial infarction. Am J Cardiol 65:119–123. 1990

142a. Smith P, Arnesen H, Holme I: The effect of warfarin on mortality and reinfarction after myocardial infarction. N Engl J Med 323:147–152, 1990

143. SPAF (Stroke Prevention in Atrial Fibrillation) Study Group: Preliminary report of the Stroke Prevention in Atrial Fibrillation Study. N Engl J Med 322:863–868, 1990

144. Stafford PJ, Strachan CJL, Vincent R, Chamberlain DA: Multiple microemboli after disintegration of clot during thrombolysis for acute myocardial infarction. Br Med J 299:1310–1312, 1989

145. Steering Committee of the Physicians Health Study: Final report on the aspirin component of the ongoing Physician Health Study. N Engl J Med 321:129–135, 1989

146. Stein B, Fuster V: Role of platelet inhibitor therapy in myocardial infarction. Cardiovasc Drugs Ther 3:797–813, 1989

147. Stein PD, Kantrowitz A: Antithrombotic therapy in mechanical and biological prosthetic heart valves and saphenous vein bypass grafts. Chest 95(suppl):107S–117S, 1989

148. Theroux P, Ouimet H, McCans J, et al: Aspirin, heparin, or both to treat acute unstable angina. N Engl J Med 319:1105–1111, 1988

149. TIMI Study Group: Comparison of invasive and conservative strategies after treatment with intravenous tissue plasminogen activator in acute myocardial infarction: Results of the thrombolysis in myocardial infarction (TIMI) Phase II Trial. N Engl J Med 320:618–627, 1989

150. Topol EJ, George BS, Kereiakes DJ, et al: A randomized controlled trial of intravenous tissue plasminogen activator and early intravenous heparin in acute myocardial infarction. Circulation 79:281–286, 1989

151. Topol EJ: Ultrathrombolysis. J Am Coll Cardiol 15:922–924, 1990

152. Turpie AGG, Robinson JG, Doyle DJ, et al: Comparison of high-dose with low-dose subcutaneous heparin to prevent left ventricular mural thrombosis in patients with transmural anterior myocardial infarction. N Engl J Med 320:352–394, 1989
153. UK-TIA Study Group: United Kingdom transient ischaemic attack (UK-TIA) aspirin trial: Interim results. Br Med J 296:316–320, 1988
154. Van de Werf F, Arnold AER: Intravenous tissue plasminogen activator and size of infarct, left ventricular function, and survival in acute myocardial infarction. Br Med J 297:1374–1379, 1988
155. Wall TC, Phillips HR, Stack RS, et al: Results of high-dose intravenous urokinase for acute myocardial infarction. Am J Cardiol 65:124–131, 1990
156. White HD, Rivers JT, Maslowski AH, et al: Effect of intravenous streptokinase as compared with that of tissue plasminogen activator on left ventricular function after first myocardial infarction. N Engl J Med 320:817–821, 1989
157. Wilcox RG, von der Lippe G, Olsson CG, et al: Trial of tissue plasminogen activator for mortality reduction in acute myocardial infarction: Anglo-Scandinavian Study of Early Thrombolysis (ASSET). Lancet 2:525–530, 1988

Reviews

158. Collen D: Coronary thrombolysis: Streptokinase or recombinant tissue-type plasminogen activator. Ann Intern Med 112:529–538, 1990
159. Coller BS: Platelets and thrombolytic therapy. N Engl J Med 322:33–42, 1990
160. Handin RI, Loscalzo J: Hemostasis, thrombosis, fibrinolysis, and cardiovascular disease. In Braunwald E (ed): Heart Disease, 3rd ed. Philadelphia, WB Saunders, 1988, pp 1758–1781
161. Marder VJ, Sherry S: Thrombolytic therapy: Current status. N Engl J Med 318:1512–1520, 1988

L.H. Opie

10

Lipid-Lowering and Antiatherosclerotic Drugs

THE CHOLESTEROL CAMPAIGN

Now that there is a national American campaign to lower blood cholesterol, American aggressiveness has been contrasted with British reservations by Kaplan, who warns against the problem of a significant number of people being misdiagnosed on too few measurements and put unnecessarily on therapies that may have adverse effects and impair their quality of life.[48] Supporting the policy of moderation is the fact that cholesterol reduction by drugs or diet reduces heart attacks but not overall mortality, as in the cholestyramine and gemfibrozil studies.[49] Real hope of an overall benefit of cholesterol reduction is given by the recently released 15-year follow-up in the niacin trial in which mortality fell by 11%.[37] Nevertheless, large prospective trials will be required to test the hypothesis that cholesterol reduction can decrease total mortality.

Quite apart from primary prevention, cholesterol reduction is an essential component of a comprehensive **secondary prevention program**, where vigorous dietary measures are the first step in post-myocardial infarction patients.[58]

IDEAL BLOOD LIPID PROFILE

Blood Cholesterol

The ideal blood cholesterol value may be about 180 to 200 mg/dl or 4.7 to 5.2 mmol/L.[1,13,20] Blood cholesterol values above 260 to 270 mg/dL or 6.7 to 7.0 mmol/L put a patient over 40 years of age at high risk for coronary heart disease.[1,19] For more modest cholesterol elevations, it is desirable to calculate the **absolute risk** of the combined impact of blood cholesterol, blood pressure levels, age, family history, and smoking habits, before making a firm decision on lipid-lowering therapy. In 1986, the European Atherosclerosis Society[4] set an ideal cholesterol value as below 200 mg/dl (<5.2 mmol/L) and advised that values of 200 to 250 mg/dl or 5.2 to 6.5 mmol/L should be treated by dietary advice and correction of other risk factors, with higher cholesterol levels sometimes requiring lipid-lowering drugs (Table 10-1). In 1988, the American National Cholesterol Education program recommended that a blood cholesterol level of above 230 mg/dl

---

This chapter was reviewed with G M Berger and B Lewis.

TABLE 10–1 BLOOD CHOLESTEROL AND TRIGLYCERIDE VALUES IN MANAGEMENT OF CARDIAC PATIENTS

Values	Management
Serum cholesterol level	
< 200 mg/dl or 5.2 mmol/L	None
200–250 mg/dl	Dietary; overall risk factor* control
> 250 mg/dl[4] or 6.5 mmol/L > 260 mg/dl[19] > 268 mg/dl[1]	As above, then consider use of lipid-lowering drugs. If response inadequate, refer to Lipid Clinic If triglycerides high, see below
Serum low-density cholesterol levels	
If total cholesterol exceeds 240 mg/dl: lipogram LDL (calculated)	
< 130 mg/dl	Ideal
130–160 mg/dl plus coronary heart disease or two risk factors	Take action
> 160 mg/dl	Diet ± drug therapy
Triglyceride level[4]	
< 200 mg/dl = 2.3 mmol/L	None
200–250 mg/dl with cholesterol < 200 mg/dl	Loss of weight, dietary therapy, look for cause of high levels, including diuretics and some β-blockers
200–500 mg/dl (2.3–5.6 mmol/L) with cholesterol 200–300 mg/dl	As above, then consider lipid-lowering drug, especially if cholesterol > 250 mg/dl
> 500 mg/dl with cholesterol > 300 mg/dl	Refer lipid clinic for active dietary and drug therapy
> 1000 mg/dl (chylomicronemia)	Urgent therapy needed, risk of pancreatitis
High-density lipoprotein level	
< 35 mg/dl or < 0.9 mmol/L	Regard as additional reason for treatment
Apolipoprotein B	
> 125 mg/dl	Regard as additional reason for treatment[35]

*Overall risk for coronary heart disease (CHD)**: Defined by European Atherosclerosis Society as family history of CHD, smoking, hypertension, diabetes mellitus, male sex, and low HDL-cholesterol (< 35 mg/dL = < 0.9 mmol/L), especially in younger patients.[4] For discussion of cut-off values for blood lipids, see ref. 4.

(6.0 mmol/L) warranted a lipogram, upon which an LDL-cholesterol of above 160 mg/dl called for active treatment, sometimes including drugs.[59]

Other Lipid Abnormalities. The atherogenic role of lipid abnormalities other than cholesterol is not so clear-cut.[1,4,23] Although high blood **triglyceride** levels are common in patients with coronary heart disease (CHD), a specific causative role for hypertriglyceridemia in CHD still remains to be proven, with the exception of some rare abnormalities. An elevated blood triglyceride level may be viewed with special concern when combined with high blood cholesterol values (Table 10-1). Hypertriglyceridemia is often part of a **cluster of risk factors** including obesity, sedentary lifestyle, alcohol use, hypertension, and diabetes mellitus. **High-density lipoproteins** (HDL) may aid in clearing cholesterol from the diseased arteries. When the HDL-cholesterol falls below 35 mg/dl (0.9 mmol/L),[1,3] there is added reason for lipid-lowering therapy, especially in view of the 20-year follow-up study in Israel in which HDL had the highest predicted value for future coronary events.[51] The **LDL-cholesterol** should be no higher than 160 mg/dl. The ratio of HDL to LDL, when high, is one component of a favorable blood lipid profile.

Secondary Hyperlipidemias. Diabetes mellitus, hypothyroidism, nephrotic syndrome, alcoholism, and the use of some cardiac drugs as well as progestogens should be excluded and remedied if present.

DIETARY AND OTHER NON-DRUG THERAPY

Non-drug dietary therapy is basic to the management of all primary hyperlipidemias and frequently suffices as basic therapy when coupled with exercise, limitation of alcohol, and treatment of other risk factors such as smoking, hypertension, or diabetes. Only 1 hour of brisk walking per week increased HDL-cholesterol in previously sedentary British women.[45] More vigorous training increases HDL-cholesterol in men with coronary heart disease.[32]

The **dietary recommendations of the American Heart Association**[1] are based on three phases, applied consecutively if needed: Phase I: 30% of calories as fat; equal amounts of saturated, monosaturated, and polyunsaturated fatty acids; under 300 mg cholesterol. Phase II: 25% as fat, equal distribution of types of fatty acids, less than 200 to 250 mg cholesterol content. Phase III: 20% of calories as fat, equal distribution of types of fatty acids, with 100 to 150 mg cholesterol content. Sodium intake should be limited, as hypertension is often associated.

The use of oleic acid, as in olive oil, and of linoleic acid,[24] as in sunflower seed oil, may be beneficial. Fish oils such as cod liver oil may also be beneficial. Increasing evidence suggests that long-chain omega-3 fatty fish oils may be protective, at least in the post-infarct period and when the benefit is largely independent of any change of blood lipid levels.[36]

There should also be an increased intake of fruit, vegetables, and cereal fiber, so that the fiber intake is high, thereby producing a high-carbohydrate, high-fiber, cholesterol-lowering diet.

DRUG-RELATED HYPERLIPIDEMIAS

Drugs Causing Hyperlipidemias

The cardiac patient with hyperlipidemia may be receiving agents such as β-blockers or diuretics that may harmfully influence blood lipid profiles (Table 10-2), especially triglyceride values. Also β-blockers specifically tend to reduce HDL-cholesterol. β-Blockers with high intrinsic sympathomimetic activity (ISA) or high cardioselectivity may have less or no effect. Among the agents with the most consistent changes in triglycerides are chlorthalidone, and propranolol, and the combination propranolol-hydrochlorothiazide. However, total blood cholesterol levels are little changed, reduced by only about 8% or less during diuretic therapy, and by even less with β-blockade. Not all effects may be measured in the blood lipid constituents. Thus α-blockers move LDL particles to a larger, less dense type of LDL, whereas β-blockers tend to move particle size in the opposite direction.[65] **A profound effect can be found when diuretics are given to those with low initial cholesterol values as in the young, when the average increase of cholesterol is twice that found in older subjects.**[6] The fact that both β-blockers and diuretics also impair glucose metabolism is an added cause for concern when giving these agents to young patients.

TABLE 10-2 EFFECTS OF ANTIHYPERTENSIVE AGENTS INCLUDING DIURETICS AND β-BLOCKERS ON BLOOD LIPID PROFILES

Agent	Daily Dose	Duration	Total Cholesterol (%)	HDL Cholesterol (%)	LDL Cholesterol (%)	Triglycerides (%)	Reference
Diuretics							
HCTZ	12.5 mg	4 wks	+11	−12	+29	(13)	55
HCTZ	40 mg	12 wks	+10	0	+11	+11	62
HCTZ	50–100 mg	6–12 wks	0 to +10	0	0 to (+9)	0 to +17	7,8 12,22
Chlorthalidone	100 mg	6 wks	+8	0	+3	+15	7
Chlorthalidone	50–100 mg	1 yr	+5	0	+10	+10	6
Loop	ND	4–12 mths	(+4)	(−15)	ND	(+15)	27
Indapamide	2.5 mg	Various	0	0	0	0	27,44
Indapamide	2.5 mg	12 wks	+9	ND	ND	ND	8
β-Blockers, non-selective							
Propranolol	160 mg	8–12 wks	0	−14	0	+37 (+25)[a]	3,12
	180–240 mg	24 wks	0	−10	0	+20	64
Oxprenolol	160 mg	5–15 wks	0	(−5)	0	+18	3,12
Nadolol	ND	12 wks	0	ND	ND	+22	29
Sotalol	160–640 mg	26–52 wks	0 to +16	−10 to −28	0 to +32	+34 to +66	10,11,60
β-Blockers, selective							
Acebutolol	400 mg	24 wks	0	ND	ND	0	10
Bisoprolol	10 mg	2 yrs	0	0	0	+21	41
Atenolol	100 mg	5 wks–2yrs	0	(−4) to −19	0	+8 to +25	3,12 25,41
Metoprolol	200 mg	8–12 wks	(−1)	0	0	+10	3,23 17,25

250

	Dose	Duration					Ref
β-Blockers, vasodilatory							
Pindolol	7.5–15 mg	10–12 wks	0	+10	0	0 (+11)[b]	12,23
	15–45 mg	24 wks	0	+25	0	–22	64
Celiprolol (cardioselective)	400 mg	2 yrs	0	0	0	0	41
α-Blockers							
Prazosin	4 mg	8 wks	–9	0	–10	–16	12
Indoramin	50–100 mg	8 wks	0	0	–10	(+9)	17
α-β-Blockers							
Labetalol	300–1200 mg	12 wks; 1 yr	0	0	0	0	5,18
ACE inhibitors							
Captopril	50–100 mg	12 wks	0	0	0	0	62
Enalapril	10–40 mg	1 yr	0	ND	ND	0	16
Ca antagonists							
Nifedipine	40 mg SR[c]	48 wks	0	ND	ND	0	9
Verapamil	240–720 mg	12 wks	0	0	0	0	14
Diltiazem	90–180 mg	<12 wks	0	0	0	0	2
Nitrendipine	10–40 mg	3 wks	0	0	0	0	47
Combination therapy							
Methyldopa + HCTZ	300/50 mg	3 yrs	0	0	0	0	12
Propranolol + HCTZ	320/50 mg	3 yrs	0	–18	0	+44	12
Pindolol + HCTZ	20/50 mg	6–18 mths	0	+17	–4	0	26
Prazosin + HCTZ	8/50 mg	14 wks	0	0	0	0	22
Prazosin + propranolol	4/160 mg	8 wks	0	–8	0	0	12
Enalapril + HCTZ	40/50 mg	1 yr	0	ND	ND	0	16
Captopril + HCTZ	100/50 mg	6 wks	0	ND	ND	ND	28

a = after 6 years of propranolol.[27]
b = after 5 years of pindolol.[27]
c = nifedipine capsules have no effect on blood lipids over 8 weeks.[27]
Changes in brackets = not significant; HCTZ = hydrochlorothiazide; ND = no data; SR = slow release form of nifedipine.

Drugs Not Causing Hyperlipidemias (Lipid-neutral Agents)

Agents appearing to have no harmful effects on blood lipids include the ACE inhibitors, the calcium antagonists, and the combined α-β-blocker labetalol, besides the high ISA-containing β-blocker pindolol and the cardioselective vasodilatory agent celiprolol. The α-blockers, prazosin and others, appear to influence blood lipid profiles favorably. Higher doses of prazosin appear to have similar effects to lower doses.[27] Hydralazine and the centrally acting agents (reserpine, methyldopa, and clonidine) have little or no effect on blood lipids.[27]

Recommendations

β-**Blockers** given for angina may be replaced by calcium antagonists when there is fear of the consequences of triglyceride elevation. During the therapy of hypertension, β-blockers could likewise be replaced by α-blockers, α-β-blockers, ACE inhibitors, calcium antagonists, hydralazine, or centrally active agents. If β-blocking therapy is deemed important, cardioselective agents such as atenolol, metoprolol, or acebutolol, or agents with intrinsic sympathomimetic activity (ISA) such as pindolol[27] or acebutolol have relatively little effect on blood lipid profiles. In a small comparative trial, the vasodilatory cardioselective β-blocker **celiprolol** was compared with atenolol in hypertensive patients with hypercholesterolemia; celiprolol caused an overall beneficial change in the blood lipid profile compared with atenolol, in that there were falls in total cholesterol, LDL-cholesterol and triglyceride, and an increase in HDL-cholesterol.[42]

Diuretic doses should be kept low. Nonetheless, the expectation that with ultra-low diuretic doses, as recommended in this book (12.5 mg hydrochlorothiazide daily, Chap. 4, p 82), few or no adverse changes in blood lipids would be found, has not been met; 12.5 mg hydrochlorothiazide causes as much lipid disturbance as 100 mg although with many fewer other metabolic side-effects.[55] Indapamide 2.5 mg daily, an antihypertensive dose, may have relatively little effect on lipids, although data are conflicting.[8,27]

When **oral contraceptives** are given to patients with ischemic heart disease or those with risk factors such as smoking, possible atherogenic effects of high-estrogen contraceptives merit attention. Women receiving oral contraceptives or postmenopausal estrogens should not smoke.[30] Progestogens may have androgenic effects and lower HDL-cholesterol.

DRUGS FOR TREATMENT OF HYPERLIPIDEMIA

Lipid-lowering drugs may be required when dietary and risk factor management fails, when cardiovascular drugs are not at fault, and when there are no underlying diseases (hypothyroidism, poorly controlled diabetes mellitus, nephrotic syndrome; for hypertriglyceridemia, an excess alcohol intake or obesity). In general, lipid-lowering drugs frequently cause side-effects, usually subjective but sometimes serious. Serial blood lipid profiles are required to confirm the benefits of therapy. Failure to improve within 3 months merits drug change or combination therapy. Sometimes doses less than those usually recommended can be used in conjunction with dietary intervention or in drug combinations. The major types of lipid-lowering drugs (Table 10-3) are the bile acid sequestrants, nicotinic acid and its derivatives, the fibrates, probucol, and the reductase inhibitors. These all act in different ways (Figs. 10–1 and 10–2) not yet fully understood; hence combination therapy may give additive results.

TABLE 10–3 EFFECTS OF VARIOUS DRUGS ON BLOOD LIPID PROFILES IN PATIENTS WITH CORONARY ARTERY DISEASE OR MILD HYPERCHOLESTEROLEMIA STUDIED FOR 1 YEAR OR MORE

Drug	Total Cholesterol (% change)	HDL cholesterol (% change)	LDL cholesterol (% change)	Triglycerides (% change)	Reference
Cholestyramine	−7	+2	−11	+5	15
Clofibrate	−4 to −11	No data	No data	−25	37,40
Gemfibrozil	−9 to −15	+9 to +17	−9 to −18	−31 to −35	43,66
Nicotinic acid	−12	No data	No data	−29	37
Bezafibrate	−17	+23	−16	−16	57
Probucol	−15	−17	−14	−2	57
Simvastatin	−21	+7	−26	−10	66
Colestipol plus niacin	−22	+35 to +41	−34 to −38	−17	34,35
Colestipol plus lovastatin	No data	+14	−48	No data	35
Exercise	No change	+15	No change	−40	63

Data expressed as percent of initial value or concurrent placebo control, adjusted for changes in placebo group.
All drugs associated with dietary modifications.

Bile Acid Sequestrants

Cholestyramine (Questran) and **colestipol** (Colestid) bind bile acids so that they interrupt the enterohepatic recirculation. Hence the hepatic LDL-receptor population increases in numbers so that the blood LDL is more rapidly removed and total cholesterol falls (Fig. 10-1); there may be a transitory compensatory rise in plasma triglyceride, which is usually ignored.[69] However, a second agent such as nicotinic acid or a fibrate may be required to lower triglyceride. In the Lipid Research Clinics Coronary Primary Prevention Trial,[15] cholestyramine modestly reduced coronary heart disease in hypercholesterolemic patients, which was statistically significant only when a one-tailed P-test was used, without any effect on overall mortality. Sequestrants are marketed as powders that must be mixed with liquid or sprinkled on food. Low initial doses are increased to cholestyramine 16 to 24 g daily (maximum 36 g) and colestipol 20 to 25 g daily, in 2 divided doses. Such high doses are seldom well tolerated, so that combination therapy (later) is often a viable alternative. The major side-effects of these agents are gastrointestinal (GI): constipation, heartburn, and flatulence; with large doses, steatorrhea may occur rarely. Many patients need positive motivation from their physician to see themselves through the GI side-effects of these agents, and some cannot manage more than a low dose, which may nevertheless be useful when synergistically combined with other types of agents.[69] A new candy bar preparation of cholestyramine is often more acceptable, though clearly more expensive. Watch for interference with the absorption of digoxin, warfarin, thyroxine, and thiazides, which need to be taken 1 hour before or 4 hours after the sequestrant.[68]

Divistyramine, currently available in Holland, Italy and Switzerland, is said to be more palatable than cholestyramine, to not have the gritty taste of the latter, and to cause fewer abdominal cramps (because divistyramine is less hygroscopic). The dose is half that of cholestyramine.

Inhibition of Liver Lipid Production

Nicotinic acid (= niacin) is the only hypolipidemic drug shown to reduce overall mortality in a group of patients who had all had previous infarcts.[37] Also, it is the cheapest compound and can be bought over the counter. On the debit side, it has numerous subjective side-effects, though these can be lessened by carefully building up the dose and keeping the top dose lower than previously recommended.[31] Nicotinic acid inhibits secretion of lipoproteins from the liver so that low-density lipoproteins are reduced, including the triglyceride-rich component (VLDL). It consistently increases HDL-cholesterol. The basic effect of nicotinic acid may be decreased mobilization of free fatty acids from adipose tissue, so that there is less substrate for hepatic synthesis of lipoprotein lipid (Fig. 10-2). Side-effects, common and often dose-limiting, include prostaglandin-mediated symptoms, such as flushing, dizziness and palpitations, as well as impaired glucose tolerance, increased blood urate, liver dysfunction, and rashes. A history of gout, peptic ulcer, or diabetes is a contraindication to the drug. The dose required for lipid-lowering is 1 to 2 g 2x daily, achieved gradually with a low starting dose (100 mg 2x daily with meals to avoid GI discomfort[31]). The target dose could be lower (1.5–2 g daily) than that previously recommended (up to 4 g daily), with still marked effect on blood lipids and better tolerability and, furthermore, need be given only in two daily doses.[31] Flushing lessens with time and may also respond to low-dose aspirin.

Nicofuranose (Bradilan in UK) resembles nicotinic acid with, however, fewer prostaglandin-related side-effects. Although more expensive than nicotinic acid, it still is cheap.

Acipimox (Olbetam in UK) is a synthetic nicotinic acid analog with

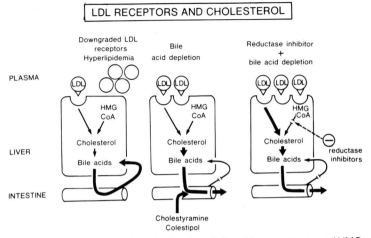

FIGURE 10–1. Proposed mode of action of bile acid sequestrants and HMG CoA reductase inhibitors, together with their combination. Bile acid sequestrants, such as cholestyramine, increase the number of LDL-receptors so that more cholesterol is cleared from the circulation (middle). Reductase inhibitors increase receptors through different mechanisms. Note the advantage of combination therapy of two different types of agents. LDL = low density lipoproteins. Figure copyright H.L. Opie.

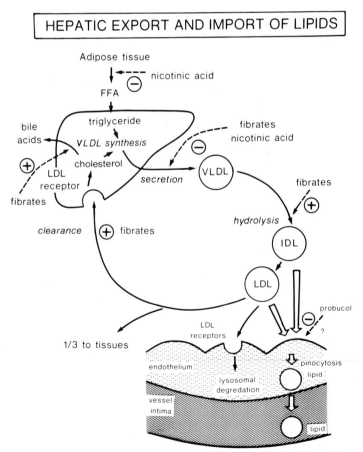

FIGURE 10–2. Proposed mechanism of action of fibrates, nicotinic acid, and probucol. LDL=low density lipoproteins; VLDL=very low density lipoproteins; IDL=intermediate density lipoproteins; and FFA=free fatty acids. Figure copyright L.H. Opie.

similar effects to nicotinic acid except that glucose tolerance may improve rather than deteriorate. Not unexpectedly, it is considerably more expensive than nicotinic acid.

The Fibrates: Activators of Plasma Lipoprotein Lipase

As a rule, none of the fibric acid derivatives reduce blood cholesterol as much as does nicotinic acid.[1] However, these agents may be preferable in conditions with high blood triglycerides. Fibrates may also reduce cholesterol and are especially effective in Type III lipidemia. They all have risk of a myositis-like syndrome, especially in patients with renal impairment or during co-therapy with the reductase inhibitors. Although all belong to the same group, structural differences between compounds seem important as judged by the very different results of large-scale trials on clofibrate (unfavorable) and gemfibrozil (favorable), stressing the requirement that each agent needs its own specific outcome trial.

Clofibrate (Atromid-S) promotes lipolysis of VLDL triglycerides by activating lipoprotein lipase, with secondary effects on blood cholesterol: also, excretion of sterols in the bile is enhanced. Among fibrates, this agent is now least used. Dose: 500 mg 2 to 3x daily after meals. Side-effects include abdominal discomfort, muscle pains, decreased libido, and cholesterol gallstones. Watch for warfarin potentiation. Initial enthusiasm for prophylaxis of coronary heart disease in the general population by clofibrate rapidly waned when it became evident that a massive European trial showed no improvement in mortality.[21] In fact, the improved cardiovascular mortality was more than offset by the increased mortality from operations required for cholesterol gallstones. Contraindications to clofibrate include biliary tract or hepatic disease, or severe renal disease. Presently, clofibrate is used chiefly for specific indications, as when hypertriglyceridemia has risk of pancreatitis.

Gemfibrozil (Lopid) is the agent used in the giant Helsinki Heart Study on 2,000 apparently healthy men with modest hypercholesterolemia, observed for 5 years.[43] Gemfibrozil in a dose of 600 mg 2x daily gave a major increase in HDL, a fall in LDL and triglyceride, and reduced coronary events by 34%. Nonetheless, the total death rate was unchanged, due to a combination of non-significant increases in intracranial hemorrhage, accidents and violence. Although there were somewhat more cataract operations and a theoretical risk of gallstone formation, no statistical significant changes were noted. The response to gemfibrozil is variable, taking up to 3 to 6 months, after which, if there is no benefit, therapy should be abandoned. Because it is highly protein bound, it potentiates warfarin. When combined with lovastatin, there is a high risk of myositis with myoglobinuria, and further risk of acute renal failure. Occasionally liver enzymes rise or there is bone marrow inhibition. Contraindications are co-therapy with lovastatin, hepatic or severe renal dysfunction, and pre-existing gallbladder disease, because of the possible risk of increased gallstones.

Bezafibrate (Bezalip, not in USA) may be more effective than clofibrate in raising HDL-cholesterol. It resembles gemfibrozil in its overall effects and side-effects. It also reduces total cholesterol, triglyceride and LDL-cholesterol.[56] Because plasma glucose tends to fall with bezafibrate, this agent may be useful in diabetics or those with abnormal glucose metabolic patterns. As with other fibrates, warfarin potentiation is possible and co-therapy with lovastatin/simvastatin should be avoided. In addition, myositis, renal failure, alopecia and loss of libido may occur. The dose is 200 mg 2 to 3x daily; however, once daily is nearly as good,[56] and there is now a slow-release formulation available (Bezalip-Mono, 400 mg once daily). Some increase in plasma creatinine is very common and of unknown consequence. The major problem with this agent is that unlike clofibrate and gemfibrozil, there are no long-term outcome trials.

Fenofibrate (Lipantil), used in Europe, is a pro-drug converted to finofibric acid in the tissues. It may reduce the cholesterol more than the other fibrates.[68]

Increased Non-receptor Mediated Cholesterol Clearance

Probucol (Lorelco in USA, Lurselle in UK) reserved for hypercholesterolemia, promotes clearance of both HDL- and LDL-cholesterol from the circulation without any effect on triglycerides, possibly acting by increased excretion of cholesterol in the bile. Its reduction of HDL may be regarded as undesirable; the package insert warns that there is a proportionately greater effect in lowering HDL than LDL-cholesterol. In addition, a non-lipid mechanism is likely: probucol has an antioxidant effect on the atherogenic process because oxidized LDL is taken up easier into the arterial wall by scavengers,[38] so that probucol can inhibit atheroma independently of effects on blood lipids. Furthermore, probucol can experimentally enhance HDL-mediated reversed cholesterol transport. These novel mechanisms need proof in man. The dose is 500 mg 2x daily with food. The side-effects, although potentially many, are usually not serious except for QT-prolongation, so that (1) the drug is contraindicated in patients with pre-existing prolonged QT; (2) it should not be given with any antiarrhythmic likely to prolong the QT or with diuretics (Fig. 8-8); (3) hypokalemia and hypomagnesemia must be excluded before therapy is started; and (4) ECGs must be taken before and during therapy. Minor side-effects include vomiting, flatulence, abdominal pain, and diarrhea; occasionally, the latter can be really troublesome. Because probucol is highly lipophilic and persists in adipose tissue for up to 6 months, pregnancy must not be embarked upon until the drug is withdrawn for that period. This is not a drug of choice for the cardiologist, particularly in view of the QT-prolongation.

HMG CoA Reductase Inhibitors: The Statins

These agents are generally regarded as an extremely exciting advance with relatively few side-effects; nonetheless, there have been no long-term outcome trials. The mechanism of action is shown in Figure 10–1.

Lovastatin (FDA approved, Mevacor) is the first commercially available hydroxymethylglutaryl coenzyme A (HMG CoA) reductase inhibitor. In a dose of 5 to 40 mg 2x daily, there is a dose response effect in reducing total cholesterol, LDL-cholesterol and triglycerides, while leaving HDL unchanged. In a dose of 20 to 40 mg 2x daily, it usually achieves the following treatment goals: total cholesterol below 240 mg/dl, LDL below 130 mg/dl, ratio LDL:HDL <3, provided it is combined with diet.[46] A single dose at night can be as effective, perhaps because cholesterol synthesis occurs largely at night.[68] In a comparative study, lovastatin 40 mg 2x daily was more effective in changing blood lipid profiles than was cholestyramine 4 to 12 mg 2x daily.[53] The most common side-effects are headache, surprisingly at about 10%, and GI problems such as flatulence, diarrhea, constipation, and nausea. Potentially serious but rare side-effects are myositis, liver damage, and lens opacification. Myositis with rhabdomyolysis and risk of acute renal failure occurs, especially during co-therapy with fibrates or nicotinic acid or with cyclosporin in transplant patients, and in the latter case up to one-third of the patients are at risk of this complication.

Cautions and contraindications in the use of HMG CoA reductase inhibitors include fertile women not on contraception, patients with pre-existing hepatic pathology or at risk of hepatic injury, patients on cyclosporin or other cytotoxic drugs, and patients on one of the fibrates or nicotinic acid or participating in severe physical exertion.[33]

Simvastatin (Zocor in UK) is a similar agent shown to work in patients with genetic hypercholesterolemia[33] with a lower dose and given once daily with supper (20-40 mg). It also increases HDL-cholesterol. It is more effective than probucol in achieving an ideal lipid profile.[61] Combination with cholestyramine causes LDL-cholesterol to fall faster. Side-effects include a rise in plasma creatine kinase (myositis) and transaminase (hepatic damage).

Several other agents soon to become available include **pravastatin** (already in Europe) and **mevastatin**.

Combination Therapy

The best combinations are those acting by different mechanisms. For example, colestipol plus lovastatin or niacin (C = 30 g/day; L = 40 mg/day; niacin = 4 g/day) decreased blood LDL, increased HDL, and decreased both measured coronary stenosis and coronary events when compared with placebo or colestipol.[35] The lipid changes achieved by colestipol plus niacin were accompanied by a decreased rate of development of angiographically demonstrated new coronary lesions.[34] In familial hypercholesterolemia, an excellent lipid-lowering triple combination was colestipol-niacin-lovastatin,[54] which decreased total cholesterol by 55%, LDL-cholesterol by 66%, triglyceride by 42%, and increased HDL-cholesterol by 35%. (Risk of myositis increased by lovastatin-niacin.) Other combinations and their effects on HDL are discussed by Witztum.[69] In general, the combination of reductase inhibitors and fibrates or nicotinic acid should not be used (risk of myositis).

Pregnancy and Lipid-lowering Drugs

As a group, lipid-lowering drugs are contraindicated during pregnancy; the bile acid sequestrants may be safest. Women desiring to become pregnant should stop other lipid-lowering drugs for about six months before conception.

Lipid Clinic Referrals

The cardiologist should consider obtaining advice from a lipid clinic if there is severe hypercholesterolemia (including the familial homozygous variety) or severe hypertriglyceridemia, or if the lipid profile remains unfavorable despite vigorous diet and eventual drug treatment.

ANTIATHEROSCLEROTIC DRUGS

The drug treatment of established coronary atherosclerosis is still in its infancy. First, it is hoped that persistent lowering of blood cholesterol will lead to an exit of cholesterol from the plaque to the circulation so that the degree of coronary stenosis is lessened, as noted in the preliminary study of Brown and colleagues.[35] Second, prophylactic aspirin, now common in use, is thought to protect by inhibiting the platelet participation in the atherosclerotic process. The evidence for this role of aspirin is still somewhat slender. Third, the calcium antagonists, and especially nifedipine, have proven beneficial in preventing formation of new coronary lesions,[67] yet without any benefit on mortality. In the INTACT study,[50] non-coronary mortality was actually increased in the nifedipine group, apparently as a chance event in the relatively small numbers included. Fourth, β-blockers may prevent some types of atheroma in highly stressed primates, presumably acting by inhibition of FFA mobilization from adipose tissue and the consequent effect of FFA in promoting platelet aggregation. Thus far, there have been no trials in humans on the use of β-blockade for this possible indication. In one relatively small study, propranolol was much less effective than nifedipine in decreasing formation of new coronary plaques.[52] Finally, early experimental data show that captopril has a potent antiatherosclerotic action.[39,67]

SUMMARY

The basis for the usual therapy of hyperlipidemias, apart from the severe and hereditary types, is strict dietary modification. Lipidemias secondary to drugs and diseases must be excluded. Among the cardiac drugs tending to cause hyperlipidemias are β-blockers (especially non-selective agents such as propranolol) and thiazide diuretics. Careful attention to all other coronary risk factors is essential. No ideal lipid-lowering drug has yet been evolved. The new HMG CoA reductase inhibitors are increasingly impressive and widely used; disadvantages are the cost and the absence of large-scale outcome trials. Each of the existing agents can be used with success for specific indications when dietary management fails or is inappropriate. The new tendency is to reason that each type of agent has a different mechanism of action, so that combination therapy is appropriate if diet plus cholestyramine/colestipol fails. A forbidden combination is that of a reductase inhibitor with fibrates because of the high risk of myositis and renal failure; combination with nicotinic acid should also be avoided. The ideal blood cholesterol level appears to be falling lower and lower, emphasizing the virtues of dietary advice for all cardiac patients. Similar principles apply to post-infarct management, where lipid-lowering is an essential part of a comprehensive program of risk factor modification.

REFERENCES

References from Previous Editions

1. AHA Special Report: Circulation 69:1067A–1090A, 1969
2. Chaffman M, Brogden RN: Drugs 29:387–454, 1985
3. Day L, Metcalfe J, Simpson CN: Br Med J 284:1145–1148, 1982
4. European Atherosclerosis Society: Eur Heart J 8:77–88, 1987
5. Frishman W, Michelson E, Johnson B, et al: Am J Cardiol 49:984, 1982
6. Goldman AI, Steele BW, Schnaper HW, et al: JAMA 244:1691–1695, 1980
7. Grimm RH Jr, Leon AS, Hunninghake DB, et al: Ann Intern Med 94:7–11, 1981
8. Kreeft JH, Langlois S, Ogilvie RI: J Cardiovasc Pharmacol 6:622–626, 1984
9. Landmark K: J Cardiovasc Pharmacol 7:12–17, 1985
10. Lehtonen A: Am Heart J 109:1192–1196, 1985
11. Lehtonen A, Viikari J: Clin Sci 57:405s–407s, 1979
12. Leren P, Eide I, Foss A, et al: Br J Clin Pharmacol 13:441S–444S, 1982
13. Lewis B, Mann JI: Lancet 1:956–959, 1986
14. Lewis GRJ: Am J Cardiol 57:35D–38D, 1986
15. Lipid Research Clinics Coronary Primary Prevention Trial Results: JAMA 251:351, 1984
16. Malini PL, Strocchi E, Ambrosioni E, et al. J Hypertens 2(suppl 2):101–105, 1984
17. Martinez TLR, Auriemo CRC, Machado AMO, et al: J Cardiovasc Pharmacol 8(suppl 2):S76–S79, 1986
18. McGonigle RJS, Williams L, Murphy MJ, et al: Lancet 1:163, 1981
19. NIH Consensus Conference: JAMA 253:2080–2086, 1985
20. Oliver MF: Lancet 2:655, 1982
21. Oliver MF, Heady JA: Lancet 2:600–604, 1984
22. Overlack A, Stumpe KO. J Cardiovasc Pharmacol 8(suppl 2):S53–S55, 1986

23. Pasotti C, Capra A, Fiorella G, et al: Br J Clin Pharmacol 13:435S–439S, 1982
24. Riemersma RA, Wood DA, Butler S, et al: Br Med J 292:1423–1427, 1986
25. Rossner S, Weiner L: Drugs 25(suppl 2):322–325, 1983
26. Samuel P, Chin B, Fenderson RW, et al: Am J Cardiol 57:24C–28C, 1986
27. Weidmann P, Uehlinger DE, Gerber A: J Hypertens 3:297–306, 1985
28. Weinberger MH: Hypertension 5(suppl III):132–138, 1983
29. Weinberger MH: Arch Intern Med 145:1102–1105, 1985
30. Wilson PWF, Garrison RJ, Castelli WP: N Engl J Med 313:1038–1043, 1985

New References

31. Alderman JD, Pasternak RC, Sacks FM, et al: Effect of a modified, well-tolerated niacin regimen on serum total cholesterol, high density lipoprotein cholesterol and the cholesterol to high density lipoprotein ratio. Am J Cardiol 64:725–729, 1989
32. Arvan S, Rueda BG: Nonselective β-receptor blocker effect on high density lipoprotein cholesterol after chronic exercise. J Am Coll Cardiol 12:662–668, 1988
33. Berger GMB, Marais AD, Seftel HC, et al: Treatment of hypercholesterolemia with the HMG CoA reductase inhibitor, simvastatin. Cardiovasc Drugs Ther 3:219–227, 1989
34. Blankenhorn DH, Nessim SA, Johnson RL, et al: Beneficial effects of combined colestipol-niacin therapy on coronary atherosclerosis and coronary venous bypass grafts. JAMA 257:3233–3240, 1987
35. Brown BG, Lin JT, Schaefer SM, et al: Niacin or lovastatin, combined with colestipol, regress coronary atherosclerosis and prevent clinical events in men with elevated apolipoprotein B (abstract). Circulation 80(suppl II):II-266, 1989
36. Burr ML, Fehily AM, Gilbert JF, et al: Effects of changes in fat, fish, and fibre intakes on death and myocardial reinfarction: Diet and reinfarction trial (DART). Lancet 2:757–761, 1989
37. Canner PL, Berge KG, Wenger NK, et al: Fifteen year mortality in coronary drug project patients: Long-term benefit with niacin. J Am Coll Cardiol 8:1245–1255, 1986
38. Carew TE: Role of biologically modified low-density lipoprotein in atherosclerosis. Am J Cardiol 64:18G–22G, 1989
39. Chobanian AV, Haudenschild CC, Nickerson C, Drago R: Antiatherogenic effect of captopril in the Watanabe heritable hyperlipidemic rabbit. Hypertension 15:327–331, 1990
40. Committee of Principal Investigators: A co-operative trial in the primary prevention of ischaemic heart disease using clofibrate. Br Heart J 40:1069-1118, 1978
41. Fogari R, Zoppi A, Pasotti C, et al: Plasma lipids during chronic antihypertensive therapy with different β-blockers. J Cardiovasc Pharmacol 14(suppl 7):S28–S32, 1989
42. Fogari R, Zoppi A, Tettamanti F, et al: The effect of celiprolol on the blood lipid profile in hypertensive patients with high cholesterol. Cardiovasc Drugs Ther, 1990 (in press)
43. Frick MH, Elo O, Haapa K, et al: Helsinki Heart Study: Primary prevention trial with gemfibrozil in middle-aged men with dyslipidemia. N Engl J Med 317:1237–1245, 1987
44. Gerber A, Weidmann P, Bianchetti MG, et al: Serum lipoproteins during treatment with the antihypertensive agent indapamide. Hypertension 7(suppl II):II164–II169, 1985
45. Hardman AE, Hudson A, Jones PRM, Norgan NG: Brisk walking and plasma high density lipoprotein cholesterol concentration in previously sedentary women. Br Med J 299:1204–1205, 1989
46. Henwood JM, Heel RC. Lovastatin: A preliminary review of its pharmacodynamic properties and therapeutic use in hyperlipidaemia. Drugs 36:429–454, 1988
47. Johnson BF, Romero L, Marwaha R: Hemodynamic and metabolic effects of the calcium channel blocking agent nitrendipine. Clin Pharmacol Ther 39:389–394, 1986
48. Kaplan NM: Critical comments on recent literature: The cholesterol campaign: American aggressiveness and British reservations. Am J Hypertens 2:941–942, 1989
49. Editorial: Secondary prevention of coronary disease with lipid lowering drugs (Anonymous). Lancet 1:473–474, 1989

50. Lichtlen PR, Hugenholtz PG, Rafflenbeul W, et al: Retardation of coronary artery disease in man by the calcium channel blocker nifedipine: Results of INTACT (International Nifedipine Trial on Antiatherosclerotic Therapy). Lancet 335:1109-1113, 1990
51. Livshits G, Weisbort J, Meshulam N, Brunner D: Multivariate analysis of the twenty-year follow-up of the Donolo-Tel Aviv Prospective Coronary Artery Disease Study and the usefulness of high density lipoprotein cholesterol percentage. Am J Cardiol 63:676–681, 1989
52. Loaldi A, Polese A, Montorsi P, et al: Comparison of nifedipine, propranolol and isosorbide dinitrate on angiographic progression and regression of coronary arterial narrowings in angina pectoris. Am J Cardiol 64:433–439, 1989
53. Lovastatin Study Group III: A multicenter comparison of lovastatin and cholestyramine in the therapy of severe primary hypercholesterolemia. JAMA 260:359–366, 1988
54. Malloy MJ, Kane JP, Kunitake ST, Tun P: Complementarity of colestipol, niacin, and lovastatin in treatment of severe familial hypercholesterolemia. Ann Intern Med 107:616–623, 1987
55. McKenney JM, Goodman RP, Wright JT, et al: The effect of low-dose hydrochlorothiazide on blood pressure, serum potassium and lipoproteins. Pharmacotherapy 6:179–184, 1986
56. Monk JP, Todd PA: Bezafibrate. A review of its pharmacodynamic and pharmacokinetic properties, and therapeutic use in hyperlipidaemia. Drugs 33:539–576, 1987
57. Mordasini R, Riesen W, Oster P, Riva G: Verhalten der high-density-lipoproteine (HDL) unter medikamentoser lipidsenkender behandlung. Schweizerische Medizinische Wochenschrift 112:95–97, 1982
58. Moss AJ, Benhorin J: Prognosis and management after a first myocardial infarction. N Engl J Med 322:743–753, 1990
59. National Cholesterol Education Program Expert Panel on Detection, Evaluation, and Treatment of High Blood Cholesterol in Adults: Arch Intern Med 148:36–69, 1988
60. Northcote RJ, Packard CJ, Ballantyne D: The effect of sotalol on plasma lipoproteins and apolipoproteins. Clin Chem Acta 158:187–192, 1986
61. Pietro DA, Alexander S, Mantell G, et al: Effects of simvastatin and probucol in hypercholesterolemia (Simvastatin Multicenter Study Group II). Am J Cardiol 63:682–686, 1989
62. Pollare T, Lithell H, Berne C: A comparison of the effects of hydrochlorothiazide and captopril on glucose and lipid metabolism in patients with hypertension. N Engl J Med 321:868–873, 1989
63. Reaven PD, McPhillips JB, Criqui MH, Barrett-Connor E: Effect of physical activity on lipid and lipoprotein levels in older men (abstract). Circulation 80(suppl II):II-509, 1989
64. Roman O, Pino ME, Pereda T, Valenzuela A: Effects of pindolol and propranolol on blood lipids in hypertensive patients. Cardiovasc Drugs Ther 3:767–770, 1989
65. Superko HR: Drug therapy and the prevention of atherosclerosis in humans. Am J Cardiol 64:31G–38G, 1989
66. Tikkanen MJ, Bocanegra TS, Walker F, Cook T: The Simvastatin Study Group: Comparison of low-dose simvastatin and gemfibrozil in the treatment of elevated plasma cholesterol. Am J Med 87(suppl 4A):4A–47S, 1989

Reviews

67. Fleckenstein A, Frey M, Zorn J, Fleckenstein-Grun G: Calcium, a neglected key factor in hypertension and arteriosclerosis: Experimental vasoprotection with calcium antagonists or ACE inhibitors. In Laragh JH, Brenner BM (eds): Hypertension: Pathophysiology, Diagnosis and Management. New York, Raven Press, 1990, pp 471–509
68. O'Connor P, Feely J, Shepherd J: Lipid lowering drugs. Br Med J 300:667–672, 1990
69. Witztum JL: Current approaches to drug therapy for the hypercholesterolemic patient. Circulation 80:1101–1114, 1989

B.J. Gersh
L.H. Opie

Which Drug for Which Condition?

ANGINA PECTORIS

For **exertional angina pectoris**, initial treatment requires attention to precipitating factors (hypertension, anemia, congestive heart failure [CHF], tachyarrhythmias, and valve disease). Sublingual nitroglycerin in combination with either a β-blocker or calcium antagonist remains standard therapy. Thereafter, the addition of long-acting nitrates is indicated. To avoid or lessen nitrate tolerance, "eccentric" dosage schedules are recommended for long-acting preparations (see Table 2-3). Alternatively, β-blockers and calcium antagonists are often combined. The superiority of this approach to optimal doses of β-blockade and nitrates alone has been challenged[86] and defended.[103] The β-blocker-calcium antagonist combination seems safest in the case of nifedipine and is pharmacokinetically simplest with β-blockers such as atenolol, which are not metabolized by the liver. The combination of verapamil or diltiazem with a β-blocker is also possible, although particular care should be taken in patients with left ventricular dysfunction or conduction defects.[72] "Triple therapy" with nitrates, calcium antagonists, and β-blockade should not be automatically equated with maximal therapy because patients' reactions vary.

In true **Prinzmetal's angina**, a relatively rare condition, β-blockers are inferior to calcium antagonists and may aggravate the condition. In refractory cases of Prinzmetal's angina associated with coronary artery disease, bypass grafting combined with cardiac sympathetic denervation (plexectomy) appears superior to bypass alone.[4]

In **combined exertional and rest angina**, it has in the past been supposed that calcium antagonists should be better than β-blockers, but that is not the case. Atenolol 100 mg daily was better than either nifedipine 20 mg 3x daily or isosorbide mononitrate 40 mg b.d. in a cross-over study.[94] Of particular note is that all three agents were equieffective for control of nocturnal angina and silent ST-changes.

In **unstable angina with threat of AMI**, the present trend is to combine anti-ischemic therapy (β-blockers and nitrates) with antithrombotic therapy (heparin or aspirin). Either heparin or aspirin induces a dramatic improvement in the outcome at 48 hours,[106] but the combination heparin-aspirin is no better. Aspirin itself does not decrease pain or associated silent ST-segment shifts,[83] whereas heparin does. Therefore treatment is initiated by heparin, and as it is stopped, aspirin is started. There are no good data indicating that β-blockade by itself is beneficial. The often quoted HINT study[63] was inconclusive when comparing the β-blocker metoprolol with placebo in unstable angina, although it clearly showed that the addition of nifedipine to pre-existing β-blocker therapy was beneficial. With the ultrashort-acting β-blocker esmolol, there are fewer episodes of anterior ischemia when compared with placebo.[43] Diltiazem, a calcium antagonist acting hemodynamically differently from nifedipine, may be used instead of a β-blocker and is equieffective;[105] once again, diltiazem has not been compared with placebo. In the HINT study, nifedipine by itself was clearly detrimental, which is why this study was stopped. **In the absence of coronary spasm, the case for routine nifedipine is very weak;** two randomized trials in unstable angina have shown that it causes harm, presumably by excess hypotensive or tachycardic effects, unless nifedipine is combined with a β-blocker. Regardless of drug therapy, many patients require coronary revascularization (bypass or PTCA) within the first few months.[89] Currently much interest centers on the possible use of thrombolytic therapy, without clarification of its precise role.[109]

Coronary Artery Bypass Surgery and PTCA for Angina Pectoris. Multiple studies over the last 20 years have provided a clear message: In patients at high risk, revascularization prolongs survival in comparison with medical therapy alone.[56] High risk patients are characterized by unstable angina, effort angina that is more than mild, left mainstem disease whether symptomatic or not, LV dysfunction, especially when combined with multivessel disease, and an age of 65 years or more.[104] **The decision about surgery must be tailored to the individual and needs to take into account all these complex factors** and, in addition, the patient's lifestyle, occupation, other medical conditions, and tolerance for medical therapy. Even in some higher risk patients, careful medical therapy may lead to clinical improvement[13] with the option for subsequent revascularization still there.

Percutaneous Transluminal Coronary Angioplasty (PTCA). PTCA is extensively employed and works well, especially for severely symptomatic single vessel disease, though there have been no randomized trials proving its efficacy when compared with medical therapy or surgery; several such trials are now in progress. Restenosis remains a significant problem and is the "Achilles heel" of angioplasty.

SILENT MYOCARDIAL ISCHEMIA

"Silent" ECG ischemia, detected by ST-segment deviations on ambulatory monitoring, constitutes part of the total ischemic burden in coronary artery disease. Yet it is not known whether therapy should specifically be directed toward the silent component, whether silent ischemia needs to be shortened in duration or totally eliminated, or whether therapy may best be guided by clinically overt features such as chest pain. In a preliminary presentation on patients with both stable angina and silent ischemia, diltiazem-SR, nifedipine, and propranolol-LA all improved exercise tolerance, but surprisingly only propranolol reduced silent ischemia.[102] However, in other preliminary reports, diltiazem, atenolol, and nifedipine were all effective against silent ischemia.[58,107] The general rule seems to be that the same agents benefiting patients with overt angina also help for silent ischemia.

ACUTE MYOCARDIAL INFARCTION (AMI)

Morphine (5–10 mg slow IV at 1 mg/min) combines a potent analgesic effect with hemodynamic actions that are particularly beneficial in reducing myocardial oxygen demand (MVO_2), namely a marked venodilator action reducing ventricular preload, an ability to decrease heart rate, and a mild arterial vasodilator action that may reduce afterload. In the presence of hypovolemia, morphine may cause profound hypotension. **Atropine** (IV 0.3 mg aliquots to maximum of 2.0 mg) has a vagolytic effect that is useful for the management of bradyarrhythmias with atrioventricular (AV) block (particularly with inferior infarction), sinus or nodal bradycardia with hypotension, or bradycardia-related ventricular ectopy. Small doses and careful monitoring are essential since the elimination of vagal overactivity may unmask latent sympathetic overactivity, producing sinus tachycardia and rarely even ventricular tachycardia (VT) or fibrillation (VF).[31] The role of prophylactic atropine for uncomplicated bradycardia is questionable.

Sinus tachycardia is a common manifestation of early phase sympathetic overactivity, which increases myocardial oxygen demand (MVO_2) and predisposes to tachyarrhythmias. **The first step is to treat the underlying cause**—for example, pain, anxiety, hypovolemia or pump failure—and then to use a β-blocker, which can be safe and effective provided that the patient is carefully observed.

Acute hypertension increases afterload and MVO_2 improves perfusion of the ischemic zone. Thus the benefits of BP reduction in AMI are not clear unless there is LV failure (frequent in severe infarcts). Nor is the ideal rate of BP reduction known; a smooth and careful reduction by IV nitroglycerin or nitroprusside seems best; other tested drugs include IV labetalol, IV esmolol, and sublingual nifedipine. The mean BP should not fall below 80 mm Hg.[66] In experimental coronary stenosis without infarction, the lower the heart rate the higher the BP that can be tolerated.[6]

Acute Reperfusion Therapy

An increase in the blood supply remains the most effective mode of preserving the ischemic myocardium and reducing infarct size. Fibrinolytic therapy has come to dominate discussions on the management of early AMI (Chap. 9). Yet pivotal questions remain unanswered. Areas of persistent controversy include the efficacy of "late" reperfusion (more than 6 hours), which agent or combination of agents is best, and the role of adjuvant therapy such as β-blockade to "widen" the therapeutic window.

Despite these reservations, IV thrombolytic therapy has become standard for patients with evolving myocardial infarction, especially when there is ST-segment elevation (ECG ischemia rather than necrosis). Numerous trials have documented a reduction in mortality compared with placebo. The greatest benefit is obtained with early administration, within 4 to 6 hours of the onset of symptoms.

Reperfusion Injury. Considerable experimental evidence points to a spectrum of reperfusion events, including ventricular arrhythmias, mechanical "stunning," and microvascular injury.[84] Evidence for reperfusion-induced cell necrosis is less clear. Nonetheless, the clinical application of reperfusion injury remains unconfirmed, although free radical formation follows successful thrombolysis.[49] Initial clinical studies with free radical scavengers, such as superoxide dismutase, have shown no benefit. At present the best means of lessening reperfusion injury is to limit the severity of ischemic injury (for example by β-blockade).[84]

Re-occlusion. Successful thrombolysis is not an end in itself. Re-occlusion occurs in 10 to 20% of patients and there are many contributory factors, including the severity of the underlying residual stenosis, the persistence of the initial thrombogenic substrate (plaque fissure), and activation of platelets and the clotting cascade. Although optimal post-thrombolytic therapy is not known, IV heparin can be replaced by aspirin-dipyridamole 24 hours post-thrombolysis without adverse effects.[82] However, in the first 18 hours it is heparin rather than aspirin that ensures higher patency rates.[60] Other studies suggest that heparin should be maintained for about 5 days (see p 240).

Post-thrombolytic PTCA. Following thrombolytic therapy, emergency PTCA is not helpful and may be harmful unless there is recurrent ischemia.[108] In the absence of thrombolytic therapy, PTCA can be a primary procedure, especially in cardiogenic shock.[71] In patients with failed thrombolytic therapy, "rescue" PTCA is logical, its efficacy being limited by the inability to determine non-invasively which patients have undergone successful reperfusion.

Prophylactic Early β-Blockade

Pooled data on trials of ten β-blockers on about 50,000 patients suggest a 15% reduction in acute phase mortality, with a 25 to 30% reduction in late phase mortality.[42,54] These benefits of early IV β-blockade, although not dramatic, are sufficiently convincing to consider β-blockade even in the absence of other indications, such as sinus tachycardia or hypertension. Heart rate reduction is required for infarct size limitation.[20] In a borderline hemodynamic situation, an "on-off" test of transient β-blockade can be achieved by titrated IV esmolol. When β-blockade needs abrupt cessation, there is no major withdrawal rebound.[9] Early β-blockade may be combined with early reperfusion, which appears to reduce recurrent infarction and ischemia,[108] to reduce the risk of cerebral hemorrhage following tPA,[110] and to lessen chest pain.[62]

Therapy of Ventricular Arrhythmias in Acute Infarction

Lidocaine (lignocaine) is widely used in the prophylaxis and therapy of early post-infarction arrhythmias. Whether prophylactic lidocaine therapy to abolish "warning arrhythmias" and to limit VF should be used remains controversial (Chap. 8). Failing lidocaine, procainamide or Class III agents are used (bretylium, amiodarone). β-Blockers also have prophylactic antiarrhythmic benefit in AMI.[28] Pacing techniques (atrial or ventricular), stellate ganglion blockade, or programmed ventricular stimulation may occasionally be lifesaving.

Treatment of LV failure is an essential adjunct to antiarrhythmic therapy, and the possibility of drug-induced VT or hypokalemia should always be borne in mind.

SUPRAVENTRICULAR ARRHYTHMIAS IN AMI

Atrial fibrillation, flutter, and paroxysmal supraventricular tachycardia are usually transient but are recurrent and troublesome. Precipitating factors requiring treatment include hypoxia, acidosis, heart failure with atrial distention, pericarditis, and sinus node ischemia. Initial therapy should be carotid sinus massage or other vagal maneuvers in the case of supraventricular tachycardia. In the absence of LV failure, verapamil or the new ultrashort-acting β-blocker esmolol are effective in controlling the ventricular rate. In the presence of LV failure, IV adenosine (just released in the USA as Adenocard) or careful use of esmolol may be tried. Cardioversion is limited to resistant cases with hemodynamic compromise. Recurrent atrial flutter may respond to atrial overdrive pacing.

LV Failure with Pulmonary Congestion

Swan-Ganz catheterization to measure LV filling pressure and cardiac output allows a rational choice between various IV agents that reduce both preload and afterload or chiefly the preload. The increasing use of bedside echocardiographic techniques to monitor LV function in AMI means that Swan-Ganz catheterization is being used less frequently. The diuretic furosemide, although standard therapy and acting by rapid vasodilation as well as by diuresis, may sometimes paradoxically induce vasoconstriction. In the patient with AMI and pulmonary edema, excess diuresis with preload reduction and relative volume depletion must be avoided. These patients have reduced ventricular compliance and require higher filling pressures to maintain cardiac output.

Where there are no intensive care facilities, IV unloading agents such as nitroprusside and nitrates are best avoided. In theory, sublingual agents that reduce the preload (short-acting nitrates) or the pre- and afterload (captopril) should be useful here. Nifedipine, still recommended for afterload reduction in AMI complicated by hypertension, is otherwise contraindicated because of the risk of hypotension and myocardial underperfusion.

Early use of ACE inhibitors is now becoming more common. Logically, captopril with its rapid onset of action and the absence of any requirement for liver metabolism, should be the agent of choice. Heart failure with recurrent angina pectoris in AMI is particularly amenable to therapy with IV nitroglycerin or nitroprusside.

"Forward Failure" in AMI

When cardiac output is low in the absence of an elevated wedge pressure or clinical and radiographic evidence of LV failure, it is crucial to exclude hypovolemia (possibly drug-induced) and right ventricular infarction. In the absence of one of these, the best strategy is to employ ACE inhibitors alone or in combination with a positively inotropic agent such as dopamine or dobutamine. Inotropic-vasodilator therapy is logical provided that arrhythmias are monitored and hypokalemia is avoided. Monitoring the hemodynamic response invasively is indispensable in this situation. Nitrates are usually contraindicated because their main effect is reduction of preload.

Inotropic support by digitalis in AMI is controversial (Chap. 6). The benefits of digoxin in AMI are probably small, so that its use is restricted to patients with frank LV failure not responding to furosemide, nitrates, or ACE inhibitors, or patients with atrial tachyarrhythmias in whom verapamil or esmolol fails or is contraindicated.

In **cardiogenic shock**, there is severe forward failure, and acute angioplasty may be of dramatic benefit.[71]

Limitation of Infarct Size

Since myocardial infarction is ultimately the consequence of an imbalance between myocardial oxygen supply and demand, it is logical and prudent to employ measures aimed at redressing this. These measures include the treatment of arrhythmias, hypoxia, heart failure, hypertension, and tachycardia. Hypokalemia should be sought and treated. Despite much experimental evidence that numerous pharmacologic agents such as β-blockers, hyaluronidase, nitrates, metabolic agents such as glucose-insulin-potassium, or free radical scavengers will reduce infarct size, clinical evidence of benefit has been difficult to obtain.

Pooled data from 10 trials of **IV nitroglycerin or nitroprusside** involving about 2,000 patients showed an average reduction of 35% in the odds of death, especially during the first week.[114] In a randomized trial, IV nitroglycerin limited infarct related complications, especially when given early with a target mean BP of <80 mm Hg.[66]

Early β-blockade may confer part of its benefits by limitation of infarct size; there is reasonable evidence for a small effect.

Calcium antagonists, on the other hand, should not be given routinely in AMI.[61] A possible exception lies in non-Q-wave infarction,[57] but the case is not immaculate.

Metabolic support by glucose-insulin-potassium (GIK) appears to reduce in-hospital mortality in patients in Killip functional classes I to III.[27] However, the absence of a really large randomized trial, and particularly the lack of any commercial backer, seems to limit interest in GIK. When combined with reperfusion in a small study, there was again benefit from GIK.[97]

LONG-TERM THERAPY AFTER AMI

Risk Factor Management. Cessation of smoking, rehabilitation exercise, and control of blood lipids are all of value in randomized trials. Until recently, there were no good data showing the benefit of control of post-infarct hypertension. Subgroup analysis of the multicenter diltiazem post-infarct trial showed that diltiazem decreased blood pressure and improved survival over 1 to 4 years;[80] however, diltiazem is contraindicated if the LV ejection fraction is <40%.

β-Blockade. Three important randomized double-blind studies show a clear-cut benefit in the secondary prevention of death following myocardial infarction in subjects treated with timolol,[24] metoprolol,[16] and propranolol.[2] With atenolol, the drug was given intravenously followed by oral therapy for 7 days and the subjects were followed for 1 year. Most of the benefit was achieved within the first week, but the groups could still be distinguished after 1 year. Obvious contraindications to β-blockade are overt heart failure, severe bradycardia, hypotension, asthma, and heart block greater than first degree. Approximately half the patients entering these trials were excluded. In patients in whom β-blockade is not started within the first few hours, it is generally commenced before hospital discharge (given with aspirin).

Several questions remain unanswered (see Chap. 1): One is whether the effect applies to all other β-blockers except those with intrinsic sympathomimetic activity;[39] if so, acebutolol is an exception (see p 16). What is the mechanism of the reduction in mortality? When should therapy be initiated and for how long? Further information about subsets of patients more likely to benefit from β-blockade is needed. There seems little point in giving β-blockade to patients with good LV function, no clinical evidence of ischemia or arrhythmias, and at low risk of mortality. In others, it would appear reasonable to give β-blockers to patients in the 30 to 70 year age group who have no contraindications. Mild to moderate compensated congestive heart failure is not a contraindication to post-infarct β-blockade, and a history of prior CHF renders β-blockade more rather than less effective.[7] The timolol and sotalol studies show that β-blockade can be discontinued abruptly.

Calcium Antagonists. Because as a group these agents do not give post-infarct protection,[61] they should not be used unless there is a specific indication such as hypertension or angina not responsive to β-blockade or in a patient with respiratory disease. The basic reason for the failure of calcium antagonists appears to be that those with LV failure do badly.[81] In a new large Danish post-infarct trial (DAVIT II, as yet unpublished) in which LV failure was prospectively excluded, verapamil 120 mg 3x daily decreased re-infarction and cardiac mortality. Verapamil is therefore a viable alternative to β-blockade in patients without LV failure.

Platelet Inhibitor Agents and Anticoagulants. Aspirin, the simplest and safest agent, is now established therapy, starting with an oral dose as soon as possible after the onset of symptoms of AMI and continuing indefinitely thereafter. It prevents re-infarction, stroke, and vascular mortality as shown by 25 trials.[40] In the past, the recommended dose was 1 tablet daily, 300 to 325 mg, but the ISIS-II trial used 160 mg daily.[65] The lower dose should have fewer side-effects. Aspirin may also be selected for those patients thought to be at risk of thromboembolism in whom oral anticoagulation is not advisable or in patients not likely to comply with the stringent requirements for prolonged oral anticoagulation therapy. Sulfinpyrazone and dipyridamole have shown marginal benefit at best, so that their routine use in post-infarction patients cannot be recommended.

Anticoagulants are usually given for 3 to 6 months post infarct to patients with prior emboli, in those with LV thrombus (echocardiographically proven) or threatened thrombus (large anterior infarcts), in those with established atrial fibrillation,[50,55] or in selected patients with overt congestive heart failure (see p 229).

Digitalis. The controversy whether digitalis contributes independently to cardiac death in the first year post infarction has not been settled (Chap. 6). Although it should not be withheld from patients with LV failure in the post-infarct phase, digitalis should not be given without careful evaluation of the risk-benefit ratio and after the use of diuretics/ACE inhibitors.

ACE Inhibitors. Apart from their use in post-infarct CHF, ACE inhibitors such as captopril may be used without concurrent diuretics in patients with low ejection fractions to prevent unfavorable remodelling[98] and, hopefully, to prevent eventual LVF. SAVE (Survival and Ventricular Enlargement Study) is a large multicenter randomized trial comparing captopril and placebo in such patients, and the results should be available in late 1991.

Nitrates. Acute IV administration of low dose nitroglycerin followed by 6 weeks of buccal therapy led to improved remodeling of the left ventricle at 6 months.[66a]

Antiarrhythmic Agents. Complex ventricular ectopy and VT in the late-hospital phase of myocardial infarction are predictors of subsequent sudden death after discharge,[30] independently of their frequent association with LV dysfunction.[32] **Nonetheless, the hoped for benefit of antiarrhythmic therapy on post-infarct mortality is still elusive** with flecainide/encainide clearly contraindicated.[45] Preliminary data with other drugs are also discouraging.[17] Signal-averaged electrocardiography identifies patients with late potentials and is a promising non-invasive means of helping to identify those at risk of sudden death. Whether antiarrhythmic therapy will help the outcome in this subgroup remains to be seen.

MANAGEMENT OF ARRHYTHMIAS

Paroxysmal Atrial Fibrillation. Severely symptomatic patients in shock or cardiac failure need immediate cardioversion. If a rapid reduction in rate is needed, for instance, when the tachycardia has precipitated ischemia, IV verapamil, IV esmolol, or IV adenosine will slow the rate pending a response to digoxin or oral verapamil. Experimentally, sinus rhythm can be restored by the use of Class I (exception: lidocaine) or Class III agents, acting through different mechanisms.[101] Clinically, a large variety of agents can be used acutely intravenously, including procainamide, disopyramide, flecainide, propafenone, encainide, or esmolol (not all available in the USA). In the prevention of paroxysmal atrial fibrillation, quinidine is most commonly used, but with mixed success. Amiodarone and the Class IC agents propafenone and flecainide may all be used in resistant cases. Nonetheless, in view of the CAST data, flecainide and encainide should be avoided in patients with atrial fibrillation on the basis of coronary artery disease. Several of these agents are still investigational. Propafenone appears very promising and has fewer side-effects than amiodarone.[59] Anticoagulation is often required (Chap. 9).

Recent-Onset Atrial Fibrillation. Patients are first given oral quinidine (or disopyramide), which will convert about one-third of patients to sinus rhythm; electrocardioversion is used for the others. Factors favoring chemical conversion include a small left atrial size and atrial fibrillation less than 6 months in duration. Digitalization is standard in combination with quinidine but usually is stopped before cardioversion. The risk of embolization at the time of rhythm conversion is about 1 to 2% when atrial fibrillation has been present for 3 days or more, so that prophylactic anticoagulation is standard. Postcardioversion quinidine may increase overall mortality (see p 181).

Chronic Atrial Fibrillation. When the ventricular rate seems not to respond to digitalis compounds, the first move is to check the patient's compliance and the digoxin blood level and to reassess for thyrotoxicosis or other systemic or cardiac diseases. Thereafter the digitalis dose may be cautiously increased; however, optimal control of exercise heart rate usually needs added oral verapamil,[1] diltiazem,[29] or β-blockade. In patients without LV failure, verapamil or diltiazem is logical first-line therapy. If it is necessary acutely to reduce the ventricular response, titrated IV verapamil or esmolol is effective. Care is required because such additional AV block can be dangerous in patients already fully digitalized. Conversely, digitalis is not given acutely to patients already receiving a β-blocker or verapamil.

Atrial Flutter. In the patient with stable atrial flutter, the ventricular rate may be controlled by digitalis, verapamil or β-blockade, or a double or triple combination of these drugs. Satisfactory control of the ventricular rate may be extremely difficult to achieve, but the rhythm is easily converted by a low-energy countershock and is highly responsive to atrial pacing techniques. The use of temporary atrial pacing electrodes for rapid atrial pacing is particularly helpful in the management of paroxysmal atrial flutter post-operatively after cardiac surgery. In the prevention of recurrent atrial flutter, one or more of these drugs are used, frequently with quinidine. In selected cases, low-dose amiodarone gives excellent results, as may propafenone. When atrial flutter complicates congenital heart disease,[12] digoxin plus quinidine or procainamide is frequently effective.

Wolff-Parkinson-White Syndrome. In the case of atrial fibrillation or flutter with antegrade **pre-excitation** via an accessory pathway (Wolff-Parkinson-White syndrome), digitalis, which shortens the refractory period of the bypass tract, is **absolutely contraindicated**. Verapamil, diltiazem, and β-blockade may sometimes be hazardous and should be avoided. The treatment of choice is cardioversion if the patient is hemodynamically compromised, or IV Class IA or IC or Class III agents (avoiding IV quinidine; lidocaine is not effective). IV disopyramide may be effective (exclude heart failure first) but is not available in the USA. The new Class IC antiarrhythmics such as flecainide, encainide, propafenone, or the Class III sotalol may all be used. In one study propafenone worked when other drugs had failed.[41] In the prevention of paroxysmal atrial fibrillation with a rapid ventricular response due to pre-excitation, low-dose amiodarone may first be tried before surgical or catheter ablation of the accessory pathway, which has been highly successful in a few specialized centers.

Supraventricular Tachycardia. Newer drugs, antitachycardia pacing techniques, and innovative surgical approaches have radically improved treatment in refractory cases. Patients with supraventricular arrhythmias that are very rapid or refractory to standard drugs, or are associated with a wide QRS complex on the standard electrocardiogram (implying either aberration, antegrade pre-excitation, or VT), warrant an invasive electrophysiologic study. Yet in the majority of patients, management can be guided by clinical principles.

Vagotonic procedures (Valsalva maneuver, facial immersion in cold water, or carotid sinus massage) may terminate the tachycardia. Always auscultate the carotid arteries before performing carotid sinus massage. If these measures fail, **IV verapamil**, **IV esmolol,** or **IV adenosine** are best (see Chap. 8). If these steps fail, vagotonic maneuvers are worth repeating. Thereafter the choice lies between IV digitalization, IV Class IC agents, of which the best may be propafenone,[59] or cardioversion and should be tempered by the clinical condition of the patient.

To prevent paroxysmal supraventricular tachycardia, the initiating ectopic beats may be inhibited by β-blockade or verapamil or by amiodarone, which is highly effective for supraventricular arrhythmias including paroxysmal atrial fibrillation and arrhythmias involving accessory pathways; severe side-effects may be limited by a low dose (see Chap. 8). The Class IC agents (propafenone, flecainide, and encainide) are all viable alternatives, but flecainide and encainide should not be used in the presence of clinical coronary artery disease.

Bradyarrhythmias. Asymptomatic sinus bradycardia does not require therapy and may be normal, especially in athletes. For **symptomatic sinus bradycardia, sick sinus syndrome,** and **sinoatrial disease**, probanthine and chronic atropine are unsatisfactory in the long run so that pacing is usually required. First, however, the effects of drugs such as β-blockers, digitalis, verapamil, diltiazem, quinidine, procainamide, amiodarone, lithium carbonate, lidocaine, methyldopa, and clonidine should be excluded. New drug approaches that may be tried when the problem is not severe include hydralazine[74] or xamoterol, which is investigational in the USA.[111]

In the **tachycardia/bradycardia syndrome**, intrinsic sinus node dysfunction is difficult to treat and once again may require pacemaking. β-Blockers aggravate the bradycardic component of the syndrome. Exceptions are pindolol or xamoterol with ISA, which may help to dampen down the tachycardia episodes while limiting the bradycardia; Holter monitoring is required to confirm the efficacy of these agents. Nonetheless, patients usually end up with a combination of a permanent pacemaker and antiarrhythmic agents.

For **AV block with syncope** or excessively slow rates, isoproterenol or transthoracic pacing is used as an emergency and temporary measure, pending pacemaker implantation.

Ventricular Arrhythmias and Pro-arrhythmic Effects. **The therapy of ventricular arrhythmias is a complex, rapidly changing area that cannot readily be simplified** (see Fig. 8–9). A full cardiologic assessment is essential together with treatment of underlying LVF, ischemia, anemia, or thyrotoxicosis. The criteria for instituting therapy are not clear-cut, although patients with sustained VT, survivors of previous arrhythmia-related cardiac arrest, and those with severely symptomatic arrhythmias all require treatment. Documentation of the efficacy of antiarrhythmics is essential prior to their long-term use. This requirement means the selection of a model, whether based on the combination of Holter monitoring and exercise testing or the inducibility of ventricular arrhythmias during an invasive electrophysiologic study. The intensive investigation and treatment of symptomatic ventricular arrhythmias is time-consuming and a task for specialized units, but the stakes are high.

Does therapy alter the **prognosis** of malignant symptomatic ventricular arrhythmias? Accumulating evidence says yes, provided that extensive investigation is followed by meticulous assessment of drug efficacy. Using programmed ventricular stimulation in patients with malignant ventricular arrhythmias or in survivors of out-of-hospital cardiac arrest, **drug suppression of inducible arrhythmias is strongly associated with a favorable long-term outcome**. In patients in whom a successful drug is not identified by electrophysiologic testing, the recurrence rate appears high.[26,35,79] Nonetheless, electrophysiologic testing may be less reliable in the case of amiodarone. There is no evidence that therapy of asymptomatic ventricular arrhythmias, even in the presence of heart disease, prolongs life or prevents sudden death. Rather, the CAST study[45] warns that the pro-arrhythmic effects of some Class IC agents can actually increase mortality in patients with ischemic heart disease.

The **choice of drug** for chronic use is ideally based on prior demonstration during acute and chronic testing that the drug actually works and on its potential for toxicity in the individual under study. Class I agents including quinidine, disopyramide, and mexiletine remain first-line drugs, with propafenone possibly the most effective and least harmful of the Class IC agents. The antiarrhythmic effect of β-blockade monotherapy has also recently been reported, and it should be considered that β-blockers are among the few anti-arrhythmic agents with positive long-term beneficial effects in post-infarct patients. Amiodarone remains the last choice because of its serious side-effects. Deciding among the agents currently available is somewhat of a personal choice and not entirely logical.

Treatment of heart failure, hypoxia, electrolyte imbalance, and ischemia is an essential adjunct to antiarrhythmic therapy. Coronary bypass surgery helps selected patients.[68] Non-pharmacologic approaches to the management of ventricular arrhythmias include sophisticated pacing modalities and surgery in conjunction with electrophysiologic mapping. Excellent results can be achieved in selected patients. The automatic implantable cardioverter defibrillator could be the harbinger of an entirely new approach to the management of patients with malignant ventricular arrhythmias. Results with this device, although confined to specialized centers, are encouraging and exciting, so that indications for implantation are widening.[67]

CONGESTIVE HEART FAILURE

Despite newer agents (particularly the ACE inhibitors), the long-term prognosis of CHF remains poor, unless a reversible cause, for instance valvular heart disease or hypertension, is present. The initial steps in a patient with heart failure are to investigate the cause and treat associated conditions including hypertension, thyrotoxicosis, and anemia. The usual policy has been to initiate treatment with diuretics, salt restriction, then digitalis before proceeding to conventional vasodilators—the current trend is toward the earlier use of ACE inhibitors. The role of digitalis remains contested; nonetheless, its benefits have now been re-established particularly in patients with more severe heart failure. As ACE inhibitors are simpler to use than digitalis, with fewer contraindications and less risk of adverse effects (except for hypotension), they are gradually becoming standard second-line therapy, although the data concerning their benefit are still lacking. Combination "triple therapy" of diuretics, ACE inhibition, and digitalis is increasingly used as standard therapy for moderate to severe heart failure.

In **severe intractable CHF**, hemodynamic monitoring by Swan-Ganz catheterization is required both to evaluate the hemodynamic status and, usually, to initiate IV therapy before going on to oral agents. Theoretically, inotropic vasodilators (inodilators, see Table 6-7) such as **amrinone** and **milrinone** should have different indications from predominant inotropes, such as dobutamine; yet a multicentered randomized study showed that **milrinone** (50 µg/kg bolus, followed by 0.5–0.625 µg/kg/min) gave very similar clinical effects to **dobutamine** with somewhat less initial chronotropic effect.[21] Once benefit has been achieved by IV inotropes, therapy should not be continued without re-evaluation because receptor downgrading is a hazard; in the case of dobutamine there is loss of a sustained effect during one week of IV infusion.[22] In the case of milrinone, long-term oral use did not give as good results as digoxin and in fact increased ventricular arrhythmias (Chap. 6). The search for an orally active and effective inotropic agent continues.

Oral Vasodilator Therapy. Oral load reduction by ACE inhibitors has become standard practice, although the large-scale VA study comparing ACE inhibitors with nitrates-hydralazine is still under way and may be decisive. In patients without pulmonary congestion, it is essential to avoid excess preload reduction, which may precipitously reduce filling pressures.

Arrhythmias in Congestive Heart Failure. Prophylactic antiarrhythmic therapy is contraindicated, especially since most antiarrhythmics inhibit the sinus node and there is a high incidence of bradyarrhythmic deaths in CHF.[76] In **significantly symptomatic arrhythmias**, it is first essential to pinpoint precipitating factors such as hypokalemia or use of sympathomimetics or phosphodiesterase inhibitors or digoxin. The hemodynamic status of the myocardium must be made optimal. Antiarrhythmics are given only after documentation of benefit by electrophysiologic studies or by ambulatory monitoring (see p 209).

β-Blockers. Their use in congestive heart failure remains highly controversial. Some patients respond dramatically to cautious addition of low-dose metoprolol, whereas others unexpectedly deteriorate. In 33 patients with dilated cardiomyopathy, metoprolol gave long-term benefit, and withdrawal of the drug was harmful in two-thirds.[112] Large randomized trials are in progress.

Diastolic Dysfunction. Traditional concepts of heart failure emphasize the primary role of systolic ventricular dysfunction. In patients with a clinical diagnosis of heart failure, there is preserved LV systolic function in about 40%, thereby emphasizing the role of "diastolic dysfunction." The role of calcium antagonists and β-blockers in this syndrome needs evaluation; either therapy is logical if combined with a mild diuretic. However, fundamental therapy is to aim for regression of massive LVH, the underlying cause of diastolic dysfunction. In the elderly with increased myocardial stiffness, therapy is still indicated even though regression is not required.

CHF: Summary. In patients with mild CHF, initial therapy is a diuretic combined with either digoxin or an ACE inhibitor. In more severe CHF, digoxin may be more effective.[91] If symptoms persist, the triple combination of diuretics, ACE inhibitors, and digitalis is now standard, also from the outset in more severe CHF. Whether an ACE inhibitor could or should be used as initial therapy is not settled. There appear to be two separate issues. Post-infarct administration of an ACE inhibitor without a diuretic can, by unloading the heart, beneficially influence remodelling and may indirectly prevent CHF. In established CHF, however, circulating renin only rises consistently after diuretic use, so that initial use of an ACE inhibitor is illogical.

ACUTE PULMONARY EDEMA

In acute pulmonary edema of cardiac origin, the initial management requires positioning the patient in an upright posture and administering oxygen. If the underlying cause is an arrhythmia, restoration of sinus rhythm takes priority. **Morphine sulfate** is highly effective in relieving symptoms. Its mechanism of action is not precisely understood, but a venodilator action and a central sedative effect are likely.[36] **IV furosemide**, which acts both as a diuretic and a vasodilator, is the other basic therapy. **Sublingual nitrates** are excellent for early unloading of the lungs and unloading the preload of the left heart. If severe hypertension is the underlying cause, **sublingual nifedipine** may be used. In complex patients in whom the afterload and preload must be meticulously controlled, IV sodium nitroprusside together with invasive monitoring of pressures may be required. Particular caution is necessary in the patient with a systolic blood pressure of less than 90 mm Hg, if **vasodilators** are contemplated. In patients with pulmonary edema secondary to severe acute or chronic mitral or aortic regurgitation, IV nitroprusside is probably the agent of choice. Once acute pulmonary edema has been relieved and in the absence of AMI, **cautious digitalization** is started (1 mg digoxin intravenously over 30 minutes, providing the patient is not already receiving digitalis) and the patient is continued on furosemide and ACE inhibitors. When there is risk of arrhythmia as in AMI, **aminophylline,** or theophylline, or the related xanthine compounds are also best avoided (bronchospasm will usually respond to diuresis or load reduction). If IV xanthine compounds must be used, they should be given slowly (side-effects on respiration and the central nervous system) with monitoring of plasma potassium and arrhythmias. These compounds have the potential to interact adversely with others used in CHF. Aminophylline may be given at 6 mg/kg intravenously over 30 minutes followed by 0.5 mg/kg/hr.

In refractory cases, resort to rotating tourniquets or intubation with mechanical ventilation. Pulmonary edema of cardiac origin must be differentiated from the adult respiratory distress syndrome, which requires specific therapy.

CARDIOMYOPATHY

Hypertrophic Cardiomyopathy (IHSS)

Although many patients are asymptomatic, there is risk of sudden cardiac death, which mandates avoidance of competitive sports even in the absence of symptoms. The cornerstone of drug therapy in symptomatic patients is to avoid agents that increase cardiac contractility, such as digitalis, or reduce ventricular preload, such as nitrates (which can, however, be given with care to patients with added angina).

Three basic therapies have been used: β-blockade, calcium antagonists (especially verapamil), and disopyramide. Each has its advocates. **High-dose propranolol** is most widely used and frequently reduces symptoms. **Verapamil** may be more useful than β-blockade in patients with asthma or other contraindications to β-blockade and is usually well tolerated. Verapamil is seen as a logical therapy to relieve the diastolic relaxation problems found in hypertrophic cardiomyopathy,[5,34] although obstructive cardiomyopathy is a relative contraindication. Occasional dangerous or even lethal side-effects with verapamil have been reported, presumably because the afterload reducing effect is more vigorous than the negative inotropic effect, so that outflow tract obstruction is precipitated. For that reason **nifedipine is contraindicated in patients with resting obstruction.**[3] **Disopyramide** (150 mg 4x daily) was hemodynamically better than propranolol 40 mg 4x daily or placebo in a small group of patients in that the subaortic pressure gradient was virtually abolished by disopyramide but not by propranolol;[93] however, the use of propranolol is better established and has other benefits, such as relief of symptoms.

Antiarrhythmics. When severe arrhythmias intervene or are feared, **amiodarone** is the antiarrhythmic of choice,[23] although controversial in "high risk" children.[78] In patients with a family history of sudden death, syncope, or severe dyspnea, or in patients in whom malignant arrhythmias are suspected for other reasons, Holter monitoring for 48 to 72 hours is required to evaluate antiarrhythmic therapy. **Disopyramide** should have antiarrhythmic as well as hemodynamic benefit.

Surgery. For refractory symptoms, septal myectomy is effective therapy, although the exact indications are not widely agreed upon or the mechanism of benefit settled.[77] The role of mitral valve replacement is even more controversial.[69]

In older patients the entity of **hypertensive hypertrophic cardio-myopathy** has now been recognized, and β-blockers or verapamil is used in therapy.[37] Digitalis, diuretics and load reducers such as nifedipine or ACE inhibitors are all contraindicated.

Dilated Cardiomyopathy

The standard therapy for CHF in this condition consists of inotropic support, diuretics, ACE inhibitors, with β-blockers only in selected patients. Arrhythmias are frequent in such patients and sudden cardiac death is often due to asystole.[76] Antiarrhythmic therapy is not as logical as previously thought because most antiarrhythmic drugs can depress the sinus node, another reason for care with β-blockade (data are needed). For atrial fibrillation, anticoagulation is usual.[11] Immunosuppressive therapy by prednisone is not part of routine treatment, as recently shown in a multicenter study.[88] A large trial, evaluating different immunosuppressives, is in progress.

Cardiac transplantation is used for selected patients with cardiomyopathy failing to respond to conservative therapy, including cautious β-blockade. Select an experienced transplant center, expert in all phases of care, and don't wait until there is deterioration in the patient's general health.

VALVULAR HEART DISEASE

Rheumatic Fever Prophylaxis. Treatment should start as soon as a definitive diagnosis of streptococcal infection has been made; the treatment is either a single dose of benzathene penicillin—1,200,000 units for adults and half dose for children—or a full 10-day course of oral penicillin-V (125–250 mg 3x daily). Thereafter, in selected patients in whom recurrences are feared, the penicillin injection is repeated monthly, or pencillin-V is given as 125 to 250 mg twice daily continuously.[99]

General Approach to Valvular Heart Disease. In most patients with symptomatic valvular regurgitation or stenosis, valve replacement or repair is indicated. As surgical techniques and the performance of prosthetic valves have improved, so have the surgical indications become less stringent. **Now most patients with LV dysfunction are operated on even if asymptomatic.** The indications for surgery for other patients with severe but asymptomatic valvular regurgitation are less clearly established. Concomitant therapy in patients with valvular heart disease may include diuretics, digitalis and, especially for certain non-stenotic lesions, vasodilators. Attention to arrhythmias, particularly atrial fibrillation, is essential and anticoagulants may be needed (see Chap. 9).

Aortic Stenosis. In valvular stenosis, the basic problem is obstruction and requires surgical relief. When heart failure or hypertension is a complication, vasodilator therapy is contraindicated except for cautious preload reduction avoiding an excess fall in the filling pressure. Sometimes excessive peripheral vasoconstriction requires relief by cautious afterload reduction. In **aortic stenosis with angina**, therapy without surgery is difficult because the angina is at least partially based on the increased demand of the hypertrophic left ventricle (there may also be accompanying coronary artery disease). In older patients with contraindications to surgery, percutaneous balloon aortic valvuloplasty offers a reasonable alternative to surgery, with, however, risk of restenosis.

Mitral Stenosis. In **mitral stenosis with sinus rhythm**, β-blockade by atenolol improves exercise capacity and is preferable to propranolol to lessen possible pulmonary symptoms. Prophylactic digitalization hopefully avoids a high ventricular rate during intermittent atrial fibrillation; good evidence for this practice is not available. Balloon valvuloplasty is increasingly used for relief of the stenosis. **Paroxysmal atrial fibrillation** precipitating left-sided failure may require carefully titrated IV verapamil or esmolol, provided that the left ventricle itself is not depressed in function (a risk of associated mitral regurgitation). In **established atrial fibrillation**, digitalization is usually not enough to prevent an excessive ventricular rate during exercise, so that digoxin should be augmented by verapamil[1] or by β-blockade to slow the ventricular rate adequately during exercise. In patients at high risk for emboli (previous thromboembolism or atrial paroxysmal arrhythmias or advanced disease) anticoagulation is required.

Mitral or Aortic Valve Regurgitation. Afterload reduction is much more effective in regurgitation than in stenosis. In severe or symptomatic regurgitation, valve replacement is required. Post-infarct mitral regurgitation can cause sudden deterioration and has long-term risks, despite optimal therapy including ACE inhibitors.

INFECTIVE ENDOCARDITIS

The management of acute or subacute endocarditis varies with the etiology and virulence of the infecting organism and the clinical manifestations of the episode. Consideration should be given to differences in the prognosis, the bacteriologic spectrum, and the response to therapy between prosthetic and native valve endocarditis.

Optimal therapy requires identification of the **causative organism**, which may delay initiation of therapy in subacute endocarditis for a short period. Definitive antibiotic therapy is based upon susceptibility testing. In culture-negative endocarditis, therapy is empiric. The causative organism is still usually a streptococcus viridans, susceptible to penicillin-gentamicin. Gentamicin enhances the activity of the penicillin. In the UK, a working party has recommended[113] that, after 14 days of IV penicillin and gentamicin, drug therapy be changed to oral amoxycillin for at least 2 weeks with 4 weeks of total treatment. When the organism is staphylococcus aureus, IV penicillin is changed to flucloxacillin.[113] Again, gentamicin is stopped after 14 days because of the risk of possible renal toxicity. The duration of antibiotic therapy is still under debate, but a 4 to 6 week period is generally accepted. In selected patients, there may be a place for short-course therapy with **two** drugs.[47] Conditions predisposing the patient to infective endocarditis, such as poor dental hygiene or genito-urinary tract pathology, must be remedied.

An increasing aggressive approach to **early cardiac surgery** has favorably influenced the outcome of infective endocarditis.[19] In patients with **native valve endocarditis**, the indications for surgery are heart failure resulting from valve dysfunction, uncontrolled infection, new conduction disturbances suggestive of ring abscess formation, fungal infection, relapse after initially successful therapy, and possibly recurrent emboli.[19,38] The approach to **prosthetic valve endocarditis**, particularly within three months of the initial operation, is also aggressive, with surgery for any signs of prosthetic valve dysfunction or any of the indications for surgery in native valves.[18] In the face of hemodynamic decompensation, surgery should not be delayed pending completion of antibiotic therapy.

Anticoagulant Therapy. The decision to initiate or continue anticoagulant therapy in patients with infective endocarditis is often difficult. In those patients already on anticoagulants (e.g., patients with mechanical prostheses or those in whom there are other indications for anticoagulation, such as thrombophlebitis) anticoagulant

TABLE 11–1 AMERICAN RECOMMENDED ANTIBIOTIC REGIMENS FOR DENTAL/RESPIRATORY TRACT PROCEDURES

Standard Regimen

For *dental procedures* that cause gingival bleeding, and oral/respiratory tract surgery	*Penicillin V 2.0 g orally 1 hr before, then 1.0 g 6 hr later.* For patients unable to take oral medications, 2 million units of aqueous penicillin G IV or IM 30–60 min before a procedure and 1 million units 6 hr later may be substituted

Special Regimens

Parenteral regimen for use when maximal protection desired; e.g., for patients with prosthetic valves	Ampicillin 1.0–2.0 g IM or IV *plus* gentamicin 1.5 mg/kg IM or IV $^{1}/_{2}$ hr before procedure, followed by 1.0 g oral penicillin V 6 hr later
Oral regimen for penicillin-allergic patients	Erythromycin 1.0 g orally 1 hr before, then 500 mg 6 hr later
Parenteral regimen for penicillin-allergic patients	Vancomycin 1.0 g IV *slowly* over 1 hr starting 1 hr before. No repeat dose is necessary

From Shulman et al.[99] Reproduced with permission of the American Heart Association.

therapy should be continued or initiated. In the event of a cerebral thromboembolic complication, the risk of anticoagulant-induced hemorrhage must be balanced against the risk of recurrent embolism.

Antibiotic Prophylaxis. American practice is based on penicillin prophylaxis, whereas amoxycillin is the drug of choice in Europe (Tables 11-1 and 11-2). Chemoprophylaxis is indicated for patients with increased susceptibility to infective endocarditis who must undergo dental or urogenital procedures that may produce a bacteremia. Cardiac conditions for which antibiotic prophylaxis is recommended are rheumatic or other acquired valvular heart disease, prosthetic heart valves or a prosthetic patch, hypertrophic obstructive cardiomyopathy, prior infective endocarditis, and congenital heart disease, with the exception of uncomplicated secundum atrial septal defects and repaired patent ductus arteriosus. In **mitral valve prolapse** with only a click, antibiotic prophylaxis is debatable; when there is a murmur, prophylaxis is definitely desirable.[48]

COR PULMONALE

Therapy of right heart failure is similar to that of left heart failure, except that digitalis appears to be less effective because of a combination of hypoxemia, electrolyte disturbances, and enhanced adrenergic discharge. Thus when atrial fibrillation develops, cautious use of verapamil may both benefit the ventricular rate in atrial fibrillation,

TABLE 11–2 EUROPEAN RECOMMENDATIONS: ANTIBIOTIC PROPHYLAXIS OF INFECTIVE ENDOCARDITIS FOR ADULTS DURING DENTAL PROCEDURES

Not Allergic to Penicillin		Allergic to Penicillin	
Oral Amoxycillin	*IV or IM Amoxycillin*	*Oral* Erythromycin*	*Oral Clindamycin*
3 g 1 hr before	1 g just before 0.5 g 6 hr later	1.5 g 1 hr before 0.5 g 6 hr later	1 g just before

*or IV erythromycin just before the procedure.
Modified from Delaye et al[10] and from Simmons et al.[100]

may cause mild bronchodilation, and may help relieve pulmonary artery pressure. Verapamil may also benefit chaotic multifocal atrial tachycardia,[73] as is sometimes caused by theophylline toxicity. However, there appear to be no formal trials regarding the use of verapamil in such conditions.

In general, β-blockers should be avoided because of the risk of bronchospasm. Bronchodilators should be β₂-selective, such as salbutamol (albuterol), which has relatively little effect on the heart rate while causing peripheral vasodilation and unloading of the left heart, which may also be compromised.

When right ventricular failure is accompanied by LV failure, and the latter is not caused by hypoxemia, digitalis is again added to diuretic therapy. For load reduction, nitrates may have a special role in reducing pulmonary vascular resistance. In cor pulmonale secondary to hypoxic lung disease, home oxygen therapy is essential.

PULMONARY HYPERTENSION

Primary pulmonary hypertension includes a variety of histologic appearances and probably pathogenic mechanisms, while excluding pulmonary hypertension secondary to chronic pulmonary disease. Diffuse pulmonary thromboembolism or pulmonary arteriolar thrombosis in situ occurs in some patients. Unless lung biopsy is performed, the pathogenesis cannot be established, and long-term anticoagulants are frequently used on the assumption that there is thromboembolism.

Calcium antagonists are increasingly being tried, with one of the best documented being nifedipine in a dose of 240 mg daily.[95] The results are unpredictable and generally disappointing unless there is hypoxic vasoconstriction as the basis of the pulmonary hypertension. Pulmonary vasodilators should only be given under stringent monitoring.[87]

PERIPHERAL VASCULAR DISEASE

The basic problem is vascular atheroma, added to which are (1) variable degrees of arterial spasm and (2) variable severities of arterial thrombosis and platelet aggregation and embolization. Thus far, the most effective attack on atheroma has been by surgery, when appropriate, with percutaneous angioplasty including lasers being used increasingly. Promising new drugs are becoming available. Correction of coronary risk factors appears to play little or no role, except smoking in most types of active peripheral vascular disease. Exercise training benefits.[51]

Pentoxifylline (Trental) protects against red cell deformability as the erythrocytes are squeezed through the narrowed arterioles. It is licensed for use in intermittent claudication[25] in the USA (600–1200 mg daily in three divided doses with meals; side-effect nausea). In a multicenter Scandinavian trial, the best response was in patients with chronic occlusive peripheral arterial disease more than one year in duration and with a resting ankle/arm pressure ratio of 0.8 or less.[75]

Platelet active agents and prostaglandin inhibitors have all been tried; only recently has objective angiographic data favoring aspirin (330 mg daily) plus dipyridamole (75 mg 3x daily) become available.[14] The serotonin antagonist, **ketanserin**, has proved to be of no benefit.[85] **Iloprost**, a prostacyclin analog, given by daily infusion for 4 to 28 days, healed ulcers and improved ischemic pain in patients with severe thromboangiitis obliterans (Buerger's disease); aspirin was much less effective.[53]

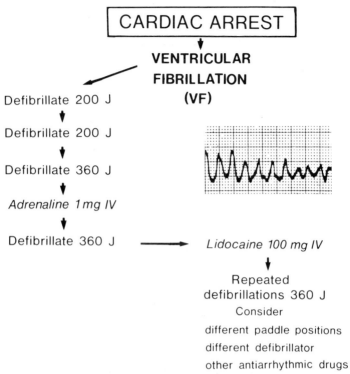

FIGURE 11–1. Algorithm for cardiopulmonary resuscitation (CPR) when there is ventricular fibrillation. Adrenaline=epinephrine. Modified from Chamberlain DA: Advanced life support: Revised recommendations of the Resuscitation Council (UK). Br Med J 299:446–448, 1989, with permission.

L-carnitine (levocarnitine, Carnitor) (2 g twice daily) improved the walking capacity of patients with intermittent claudication without hemodynamic effects, probably acting through a metabolic mechanism;[44] further confirmatory trials are required.

For peripheral vascular disease plus angina or hypertension, calcium antagonists are preferred therapy. These agents are now being evaluated for their possible role in improvement of arterial blood flow. Experimentally, all calcium antagonists, including verapamil, nifedipine, and diltiazem, can stop the progression of atheroma and have complex effects including enhancement of cholesteryl ester hydrolysis,[52] but cannot yet routinely be advised. β-Blockers are generally contraindicated in the presence of active peripheral vascular disease, although the evidence is not firm.[15] When used, the vasodilatory types might be preferable.

In summary, the basis of medical therapy lies in cessation of smoking and exercise training. Pentoxifylline, aspirin, and, possibly in selected patients, L-carnitine may all be useful.

RAYNAUD'S PHENOMENON

Once a secondary cause has been excluded (for example vasculitis, scleroderma, or lupus erythematosus), then **calcium channel antagonists** are logical. Nifedipine is best tested.[96] β-Blockers are traditionally contraindicated in Raynaud's phenomenon, although low-dose propranolol or metoprolol do not exaggerate primary Raynaud's phenomenon.[8]

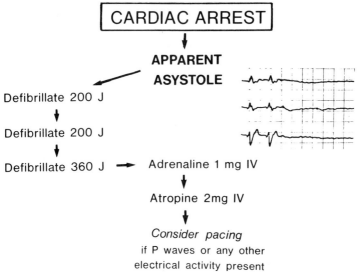

FIGURE 11–2. Algorithm for CPR in a patient with asystole. Adrenaline= epinephrine. Modified from Chamberlain DA: Advanced life support: Revised recommendations of the Resuscitation Council (UK). Br Med J 299:446–448, 1989, with permission.

BERI-BERI HEART DISEASE

This condition is characterized by high output CHF due to thiamine deficiency. Common in Africa and Asia, in western countries it is under-diagnosed, especially in alcoholics.[70] The basis of treatment is thiamine 100 mg parenterally followed by 50 to 100 mg daily with vitamin supplements, a balanced diet, and abstinence from alcohol. Even in Shoshin beri-beri with peripheral circulatory shock and severe metabolic acidosis, thiamine remains the mainstay of treatment because the acidosis responds poorly to treatment. Diuretics are needed when diuresis is delayed beyond 48 hours (comment by courtesy of Dr. D.P. Naidoo, University of Natal, South Africa).

HEART DISEASE IN DIABETICS

There are several important aspects of the association between ischemic heart disease, hypertension, and diabetes mellitus. First, diuretic therapy is still commonly used in mild heart failure and in hypertension. Diuretic therapy helps to upset glucose metabolism even without changing the fasting blood sugar.[64] Thiazides, even in low doses, can induce unfavorable blood lipid changes. Therefore, all diuretics, including indapamide and the loop diuretics, are relatively contraindicated in diabetic patients (non-insulin requiring) or, if used, should be in as low a dose as possible. However, this constraint does not apply to spironolactone (although risking potassium retention).

Secondly, because diabetes mellitus is a major risk factor for ischemic heart disease and often is an associated factor with hypertension, strict control of diabetes in these conditions is required. It makes little sense that cardiologists carefully regulate blood pressure and angina, while being relatively lax on diabetic control.

The preferential use of ACE inhibitors in **diabetic renal disease** is becoming established even in the absence of hypertension,[90] and some would argue that these agents are first choice in all **diabetic hypertensives**. Both the ACE inhibitors and calcium antagonists are

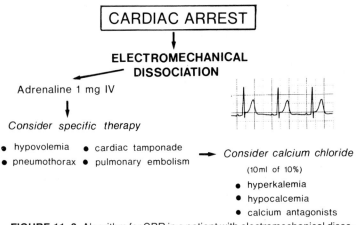

FIGURE 11–3. Algorithm for CPR in a patient with electromechanical dissociation. Adrenaline=epinephrine. Modified from Chamberlain DA: Advanced life support: Revised recommendations of the Resuscitation Council (UK). Br Med J 299:446–448, 1989, with permission.

free of adverse side-effects on glucose metabolism and on blood lipid profiles. β-Blockers, previously thought not to impair glucose tolerance, are now established villains.[92]

CARDIOPULMONARY RESUSCITATION

The recommendations of the UK Resuscitation Council have recently been published.[46] In the algorithm for ventricular fibrillation (Figs. 11–1 to 11–3), the important change from conventional recommendation is the earlier use of adrenaline to maintain cerebral perfusion. Sodium bicarbonate is not recommended except in prolonged resuscitation, because in the absence of adequate respiration the CO_2 formed from the bicarbonate permeates into the cell to increase intracellular acidosis. During prolonged resuscitation it is assumed that respiration will have been established.

In apparent asystole, adrenaline is given again to maintain cerebral perfusion, even before lidocaine. In electromechanical dissociation, adrenaline is again given early. Calcium chloride is thought to have specific value in the presence of hyperkalemia, hypocalcemia, or calcium antagonist excess.

REFERENCES

References from Previous Editions

1. Beasley R, Smith DA, McHaffie DJ: Br Med J 290:9–11, 1985
2. β-Blocker Heart Attack Study Group: JAMA 246:2073–2074, 1981
3. Betocchi S, Cannon RO, Watson RM, et al: Circulation 72:1001–1007, 1985
4. Betriu A, Pomar JL, Bourassa MG, et al: Am J Cardiol 51:661–667, 1983
5. Bonow RO, Dilsiziam V, Rosing DR, et al: Circulation 72:853–864, 1985
6. Buffington CW: Anesthesiology 63:651–662, 1985
7. Chadda K, Goldstein S, Byington R, et al: Circulation 73:503–510, 1986
8. Coffman JD, Rasmussen HM: Circulation 72:466–470, 1985
9. Croft CH, Rude RE, Gustafson N, et al: Circulation 73:1281–1290, 1986
10. Delaye J, Etienne J, Feruglio GA, et al: Eur Heart J 6:826–828, 1985
11. Fuster V, Gersh BJ, Giuliani ER, et al: Am J Cardiol 47:525–531, 1981
12. Garson A Jr, Bink-Boelkens M, Hesslein PS, et al: J Am Coll Cardiol 6:871–878, 1985

13. Gersh BJ, Kronmal RA, Schaff HV, et al: N Engl J Med 71:217–224, 1985
14. Hess H, Mietaschik A, Deichsel G: Lancet 1:415–419, 1985
15. Hiatt WR, Stoll S, Nies AS: Circulation 72:1226–1231, 1985
16. Hjalmarson A, Hurlitz J, Malik I, et al: Lancet 2:823–827, 1981
17. IMPACT Research Group: J Am Coll Cardiol 4:1148–1163, 1984
18. Karchmer AW, Swartz MN: In Kaplan EL, Taranta AV (eds): Infective Endocarditis. American Heart Association Monograph Number 52, 1977
19. Karchmer AW, Stinson EB: In Remmington JS, Swartz MN (eds): Current Clinical Topics in Infectious Diseases. New York, McGraw-Hill, 1980
20. Kjekshus JK: Am J Cardiol 57:43F–49F, 1986
21. Konstam A, Benotti JR, Biddle T, et al: Circulation 72(suppl III):III-201, 1985
22. Kupper W, Erelemeier HH, Hamm CW: Circulation 72(suppl III):III-405, 1985
23. McKenna WJ, Harris L, Rowland E, et al: Am J Cardiol 54:802–810, 1984
24. Norwegian Multicenter Study Group: N Engl J Med 304:801–807, 1981
25. Porter JM, Cutler BS, Lee BY, et al: Am Heart J 104:66–72, 1982
26. Rae AP, Greenspan AM, Spielman SR, et al: Am J Cardiol 55:1494–1499, 1985
27. Rogers WJ, Segall PH, McDaniel HG, et al: Am J Cardiol 43:801–809, 1979
28. Rossi PRF, Yusuf S, Ramsdale D, et al: Br Med J 286:506–510, 1983
29. Roth A, Harrison E, Mitani G, et al: Circulation 73:316–324, 1986
30. Ruberman W, Weinblatt E, Goldberg JD, et al: Circulation 64:297–305, 1981
31. Scheinman MM, Thorburn D, Abbott JA: Circulation 52:627–633, 1975
32. Schulze RA Jr, Strauss HW, Pitt B: Am J Med 62:192–199, 1977
33. Spielman SR, Kay HR, Morganroth J, et al: Circulation 72(suppl III):III-57, 1985
34. Suwa M, Hirota Y, Kawamura K: Am J Cardiol 54:1047–1053, 1984
35. Swerdlow CD, Winkle RA, Mason JW: N Engl J Med 308:1436–1442, 1983
36. Timmis AD, Rothman MT, Henderson MA, et al: Br Med J 280:980–982, 1980
37. Topol EJ, Traill TA, Fortuin NJ: N Engl J Med 312:277–283, 1985
38. Wilson WR, Danielson GK, Giuliani ER, et al: Mayo Clin Proc 54:223, 1979
39. Yusuf S, Peto R, Lewis JA, et al: Prog Cardiovasc Dis 27:335–371, 1985

New References

40. Anti-Platelet Trialists' Collaboration: Secondary prevention of vascular disease by prolonged anti-platelet therapy. Br Med J 296:320–331, 1988
41. Antman EM, Beamer AD, Cantillon C, et al: Long-term oral propafenone therapy for suppression of refractory symptomatic atrial fibrillation and atrial flutter. J Am Coll Cardiol 12: 1005–1011, 1988
42. β-Blocker Pooling Project Research Group: The β-blocker pooling project (BBPP): Sub-group findings from randomized trials in post-infarction patients. Eur Heart J 9:8-16, 1988
43. Boden WE, Ruble P, Mamby S, and Multicenter Collaborating Investigators: Esmolol improves anterior myocardial ischemia in unstable angina: Multicenter esmolol unstable angina trial (abstract). Circulation 80:II-267, 1989
44. Brevetti G, Chiariello M, Ferulano G, et al: Increases in walking distance in patients with peripheral vascular disease treated with L-carnitine: A double-blind, cross-over study. Circulation 77:767–773, 1988
45. CAST Investigators (Cardiac Arrhythmia Suppression Trial): Preliminary report: Effect of encainide and flecainide on mortality in a randomized trial of arrhythmia suppression after myocardial infarction. N Engl J Med 321:406–412, 1989
46. Chamberlain DA. Advanced life support: Revised recommendations of the Resuscitation Council (UK). Br Med J 299:446–448, 1989
47. Chambers HF, Miller RT, Newman MD: Right-sided staphylococcus aureus endocarditis in intravenous drug abusers: Two-week combination therapy. Ann Intern Med 109: 614–619, 1988
48. Danchin N, Voiriot P, Briancon S, et al: Mitral valve prolapse as a risk factor for infective endocarditis. Lancet 1:743–745, 1989
49. Davies SW, Ranjadayalan K, Wickens DG, et al: Lipid peroxidation associated with successful thrombolysis. Lancet 335:741–743, 1990
50. Douglas AS, Colwell L, Rose G: Twenty-year follow-up of patients in the Medical Research Council Trial of anticoagulants in acute myocardial infarction. Br Heart J 57:413–415, 1987

51. Ernst EEW, Matrai A: Intermittent claudication, exercise, and blood rheology. Circulation 76:1110–1114, 1987
52. Etingin OR, Hajjar DP: Calcium channel blockers enhance cholesteryl ester hydrolysis and decrease total cholesterol accumulation in human aortic tissue. Circ Res 66:185–190, 1990
53. Fiessinger JN, Schafer M: Trial of iloprost versus aspirin treatment for critical limb ischemia of thromboangiitis obliterans. Lancet 335:555–557, 1990
54. Furberg CD: Secondary prevention trials after acute myocardial infarction. Am J Cardiol 60:28A–32A, 1987
55. Fuster V, Halperin JL: Left ventricular thrombi and cerebral embolism (editorial). N Engl J Med 320:392–394, 1989
56. Gersh BJ, Califf RM, Loop FD, et al: Coronary bypass surgery and chronic stable angina. Circulation 79(suppl I):I46–I59, 1989
57. Gibson RS, Boden WE, Theroux P, et al: Diltiazem and reinfarction in patients with non-Q-wave myocardial infarction: Results of a double-blind randomized multicenter trial. N Engl J Med 315:423–429, 1986
58. Gonzalez JI, Hill JA, Kolb R, et al: Effects of atenolol and nifedipine alone and in combination on ambulant myocardial ischemia in minimally symptomatic patients (abstract). J Am Coll Cardiol 15:120A, 1990
59. Hammill SC, Wood DL, Gersh BJ: Propafenone for paroxysmal atrial fibrillation. Am J Cardiol 61:473–474, 1988
60. HART Study: Heparin versus aspirin reperfusion trial. Preliminary data presented by Ross at the American Heart Association Meeting, New Orleans, 1989
61. Held PH, Yusuf S, Furberg CD: Calcium channel blockers in acute myocardial infarction and unstable angina: An overview. Br Med J 299:1187–1192, 1989
62. Herlitz J, Hjalmarson A, Waagstein F: Treatment of pain in acute myocardial infarction. Br Heart J 61:9–13, 1989
63. HINT Research Group (Holland Interuniversity Nifedipine/Metoprolol Trial): Early treatment of unstable angina in the coronary care unit: A randomised double-blind placebo-controlled comparison of recurrent ischaemia in patients treated with nifedipine or metoprolol or both. Br Heart J 56:400–413, 1986
64. Houston MC: Treatment of hypertension in diabetes mellitus. Am Heart J 118:819–829, 1989
65. ISIS-II (Second International Study of Infarct Survival) Collaborative Group: Randomized trial of intravenous streptokinase, oral aspirin, both, or neither among 17,187 cases of suspected acute myocardial infarction: ISIS-II. Lancet 2:350–360, 1988
66. Jugdutt BI, Warnica JW: Intravenous nitroglycerin therapy to limit myocardial infarct size, expansion, and complications: Effect of timing, dosage, and infarct location. Circulation 78:906–919, 1988
66a. Jugdutt BI, Neiman JC, Michorowski BL, et al: Persistent improvement in left ventricular geometry and function by prolonged nitroglycerin therapy after acute transmural anterior myocardial infarction. J Am Coll Cardiol 15:214A, 1990
67. Kelly PA, Cannom DS, Garan H, et al: The automatic implantable cardioverter defibrillator: efficacy, complications, and survival in patients with malignant ventricular arrhythmias. J Am Coll Cardiol 11:1278–1286, 1988
68. Kelly P, Ruskin JN, Vlahakes GJ, et al: Surgical coronary revascularization in survivors of prehospital cardiac arrest: Its effect on inducible ventricular arrhythmias and long-term survival. J Am Coll Cardiol 15:267–273, 1990
69. Krajcer Z, Leachman RD, Colley DA, et al: Mitral valve replacement and septal myomectomy in hypertrophic cardiomyopathy: 10 year follow-up in 80 patients. Circulation 78(suppl I):I35–I43, 1988
70. Editorial: Cardiovascular Beriberi. Lancet 1:1287, 1982
71. Lee L, Bates ER, Pitt B, et al: Percutaneous transluminal coronary angioplasty improves survival in acute myocardial infarction complicated by cardiogenic shock. Circulation 78:1345–1351, 1988
72. Lessem JN, Singh BN: Calcium channel antagonism and β-blockade in combination: A therapeutic alternative and cardiovascular disorder (a review). Cardiovasc Drugs Ther 3:355–373, 1989
73. Levine JH, Michael JR, Guarnieri T: Treatment of multifocal atrial tachycardia with verapamil. N Engl J Med 3123:21–25, 1985
74. Lewis BS, Rozenman Y, Merdler A, et al: Chronotropic effect of hydralazine and its mechanism in symptomatic sinus bradycardia. Am J Cardiol 59:93–96, 1987

75. Lindgarde F, Jelnes R, Bjorkman H, et al: Conservative drug treatment in patients with moderately severe chronic occlusive peripheral arterial disease. Circulation 80:1549–1556, 1989
76. Luu M, Stevenson WG, Stevenson LW, et al: Diverse mechanisms of unexpected cardiac arrest in advanced heart failure. Circulation 80:1675–1680, 1989
77. McIntosh CL, Maron BJ: Current operative treatment of obstructive hypertrophic cardiomyopathy. Circulation 78:487–495, 1988
78. McKenna WJ, Franklin RCG, Nihowannopoulos P, et al: Arrhythmia and prognosis in infants, children, and adolescents with hypertrophic cardiomyopathy. J Am Coll Cardiol 11:147–153, 1988
79. McLaran CJ, Gersh BJ, Sugrue DD, et al: Out-of-hospital cardiac arrest in patients without clinically significant coronary artery disease: Comparison of clinical, electrophysiological, and survival characteristics with those in similar patients who have clinically significant coronary artery disease. Br Heart J 58:583–591, 1987
80. Moss AJ, Rubison M, Oakes D, et al. Effect of diltiazem on long-term outcome in post-infarction patients with a history of hypertension (abstract). Circulation 80(suppl II):II-268, 1989
81. Multicenter Diltiazem Postinfarction Trial Research Group: The effect of diltiazem on mortality and reinfarction after myocardial infarction. N Engl J Med 319:385–392, 1988
82. National Heart Foundation of Australia Coronary Thrombolysis Group: A randomized comparison of oral aspirin/dipyridamole versus intravenous heparin after rTPA for acute myocardial infarction (abstract). Circulation 80(suppl II):II-114, 1989
83. Neri Serneri G, Gensini GF, Poggesi L, et al: Effect of heparin, aspirin, or alteplase in reduction of myocardial ischaemia in refractory unstable angina. Lancet 335:615–618, 1990
84. Opie LH: Reperfusion injury and its pharmacologic modification. Circulation 80:1049–1062, 1989
85. PACK Claudication Substudy Investigators: Randomized placebo-controlled, double-blind trial of ketanserin in claudicants: Changes in claudication distance and ankle systolic pressure. Circulation 80:1544–1548, 1989
86. Packer M: Combined β-adrenergic and calcium entry blockade in angina pectoris. N Engl J Med 320:709–718, 1989
87. Packer M: Is it ethical to administer vasodilator drugs to patients with primary pulmonary hypertension (editorial)? Chest 95:1173–1175, 1989
88. Parillo JE, Cunnion RE, Epstein SE: A prospective, randomized, controlled trial of prednisone for dilated cardiomyopathy. N Engl J Med 321:1061–1068, 1989
89. Parisi AF, Khuri S, Depree RH, et al: Medical compared with surgical management of unstable angina: 5-year mortality and morbidity in the Veterans Administration study. Circulation 80:1176–1189, 1989
90. Parving H-H, Hommel E, Nielsen MD, Giese J: Effect of captopril on blood pressure and kidney function in normotensive insulin dependent diabetics with nephropathy. Br Med J 299:533–536, 1989
91. Pitt B: Should digoxin be the drug of first choice after diuretics and chronic congestive heart failure? III: Antagonists viewpoint. J Am Coll Cardiol 12:271–273, 1988
92. Pollare T, Lithell H, Selinus I, Berne C: Sensitivity to insulin during treatment with atenolol and metoprolol: A randomized, double-blind study of effects on carbohydrate and lipoprotein metabolism in hypertensive patients. Br Med J 298:1152–1157, 1989
93. Pollick C: Disopyramide in hypertrophic cardiomyopathy. II: Noninvasive assessment after oral administration. Am J Cardiol 62:1252–1255, 1988
94. Quyyumi AA, Crake T, Wright CM, et al: Medical treatment of patients with severe exertional and rest angina: Double-blind comparison of β-blocker, calcium antagonist, and nitrate. Br Heart J 57:505–511, 1987
95. Rich S, Brundage BH: High-dose calcium channel-blocking therapy for primary pulmonary hypertension: Evidence for long-term reduction in pulmonary arterial pressure and regression of right ventricular hypertrophy. Circulation 76:135–141, 1986
96. Roath S: Management of Raynaud's phenomenon. Drugs 37:700–712, 1989
97. Satler LF, Green CE, Kent KM, et al: Metabolic support during coronary reperfusion. Am Heart J 114:54–58, 1987
98. Sharp EN, Murphy J, Smith H, et al: Treatment of patients with symptomless left ventricular dysfunction after myocardial infarction. Lancet 1:255–258, 1988

99. Shulman ST, Amren DP, Bisno AL, et al: Prevention of rheumatic fever: A statement for health professionals by the Committee on Rheumatic Fever and Infective Endocarditis of the Council on Cardiovascular Disease in the Young. Circulation 70:1118A–1122A, 1984

100. Simmons NA, Cawson RA, Eykyn SJ, et al: Antibiotic prophylaxis of infective endocarditis: Recommendations from the Endocarditis Working Party of the British Society for Antimicrobial Chemotherapy. Lancet 335:88–89, 1990

101. Spinelli W, Hoffman BF: Mechanisms of termination of reentrant atrial arrhythmias by Class I and Class III antiarrhythmic agents. Circ Res 65:1565–1579, 1989

102. Stone PH, Gibson RS, Glasser SP, et al: Comparison of diltiazem, nifedipine, and propranolol in the therapy of silent ischemia. Circulation 80(suppl II):II2–II267, 1989

103. Strauss WE, Parisi AF: Combined use of calcium channel and β-adrenergic blockers for the treatment of chronic stable angina: Rationale, efficacy, and adverse effects. Ann Intern Med October:570–581, 1988

104. Taylor HA, Deumite J, Chaitman BR, et al: Asymptomatic left main coronary artery disease in the coronary artery surgery study (CASS) registry. Circulation 79:1171–1179, 1989

105. Theroux P, Taeymans Y, Morissette D, et al: A randomized study comparing propranolol and diltiazem in the treatment of unstable angina. J Am Coll Cardiol 5:717–722, 1985

106. Theroux P, Ouiment H, McCans J, et al: Aspirin, heparin, or both to treat acute unstable angina. N Engl J Med 319:1105–1111, 1988

107. Theroux P, Baird M, Juneau M, et al: Effect of diltiazem upon episodes of silent myocardial ischemia during daily life (abstract). J Am Coll Cardiol 15:120A, 1990

108. TIMI Study Group: Comparison of invasive and conservative strategies after treatment with intravenous tissue plasminogen activator in acute myocardial infarction: Results of the thrombolysis in myocardial infarction (TIMI) Phase II Trial. N Engl J Med 320:618–627, 1989

109. Topol EJ, Nicklas JM, Kander MH, et al: Coronary revascularization after intravenous tissue plasminogen activator for unstable angina pectoris: Results of a randomized, double-blind placebo-controlled trial. Am J Cardiol 62:368–371, 1988

110. Topol EJ: Ultrathrombolysis. J Am Coll Cardiol 15:922–924, 1990

111. Tseu FL, Morley CA, MacKintosh AF: Oral xamoterol in patients with sinoatrial disease. Br Heart J 56:469–472, 1986

112. Waagstein F, Caidahl K, Wallentin I, et al: Long-term β-blockade in dilated cardiomyopathy: Effects of short- and long-term metoprolol treatment followed by withdrawal and re-administration of metoprolol. Circulation 80:551–563, 1989

113. Working Party of the British Society for Antimicrobial Chemotherapy: The antibiotic prophylaxis of infective endocarditis. Lancet 2:1323–1326, 1982

114. Yusuf S, McMahon S, Collins R, et al: Effect of intravenous nitrates on mortality and acute myocardial infarction: An overview of the randomized trials. Lancet 1:1088–1092, 1988

Index

Note: Page numbers in *italics* refer to illustrations; page numbers
followed by t refer to tables.